Recent Advances in

Paediatrics 21

Edited by

Timothy J. David MB ChB MD PhD FRCP FRCPCH DCH

Professor of Child Health and Paediatrics,
University of Manchester;
Honorary Consultant Paediatrician,
Booth Hall Children's Hospital,
Royal Manchester Children's Hospital and St Mary's Hospital,
Manchester, UK

© 2004 Royal Society of Medicine Press Ltd

Published by the Royal Society of Medicine Press Ltd
1 Wimpole Street, London W1G 0AE, UK
Tel: +44 (0) 20 7290 2921; Fax: +44 (0) 20 7290 2929
E-mail: publishing@rsm.ac.uk
Website: www.rsmpress.co.uk

The contributors are responsible for the scientific content and for the views expressed, which are not necessarily those of the Royal Society of Medicine or of the Royal Society of Medicine Press Ltd. Although every effort has been made to ensure that drug dosages, procedures, use of equipment and drugs, and other information are accurate, the ultimate responsibility rests with the prescribing physician and neither the publishers nor the authors can be held responsible for errors or for any consequences arising from the use of information contained herein. For any product or type of product, whether a drug or device, physicians should consult the detailed prescribing information or instructions issued by the manufacturer.

British Library Cataloguing in Publication Data
A catalogue record for this book is available from the British Library

ISBN 1-85315-572-1

ISSN 0-309-0140

Distribution in Europe and Rest of World:
Marston Book Services Ltd, PO Box 269, Abingdon, Oxon OX14 4YN, UK
Tel: +44 (0) 1235 465500; Fax: +44 (0) 1235 465555

Distribution in the USA and Canada:
Royal Society of Medicine Press Ltd, c/o Jamco Distribution Inc
1401 Lakeway Drive, Lewisville, TX 75057, USA
Tel: +1 800 538 1287; Fax: +1 972 353 1303
E-mail: jamco@majors.com

Distribution in Australia and New Zealand:
Elsevier Australia
30-52 Smidmore Street, Marrickville NSW 2204, Australia
Tel: +61 2 9517 8999; Fax: +61 2 9517 2249
E-mail: service@elsevier.com.au

Commissioning editor: Peter Richardson
Editorial assistant: Shirley Mukisa
Production by GM & BA Haddock, Midlothian, UK
Printed in Great Britain by Bell & Bain, Glasgow, UK

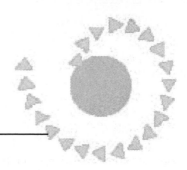

Contents

Contents

Preface

The aim of *Recent Advances in Paediatrics* is to provide a review of important topics and help doctors keep abreast of developments in the subject. The book is intended for the practising clinician, those in specialty training, and doctors preparing for specialty examinations. The book is sold very widely in Britain, Europe, North America and Asia, and the contents and authorship are selected with this very broad readership in mind. There are 14 chapters which cover a variety of general paediatric, neonatal and community paediatric areas. As usual, the selection of topics has veered towards those of general rather than special interest.

The final chapter, an annotated literature review, is a personal selection of key articles and useful reviews published in 2002. Comment about a paper is sometimes as important as the original article, so when a paper has been followed by interesting or important correspondence, or accompanied by a useful editorial, this is also referred to. As with the choice of subjects for the main chapters, the selection of articles has inclined towards those of general rather than special interest. There is, however, special emphasis on community paediatrics and medicine in the tropics, as these two important areas tend to be less well covered in general paediatric journals. Trying to reduce to an acceptable size the short-list of particularly interesting articles is an especially difficult task. Each topic in the literature review section is asterisked in the index, so selected publications on (for example) child abuse can be identified easily, as can any parts of the book that touch on the topic.

I am indebted to the authors for their hard work, prompt delivery of manuscripts and patience in dealing with my queries and requests. I would also like to thank my secretaries Angela Smithies and Val Smith, and Gill Haddock of the RSM Press, for all their help. Working on a book such as this makes huge inroads into one's spare time, and my special thanks go to my wife and sons for all their support.

2003

Professor Timothy J. David
E-mail: t.david@netcomuk.co.uk
University Department of Child Health, Booth Hall Children's Hospital, Manchester M9 7AA, UK

Paul Brogan

Recognition, diagnosis and management of Kawasaki disease

In 1967, Tomisaku Kawasaki described 50 Japanese children with an illness characterised by fever, rash, conjunctival injection, erythema and swelling of hands and feet, and cervical lymphadenopathy,[1] although it was not until 1974 that the first English language report form Professor Kawasaki was published. The mucocutaneous lymph node syndrome that he described is now recognised as Kawasaki disease, and is the second commonest vasculitic illnesses of childhood (Henoch-Schonlein purpura being the commonest).

Kawasaki disease is associated with the development of systemic vasculitis complicated by coronary and peripheral arterial aneurysms, and myocardial infarction in some patients.[2] It has superseded rheumatic fever in that Kawasaki disease is now the commonest cause of acquired heart disease in children in the UK and the US.[2]

Despite intensive research into the illness, the cause remains unknown; although there have been significant improvements in diagnosis and treatment of children with the disease, there are still a number of important unanswered questions regarding therapy. Furthermore, there is still no diagnostic test available for Kawasaki disease.

This review focuses on recent advances in Kawasaki disease with specific reference to recognition, diagnosis (including novel surrogate markers of endothelial injury), and treatment. Areas of controversy will be discussed, and key points for clinical practice will be highlighted.

EPIDEMIOLOGY

Kawasaki disease is commonest in Japan where, by the end of 2001, 168,394 cases had been reported. The disease is also commoner in Japanese and other Oriental children living abroad.[2] Children aged 6 months to 5 years are most susceptible,

Paul Brogan BSc MBChB MRCP MSc PhD
Specialist Registrar in Paediatric Nephrology, Victoria Ward, Level 8 Southwood Building, Great
Ormond Street Hospital for Children, London WC1N 3JH, UK. E-mail: brogap@gosh.nhs.uk

with peak incidence in children aged 9–11 months.[3] Seasonal variation in the disease incidence has been reported, with peak occurrence in the winter and spring months.[2] Outbreaks of Kawasaki disease have been linked to weather patterns with clusters of cases occurring in association with precipitation.[4] Direct person-to-person spread is not observed, although in Japan the disease occurs more commonly in siblings of index cases with an estimated peak incidence of 8–9% in siblings under the age of 2 years.[5] Currently, the estimated incidence of Kawasaki disease in the UK is 8.1 per 100,000 children under the age of 5 years – an incidence which has doubled since 1991.[6] This increase may truly reflect a rising incidence, although increased case recognition may partly account for this observation.

AETIOLOGY – RECENT ADVANCES AND CONTROVERSIES

Although Kawasaki disease is believed to be caused by an infectious agent in an immunologically susceptible individual, the causative agent remains elusive. Many infectious agents have been proposed to cause Kawasaki disease in the past, but none unequivocally proven as the sole agent responsible for all cases. It appears increasingly likely that many infectious insults may culminate in common immunological pathways resulting in the clinical phenotype of Kawasaki disease in genetically susceptible individuals. Perhaps the most important controversy is the on-going debate regarding superantigens versus conventional antigens in the aetio-pathogenesis of Kawasaki disease.

There are striking similarities between the clinical and immunological features of Kawasaki disease and the superantigen toxin mediated staphylococcal and streptococcal toxic shock syndrome and scarlet fever.[7–9] The difficulty in distinguishing these diseases has been extensively documented,[10–12] and the exclusion of staphylococcal disease has been one of the criteria for the diagnosis of Kawasaki disease. The similarities between these diseases led to the suggestion that Kawasaki disease is also caused by a bacterial superantigen toxin.[3,13] This theory remains controversial with several studies supporting the notion, and an equal number refuting the superantigen theory. The epidemiology of Kawasaki disease is characteristic of an infectious disease and suggests that it is caused by an infectious agent to which everyone is exposed and to which most acquire immunity in childhood. Those individuals who succumb to Kawasaki disease may be genetically predisposed.

The study by Abe et al.[14] in 1992 was the first to describe selective expansion of Vβ2 and Vβ8.1 T cells in Kawasaki disease, indicating T cell Vβ skewing – the hallmark of a superantigen-mediated process. Since then, many similar studies have examined T cell Vβ repertoires in Kawasaki disease using a variety of techniques (mainly flow cytometry or semi-quantitative polymerase chain reaction), or examined the prevalence of serological conversion or colonisation with superantigen-producing organisms. So far, data are conflicting and the jury is still out regarding whether or not superantigens are involved in the aetio-pathogenesis of Kawasaki disease.

RECOGNITION AND DIAGNOSIS

There is no diagnostic test for Kawasaki disease; therefore, diagnosis is based on clinical criteria (Table 1)[15] and the exclusion of other diseases, particularly

Table 1 Kawasaki disease: diagnostic criteria[15]

Criterion	Description
Fever	Duration of 5 days or more PLUS 4 of 5 of the following:
1. Conjunctivitis	Bilateral, bulbar, non-suppurative
2. Lymphadenopathy	Cervical, > 1.5 cm
3. Rash	Polymorphous, no vesicles or crusts
4. Changes of lips or oral mucosa	Red cracked lips; 'strawberry' tongue; or diffuse erythema of oropharynx
5. Changes of extremities	Initial stage: erythema and oedema of palms and soles
	Convalescent stage: peeling of skin from fingertips

Kawasaki disease may be diagnosed with fewer than 4 of these features if coronary artery abnormalities are detected.

sepsis. The differential diagnosis includes toxic shock syndrome (streptococcal and staphylococcal), staphylococcal scalded skin syndrome, scarlet fever, and infection with enterovirus, adenovirus, measles, parvovirus, Epstein-Barr virus, cytomegalovirus, *Mycoplasma pneumoniae*, rickettsiae, and leptospirosis.[16] The differential diagnosis of intravenous immunoglobulin (IVIG) resistant Kawasaki disease includes polyarteritis nodosa, systemic-onset juvenile idiopathic arthritis, and malignancy (particularly lymphoma).

Fever of 5 days duration plus 4 of the 5 remaining criteria or the presence of fever and coronary artery abnormalities with 3 additional criteria are required for the diagnosis of 'complete' cases.[17] 'Incomplete' cases comprise those with less than the prerequisite number of criteria. Irritability is an important sign, which is usually present, although not included as one of the diagnostic criteria.[16] The exact mechanism of the irritability is unclear, but it may be related to the presence of aseptic meningitis. Another clinical sign not incorporated into the diagnostic criteria but which is relatively specific to Kawasaki disease is the development of erythema and induration at sites of BCG immunisations.[16] The mechanism of this clinical sign is cross-reactivity of T cells in Kawasaki disease patients between specific epitopes of mycobacterial and human heat-shock proteins.[18] With an increasing number of infants receiving the BCG in the UK, it is likely that this sign will become more common, and awareness of it could result in earlier diagnosis and treatment.

Other relatively common clinical findings in Kawasaki disease include arthritis, aseptic meningitis, pneumonitis, uveitis, gastroenteritis, meatitis and dysuria, and otitis.[19] Relatively uncommon abnormalities include hydrops of the gallbladder, gastrointestinal ischaemia, jaundice, petechial rash, febrile convulsions, and encephalopathy or ataxia.[19] Cardiac complications other than coronary arterial abnormalities include cardiac tamponade, cardiac failure, myocarditis, and pericarditis.[19]

Increasingly, 'atypical' or incomplete presentations of Kawasaki disease are identified, in which full diagnostic criteria are not met. This makes the recognition of Kawasaki disease all the more difficult, especially in countries where measles is still endemic. Nonetheless, children with atypical or incomplete Kawasaki disease are at risk from coronary arterial abnormalities – in Japan, the incidence of coronary involvement at day 30 in children with atypical Kawasaki disease in one series was 12%.[20]

An important point worthy of emphasis which is key to the recognition of Kawasaki disease is that the clinical criteria may present sequentially such that a so-called 'incomplete' case can evolve with time into a 'complete' case. Thus, the diagnosis of Kawasaki disease must be considered in any child with a febrile exanthematous illness, particularly if it persists longer than 4–5 days, and it is imperative to ask specifically about previous symptoms and signs which may have resolved by the time of presentation.

LABORATORY FINDINGS

Kawasaki disease is associated with many non-specific laboratory findings. Acute phase proteins, neutrophils, and erythrocyte sedimentation rate are usually elevated. Thrombocytosis occurs towards the end of the second week of the illness and, therefore, may not be helpful diagnostically.[19] Liver function may be deranged. Sterile pyuria is occasionally observed, and also CSF pleocytosis (predominantly lymphocytes) representing aseptic meningitis.[2]

TOWARDS A DIAGNOSTIC TEST

At the Seventh International Kawasaki Disease Symposium in Japan in 2001, one of the key issues was lack of a gold standard diagnostic test for the disease.[21] A number of exciting novel markers of endothelial injury and surrogate markers of disease activity have been described in recent years, but none as yet with sufficiently robust test characteristics to be of use to clinicians.

Very recently, circulating endothelial cells have been shown to be increased in the peripheral blood of 20 children with Kawasaki disease.[22] The authors suggest that this observation may be a reflection of endothelial injury associated with Kawasaki disease. In support of this hypothesis, they observed higher numbers of circulating endothelial cells in those affected by coronary arterial aneurysms (n = 6) than those without aneurysms.

Recently, we have been investigating circulating endothelial microparticles as a novel marker for endothelial damage in childhood vasculitides including 15 children with Kawasaki disease. Endothelial microparticles are fragments of the endothelial bilipid membrane released into the peripheral circulation in a number of diseases associated with endothelial injury including acute coronary events, multiple sclerosis, and systemic lupus erythematosus. So far, the diagnostic test characteristics are promising for the differentiation of Kawasaki disease from other febrile exanthemata of childhood, although at the moment this remains a research tool.

Another laboratory approach to diagnosis has utilised the observation of many others that there may be skewing of the T cell Vβ repertoire (the hallmark of superantigen mediated diseases such as toxic shock syndrome) during the acute phase of Kawasaki disease. Reichardt *et al.*[23] recently examined T-cell subsets in 20 children with suspected Kawasaki disease (7 ultimately proven), 24 febrile controls, and 184 healthy controls. They observed increased levels of T cells expressing Vβ2.1 in the 7 proven Kawasaki disease patients and suggested that this observation may be useful diagnostically.

Other proposals to improve upon the sensitivity of clinical criteria currently used to diagnose Kawasaki disease have included the incorporation of laboratory markers (such as acute phase reactants) and inclusion of important non-principal symptoms and signs (such as irritability or BCG scar activation).[21] Lastly, inclusion of subtle non-aneurysmal echocardiographic findings such as coronary perivascular brightness seen in the coronary arterial wall in the acute phase of the disease may prove diagnostically helpful in the future.[21]

TREATMENT

Treatment of Kawasaki disease is aimed at reducing inflammation, and preventing the occurrence of coronary artery aneurysms and arterial thrombosis. The optimal doses of aspirin and IVIG are discussed, and the treatment of refractory Kawasaki disease is considered. Recent advances relating to novel therapeutic approaches will be highlighted.

ASPIRIN

It is worthy of note that treatment of Kawasaki disease with aspirin alone has never been subject to a randomised controlled trial, although aspirin versus aspirin plus IVIG has been studied. Aspirin is given in the acute phase of the illness at relatively high 'anti-inflammatory' doses (30–100 mg/kg/day). When the child is afebrile for 48 h (so-called defervescence of the disease), aspirin is given as an anti-platelet agent in a dose of 2–5 mg/kg/OD, the duration being dependent on the subsequent findings on echocardiography, but usually for a minimum of 6 weeks. If there are no coronary arterial abnormalities detected on echocardiography at 6 weeks, the aspirin can be stopped. If aneurysms are detected at 6 weeks, the aspirin is continued until they resolve. In the case of coronary aneurysms greater than 8 mm (which rarely resolve), life-long therapy with aspirin is recommended (see below).

Recent reviews have recommended the higher anti-inflammatory dose of 100 mg/kg/day in the acute phase of the illness[17] on the basis of reducing duration of fever and length of hospitalisation compared with low dose aspirin (3–8 mg/kg/day).[24] Certainly, this is the current practice in many centres in the US, although the Japanese favour more moderate doses of aspirin (30–50 mg/kg/day). No comparative data on fever and hospitalisation exists regarding high dose aspirin versus moderate doses (30–50 mg/kg/day).

Meta-analysis comparing moderate anti-inflammatory doses of aspirin (30–50 mg/kg/day) with IVIG versus high dose aspirin (80–120 mg/kg/day) with IVIG found no significant difference in the incidence of coronary arterial abnormalities between the groups.[25] Currently, it is our practice in the UK to administer aspirin at a dose of 30 mg/kg/day during the acute phase of the illness,[16] since this may be better tolerated in terms of gastrointestinal and other side effects.[26] Some have advocated the use of dipyridamole in addition to moderate dose aspirin as a synergistic anti-platelet agent. The evidence for the effectiveness of this in this situation is, however, lacking.

INTRAVENOUS IMMUNOGLOBULIN

Early recognition and treatment of Kawasaki disease with aspirin and IVIG has been shown unequivocally by meta-analysis to reduce the occurrence of coronary artery abnormalities.[25,27] Moreover, the prevalence of coronary artery abnormalities in Kawasaki disease is highly dependent on total IVIG dose, but independent of aspirin dose.[25] Treated with aspirin alone, 20–40% of children develop coronary artery abnormalities.[25,27] Combined therapy with aspirin and high dose IVIG given as a single infusion reduces the occurrence of coronary artery abnormalities to 9% at 30 days, and 4% at 60 days after the onset of the illness.[27] The prevalence of coronary artery abnormalities is inversely related to the total dose of IVIG, 2 g/kg of IVIG being the optimal dose, usually given as a single infusion.[25,27] Meta-analysis of randomised controlled trials comparing divided lower doses of IVIG (400 mg/kg/day for 4 consecutive days) versus a single infusion of high dose IVIG (2 g/kg over 10 h) has clearly demonstrated the therapeutic benefits in the prevention of coronary artery abnormalities with the latter regimen.[27] One important practical point, however, is that infants who have cardiac compromise may not be able to tolerate the fluid challenge associated with the high-dose, single infusion, and consideration of divided doses given over several days may be appropriate for this patient group.

IVIG treatment should be started early in the disease, preferably within the first 10 days of the illness.[25,27] Importantly, however, clinicians should not hesitate to give IVIG to patients who present after 10 days if there are signs of persisting inflammation.

Not all patients respond to a single dose of IVIG, and some require a second dose. It has been observed by many that those children who received IVIG before day 5 of the illness may require a second infusion of IVIG for primary treatment failure or disease recrudescence.[21] Thus, the timing of IVIG administration appears to be important, although this latter point should not dissuade clinicians from giving IVIG before day 5 of fever if the diagnosis of Kawasaki disease is suspected.

Lastly, one question that remains unanswered is whether the type of IVIG administered is important, perhaps as a result of the presence of antibodies to epitopes derived from different donor pools. There are currently, however, no data to suggest that particular preparations derived from populations of different ethnicity is superior.

THE ROLE OF CORTICOSTEROIDS

The use of corticosteroids in Kawasaki disease remains controversial. Unlike other vasculitic conditions, where corticosteroid remains the mainstay of treatment, early anecdotal observations suggested that the incidence of coronary artery abnormalities was greater in those treated with prednisolone compared with those treated with aspirin alone. Other workers have suggested that the use of pulsed methylprednisolone is effective in treating patients with Kawasaki disease resistant to IVIG.[28] Currently, there is a role for corticosteroid in patients with Kawasaki disease refractory to treatment with IVIG,[29] and also for those patients who may refuse IVIG because of religious beliefs, such as Jehovah's Witnesses. However, treatment of refractory Kawasaki disease with corticosteroid should be undertaken in specialised centres.

RECENT THERAPEUTIC ADVANCES

Comparisons of IVIG products and different dose regimens were the subject of several papers at the Seventh International Kawasaki Disease Symposium. Iwasa et al.[21] suggested that IVIG prepared using propylene glycol was associated with better outcomes than sulphonated IVIG, a finding also confirmed independently by other workers. In the study by Muta et al.,[21] the incidence of coronary artery complications was 10% with sulphonated IVIG, versus 2.8% with a polyethylene glycol-treated product.

Recent studies have confirmed the optimum dosage of IVIG to be 2 g/kg given as a single infusion. Lower doses (1 g/kg) are associated with an increased need for re-treatment, and increased incidence of coronary arterial involvement.[21,30]

Risk factors to identify those more likely to require re-treatment with IVIG have been proposed by Durongpisitkul et al.[31] They observed that 11.6% of 120 Kawasaki disease patients in Thailand failed treatment with a single dose of IVIG. They found that a haemoglobin less than 10 g/dl, high neutrophil count, and low serum albumin were associated with the need for re-treatment with IVIG. These factors were also predictive of coronary artery abnormalities.

Sundel et al.[32] recently conducted a prospective randomised open-label trial to determine whether the addition of a single intravenous pulse of methyl-prednisolone (30 mg/kg) to standard IVIG/aspirin therapy might improve outcome. They demonstrated that treatment with methylprednisolone plus IVIG/aspirin resulted in faster resolution of fever, more rapid improvement in acute phase markers, and shorter length of hospitalisation. Adverse effects related to methylprednisolone were rare. This study was, however, underpowered to detect a difference in coronary artery abnormalities. Similarly, Jibiki et al.[21] reported shortened fever course when combining dexamethasone with IVIG, but no change in coronary artery abnormalities.

Therapy for giant coronary arterial aneurysms with the anti-platelet monoclonal antibody abciximab (anti-platelet GPIIb/IIIa receptor antibody) has been reported in a small series of patients with Kawasaki disease, although despite previous suggestions of efficacy little regression of coronary arterial aneurysms was observed.[21]

Data regarding the efficacy of ulinastatin, a urinary trypsin inhibitor that inhibits neutrophil elastase activity, have so far remained inconclusive. Lastly, add-on treatment with plasma exchange has been attempted in selected high-risk patients with Kawasaki disease with apparent benefit, although the level of evidence is not yet sufficient to recommend this mode of therapy routinely.[21]

CURRENT UK TREATMENT GUIDELINE

The current UK guideline for the treatment of Kawasaki disease (KD) is given in Figure 1.[16] It is proposed that complete cases are treated, and additionally incomplete cases are treated at the discretion of the admitting clinician. Clinicians should have a lower threshold for treatment of incomplete cases under the age of 1 year. For older children with incomplete Kawasaki disease, the decision to treat will be influenced by factors such as the small, but theoretical, risk of blood-borne virus infection from IVIG.

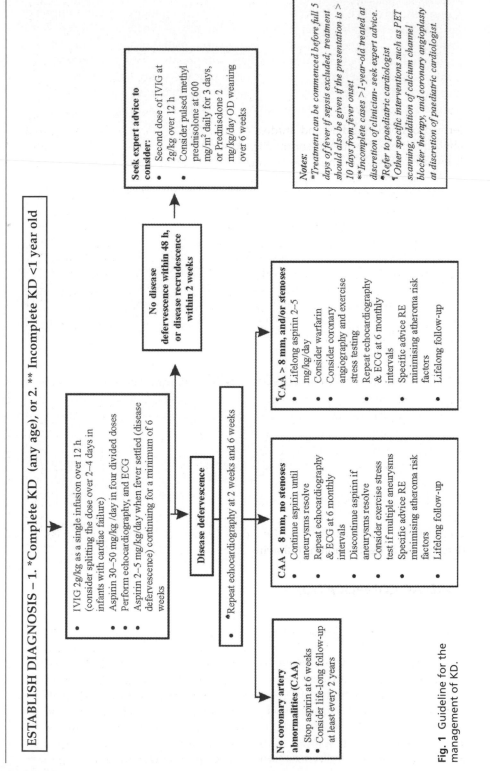

ESTABLISH DIAGNOSIS – 1. *Complete KD (any age), or 2. ** Incomplete KD <1 year old

- IVIG 2g/kg as a single infusion over 12 h (consider splitting the dose over 2–4 days in infants with cardiac failure)
- Aspirin 30–50 mg/kg /day in four divided doses
- Perform echocardiography, and ECG
- Aspirin 2–5 mg/kg/day when fever settled (disease defervescence) continuing for a minimum of 6 weeks

Disease defervescence

- *Repeat echocardiography at 2 weeks and 6 weeks

No disease defervescence within 48 h, or disease recrudescence within 2 weeks

Seek expert advice to consider:
- Second dose of IVIG at 2g/kg over 12 h
- Consider pulsed methyl prednisolone at 600 mg/m² daily for 3 days, or Prednisolone 2 mg/kg/day OD weaning over 6 weeks

No coronary artery abnormalities (CAA)
- Stop aspirin at 6 weeks
- Consider life-long follow-up at least every 2 years

CAA < 8 mm, no stenoses
- Continue aspirin until aneurysms resolve
- Repeat echocardiography & ECG at 6 monthly intervals
- Discontinue aspirin if aneurysms resolve
- Consider exercise stress test if multiple aneurysms
- Specific advice RE minimising atheroma risk factors
- Lifelong follow-up

ᶠCAA > 8 mm, and/or stenoses
- Lifelong aspirin 2–5 mg/kg/day
- Consider warfarin
- Consider coronary angiography and exercise stress testing
- Repeat echocardiography & ECG at 6 monthly intervals
- Specific advice RE minimising atheroma risk factors
- Lifelong follow-up

Notes:
*Treatment can be commenced before full 5 days of fever if sepsis excluded; treatment should also be given if the presentation is > 10 days from fever onset
**Incomplete cases >1-year-old treated at discretion of clinician- seek expert advice.
ᵃRefer to paediatric cardiologist
ᶠOther specific interventions such as PET scanning, addition of calcium channel blocker therapy, and coronary angioplasty at discretion of paediatric cardiologist.

Fig. 1 Guideline for the management of KD.

Life-long follow-up of all children following an episode of Kawasaki disease is recommended. The purpose of this is to document the blood pressure, and provide general advice regarding other cardiac risk factors and life-style measures. Since the publication of this guideline, there have been valid concerns relating to this proposal for follow-up. Specifically, concerns regarding the potential adverse effects of long-term follow-up in children without coronary involvement such as unnecessary anxiety and inappropriate restriction of activity have been raised. Others argue that the long-term vascular damage from Kawasaki disease is uncertain with several recent long-term prognostic studies and studies of endothelial function suggesting that abnormalities of systemic endothelial function are present many years after Kawasaki disease, even in the absence of overt coronary involvement in the acute phase of the disease (see below). For this reason, the guideline advocates long-term annual review to monitor for and minimise risk factors for coronary vascular disease in adolescent and adult life. This could be performed in the primary care setting; since Kawasaki disease is still relatively rare in the UK, such follow-up would not necessarily pose an undue burden on health care resources. Moreover, it is the experience of the author that such follow-up is re-assuring for patients and families, and rather than imposing inappropriate restriction of activity actually re-assures patients more often than not that they can adopt an entirely normal level of exercise activity. Lastly, prospective follow-up of children with Kawasaki disease will also be important in estimating the long-term cardiac risk of this disorder.

VACCINATION AFTER KAWASAKI DISEASE

There are two important issues relating to vaccination following an episode of Kawasaki disease. Firstly, IVIG can block replication of live viral vaccines and subsequent actively acquired immunity.[33] Consequently, it is currently recommended that live vaccines be deferred for at least 3 months following treatment with IVIG. Second, an important question remaining unanswered is the safety of live or other vaccines in children recovering from Kawasaki disease. It has been the experience of the author that some autoimmune disease states, including the systemic vasculitides, flare in response to live and non-live vaccine preparations. It is, therefore, advised that immunisation with all vaccines be deferred for at least 3 months following an episode of Kawasaki disease.[16]

CARDIAC COMPLICATIONS

Echocardiography and cardiac angiographic data indicate that 20–40% of untreated Kawasaki disease patients develop coronary artery abnormalities. Approximately 50% of these lesions regress within 5 years, and in most with mild coronary arterial aneurysms (3–4 mm) regression occurs within 2 years.[2] Giant aneurysms (> 8 mm) are unlikely to resolve, and some may develop stenosis with risk of coronary thrombosis, myocardial infarction, and death. In 1993, a report from the British Paediatric Surveillance Unit (BPSU) indicated a mortality rate of 3.7% in the UK for Kawasaki disease.[34] Current mortality rates reported from Japan are much lower at 0.14%.[17] The reasons for this difference include improved therapy, and better case recognition. Long-term sequelae may include the early development of coronary atherosclerosis.[35]

All patients with Kawasaki disease should undergo echocardiography on diagnosis and 6–8 weeks after the onset of the disease.[16] Some also advocate an intermediate echocardiograph at 10–14 days of disease onset to pick up any missed pathology.[16] Additionally, it is good practice to perform echocardiography at least weekly (and occasionally 48 hourly in the acute stages with on-going active inflammation) for those who develop coronary artery abnormalities to monitor aneurysm size progression, or the development of thrombus formation. Aspirin is continued for a minimum of 6 weeks, and long-term aspirin at 2–5 mg/kg/day is recommended for those with persisting aneurysms on echocardiography.[17] This can be discontinued if the aneurysms resolve. Depending on the size of the aneurysms, ECG and echocardiography performed 6–12 monthly is recommended.

Patients with aneurysms greater than 8 mm may require stress testing and possibly coronary angiography to identify stenotic lesions. Most experts recommend the addition of warfarin to aspirin therapy for those with giant (> 8 mm) coronary aneurysms,[36] though randomised controlled trials supporting this practice are lacking. If warfarin is to be commenced, it is imperative to cover the initial warfarinisation period with intravenous heparin to counteract the paradoxical prothrombotic state which can occur soon after starting warfarin in some patients.[37] It has been suggested that platelet glycoprotein IIb/IIIa receptor blockade therapy (abciximab, see above) may be a useful addition to the therapeutic armamentarium for those with giant aneurysms,[38] though more recently doubt has been cast regarding the efficacy of such therapy.[21]

Limitation of strenuous activity is recommended in all patients with giant coronary aneurysms and/or stenoses. Some patients with coronary artery stenoses may require surgical revascularisation. In those patients who develop myocardial infarction, treatment with streptokinase or tissue plasminogen activator (TPA) is indicated.[2]

A rare, but serious, complication of Kawasaki disease is the development of peripheral ischaemia and gangrene. This particular complication is associated with peripheral arterial aneurysm formation, particularly axillary aneurysms. Treatment with thrombolytic agents, anticoagulants, and intravenous prostacyclin may be indicated in such patients.[2,16]

PROGNOSIS

The overall outlook for children with Kawasaki disease is good, although coronary artery abnormalities are present in 4% of treated cases 60 days after the acute illness.[27] A 1–2% acute mortality rate due to myocardial infarction has been reduced further in many countries by alertness of clinicians to the diagnosis and early use of gamma globulin with anti-platelet therapy- the mortality for the disease in Japan is currently 0.14%.[17] Nonetheless, it has been postulated that adult atheromatous coronary disease in some cases may have its origins in childhood due to covert or overt Kawasaki disease.[39]

DOES KAWASAKI DISEASE CAUSE PREMATURE ATHEROSCLEROSIS?

Several key aspects of long-term outcome remain of ongoing concern. Most importantly controversy continues as to whether Kawasaki disease constitutes a risk factor for premature atherosclerosis. Dhillon *et al.*[40] studied vascular responses to reactive hyperaemia in the brachial artery using high-resolution ultrasound. Flow-mediated dilation (an endothelial-dependent response) was markedly reduced in Kawasaki disease patients compared with control subjects many years after the illness, even in patients without detectable early coronary artery involvement. McCrindle *et al.*[21] showed in a long-term case control study that Kawasaki disease patients were more likely to have impairment of the fibrinolytic system, another marker of endothelial dysfunction, and this again was unrelated to the degree of coronary artery involvement. Pilla *et al.*[41] demonstrated reduced arterial distensibility (an independent risk factor for cardiovascular morbidity and mortality in adults) as assessed using ultrasound pulse wave velocity in the brachio-radial arterial segments of 43 children who had Kawasaki disease a median of 3 years previously. Additionally, diastolic blood pressure was found to be significantly higher in the Kawasaki disease group as compared with 166 healthy age-matched controls.

In contrast, another recent cross-sectional study by McCrindle failed to demonstrate differences in brachial artery reactivity or carotid intima-media thickness following Kawasaki disease, although there was some degree of impaired blood pressure control documented on 24-h ambulatory blood pressure monitoring in Kawasaki disease cases.[21]

Perhaps more important than these studies of novel surrogate markers for vascular injury are the long-term epidemiological data from Japan. In the fifth look at long-term outcomes of a cohort of 6576 patients with Kawasaki disease enrolled between 1982 and 1992, the mortality rate for patients without cardiac sequelae in the acute phase of the disease and female patients with sequelae did not differ from the normal population. The mortality rate of males with cardiac sequelae was, however, 2.4 times higher than the normal population. Thus, the long-term outlook for patients with coronary involvement, particularly males, must remain guarded at the present time.

Key points for clinical practice

- The cause of Kawasaki disease is still unknown; the conventional antigen versus superantigen controversy regarding aetiopatho-genesis has not yet been resolved.

- The incidence of Kawasaki disease is rising world-wide, including the UK. This may reflect a truly rising incidence or increased clinician awareness.

- Siblings of index cases are at increased risk of Kawasaki disease, especially if under the age of 5 years.

- There is no gold-standard diagnostic test, although recently a number of novel surrogate markers of endothelial injury and/or immune markers have been proposed as being useful diagnostically. Diagnosis remains clinical, therefore.

(Continued on next page)

Key points for clinical practice (continued)

- The principal symptoms and signs may present sequentially such that the full set of criteria may not be present at any one time. Awareness of other non-principal signs (such as BCG re-activation) may improve the diagnostic pick-up rate.

- Atypical or incomplete Kawasaki disease has a significant risk of coronary arterial involvement.

- Intravenous immunoglobulin given as a single infusion of 2 g/kg over 12 h remains as the most efficacious treatment.

- The dose of aspirin during the acute febrile phase is 30–50 mg/kg in 4 divided doses, followed by 2–5 mg/kg when the fever settles. Aspirin at anti-platelet doses is continued for a minimum of 6 weeks. If there are no coronary artery abnormalities detected on echocardiography at 6 weeks, the aspirin can be stopped. If coronary artery abnormalities persist, the aspirin is continued. Aneurysms greater than 8 mm rarely resolve, and aspirin is then continued indefinitely; warfarin is usually added in addition in this situation.

- A number of studies have suggested that there may be long-term endothelial damage after Kawasaki disease, even in the absence of coronary arterial abnormalities in the acute stage of the disease. Whether Kawasaki disease causes premature atherosclerosis or not remains controversial. Until this issue is resolved long-term follow up is recommended.

References

1. Kawasaki T. [Acute febrile mucocutaneous syndrome with lymphoid involvement with specific desquamation of the fingers and toes in children]. *Arerugi* 1967; **16**: 178–222.
2. Shulman ST, De Inocencio J, Hirsch R. Kawasaki disease. *Pediatr Clin North Am* 1995; **42**: 1205–1222.
3. Levin M, Tizard EJ, Dillon MJ. Kawasaki disease: recent advances. *Arch Dis Child* 1991; **66**: 1369–1372.
4. Bronstein DE, Dille AN, Austin JP, Williams CM, Palinkas LA, Burns JC. Relationship of climate, ethnicity and socioeconomic status to Kawasaki disease in San Diego County, 1994 through 1998. *Pediatr Infect Dis J* 2000; **19**: 1087–1091.
5. Fujita Y, Nakamura Y, Sakata K *et al.* Kawasaki disease in families. *Pediatrics* 1989; **84**: 666–669.
6. Harnden A, Alves B, Sheikh A. Rising incidence of Kawasaki disease in England: analysis of hospital admission data. *BMJ* 2002; **324**: 1424–1425.
7. Curtis N, Zheng R, Lamb JR, Levin M. Evidence for a superantigen mediated process in Kawasaki disease. *Arch Dis Child* 1995; **72**: 308–311.
8. Leung DY, Giorno RC, Kazemi LV, Flynn PA, Busse JB. Evidence for superantigen involvement in cardiovascular injury due to Kawasaki syndrome. *J Immunol* 1995; **155**: 5018–5021.
9. Leung DY, Meissner C, Fulton D, Schlievert PM. The potential role of bacterial superantigens in the pathogenesis of Kawasaki syndrome. *J Clin Immunol* 1995; **15**: 11S–17S.
10. Hansen RC. Staphylococcal scalded skin syndrome, toxic shock syndrome, and Kawasaki disease. *Pediatr Clin North Am* 1983; **30**: 533–544.
11. Raimer SS, Tschen EH, Walker MK. Toxic shock syndrome. Possible confusion with Kawasaki's disease. *Cutis* 1981; **28**: 33–35.

12. Hall M, Hoyt L, Ferrieri P, Schlievert PM, Jenson HB. Kawasaki syndrome-like illness associated with infection caused by enterotoxin B-secreting *Staphylococcus aureus*. *Clin Infect Dis* 1999; **29**: 586–589.

13. Furukawa S, Matsubara T, Yabuta K. Superantigens and Kawasaki disease. *Immunol Today* 1991; **12**: 464.

14. Abe J, Kotzin BL, Jujo K *et al*. Selective expansion of T cells expressing T-cell receptor variable regions V beta 2 and V beta 8 in Kawasaki disease. *Proc Natl Acad Sci USA* 1992; **89**: 4066–4070.

15. Dajani AS, Taubert KA, Gerber MA *et al*. Diagnosis and therapy of Kawasaki disease in children. *Circulation* 1993; **87**: 1776–1780.

16. Brogan PA, Bose A, Burgner D *et al*. Kawasaki disease: an evidence based approach to diagnosis, treatment, and proposals for future research. *Arch Dis Child* 2002; **86**: 286–290.

17. Tizard EJ. Recognition and management of Kawasaki disease. *Curr Paediatr* 1999; **8**: 97–101.

18. Sireci G, Dieli F, Salerno A. T cells recognize an immunodominant epitope of heat shock protein 65 in Kawasaki disease. *Mol Med* 2000; **6**: 581–590.

19. Petty RE, Cassidy JT. Kawasaki disease. In: Cassidy RE, Petty JT. (eds) *Textbook of Pediatric Rheumatology*. Philadelphia, PA: WB Saunders, 2001; 580–594.

20. Sonobe T, Aso S, Imada Y, Tsuchiya K, Nakamura Y, Yanagawa H. The incidence of coronary artery abnormality in incomplete Kawasaki disease [Abstract]. *Proceedings of the 7th International Kawasaki Disease Symposium*, 2001 48.

21. Newburger JW, Taubert KA, Shulman ST *et al*. Summary and abstracts of the Seventh International Kawasaki Disease Symposium: December 4–7, 2001, Hakone, Japan. *Pediatr Res* 2003; **53**: 153–157.

22. Nakatani K, Takeshita S, Tsujimoto H, Kawamura Y, Tokutomi T, Sekine I. Circulating endothelial cells in Kawasaki disease. *Clin Exp Immunol* 2003; **131**: 536–540.

23. Reichardt P, Lehmann I, Sierig G, Borte M. Analysis of T-cell receptor V-beta 2 in peripheral blood lymphocytes as a diagnostic marker for Kawasaki disease. *Infection* 2002; **30**: 360–364.

24. Melish ME, Takahashi M, Shulman ST. Comparison of low dose aspirin (LDA) versus high dose aspirin (HDA) as an adjunct to intravenous gamma globulin (IVIG) in the treatment of Kawasaki syndrome (KS). *Pediatr Res* 1992; **31**: 170A (abstract).

25. Terai M, Shulman ST. Prevalence of coronary artery abnormalities in Kawasaki disease is highly dependent on gamma globulin dose but independent of salicylate dose. *J Pediatr* 1997; **131**: 888–893.

26. Matsubara T, Mason W, Kashani IA, Kligerman M, Burns JC. Gastrointestinal hemorrhage complicating aspirin therapy in acute Kawasaki disease. *J Pediatr* 1996; **128**: 701–703.

27. Durongpisitkul K, Gururaj VJ, Park JM, Martin CF. The prevention of coronary artery aneurysm in Kawasaki disease: a meta-analysis on the efficacy of aspirin and immunoglobulin treatment. *Pediatrics* 1995; **96**: 1057–1061.

28. Wright DA, Newburger JW, Baker A, Sundel RP. Treatment of immune globulin-resistant Kawasaki disease with pulsed doses of corticosteroids. *J Pediatr* 1996; **128**: 146–149.

29. Dale RC, Saleem MA, Daw S, Dillon MJ. Treatment of severe complicated Kawasaki disease with oral prednisolone and aspirin. *J Pediatr* 2000; **137**: 723–726.

30. Khowsathit P, Hong-Hgam C, Khositseth A, Wanitkun S. Treatment of Kawasaki disease with a moderate dose (1 g/kg) of intravenous immunoglobulin. *J Med Assoc Thai* 2002; **85 (Suppl 4)**: S1121–S1126.

31. Durongpisitkul K, Soongswang J, Laohaprasitiporn D, Nana A, Prachuabmoh C, Kangkagate C. Immunoglobulin failure and retreatment in Kawasaki disease. *Pediatr Cardiol* 2003; **24**: 145–148.

32. Sundel RP. Update on the treatment of Kawasaki disease in childhood. *Curr Rheumatol Rep* 2002; **4**: 474–482.

33. Siber GR, Werner BG, Halsey NA *et al*. Interference of immune globulin with measles and rubella immunization. *J Pediatr* 1993; **122**: 204–211.

34. Dhillon R, Newton L, Rudd PT, Hall SM. Management of Kawasaki disease in the British Isles. *Arch Dis Child* 1993; **69**: 631–636.

35. Burns JC, Shike H, Gordon JB, Malhotra A, Schoenwetter M, Kawasaki T. Sequelae of Kawasaki disease in adolescents and young adults. *J Am Coll Cardiol* 1996; **28**: 253–257.

36. Newburger JW. Kawasaki disease. Current treatment options. *Cardiovasc Med* 2000; **2**: 227–236.
37. Weiss P, Soff GA, Halkin H, Seligsohn U. Decline of proteins C and S and factors II, VII, IX and X during the initiation of warfarin therapy. *Thromb Res* 1987; **45**: 783–790.
38. Etheridge SP, Tani LY, Minich LL, Revenaugh JR. Platelet glycoprotein IIb/IIIa receptor blockade therapy for large coronary aneurysms and thrombi in Kawasaki disease. *Cathet Cardiovasc Diagn* 1998; **45**: 264–268.
39. Brecker SJ, Gray HH, Oldershaw PJ. Coronary artery aneurysms and myocardial infarction: adult sequelae of Kawasaki disease? *Br Heart J* 1988; **59**: 509–512.
40. Dhillon R, Clarkson P, Donald AE *et al*. Endothelial dysfunction late after Kawasaki disease. *Circulation* 1996; **94**: 2103–2106.
41. Pilla C, Cheung YF, Brogan PA, Dillon MJ, Redington AN. Chronically reduced arterial distensibility in Kawasaki disease: further evidence for the beneficial effects of immunoglobulin. *Circulation* 2000; **102** (1Suppl II), 830–831.

James Y. Paton

2

Developments in the management of asthma

It was the best of times, it was the worst of times...

A Tale of Two Cities by Charles Dickens

It would be difficult to think of a more interesting time to review developments in the management of childhood asthma. This is a time when the global burden of childhood asthma is enormous. At the same time, there has been an exponential increase in our understanding about asthma, reflected in the explosion of research articles published every year. Effective treatments are widely available. Guidelines about the management of asthma have been published and are regularly updated, making the best evidence about asthma management readily accessible. Nevertheless, asthma control remains poor for many (Table 1).[1]

This article outlines some of the important recent developments in the management of childhood asthma. It does not attempt to be encyclopaedic but reflects one specialist paediatrician's viewpoint. Readers looking for more detail are referred to recently published guidelines[2] and the Cochrane Database of Systematic Reviews.

CHILDHOOD ASTHMA TODAY

Throughout the world, asthma is amongst the commonest chronic diseases of childhood. In the UK, asthma affects between 10–20% of children depending on the disease measure used.[3]

Evidence is consistent in showing a substantial increase in the burden of childhood asthma over the past 30 years,[3] a time when the prevalence and

Dr James Y. Paton MD FRCPCH
Reader in Paediatric Respiratory Disease, Department of Child Health, Royal Hospital for Sick Children, Yorkhill NHS Trust Hospital, Glasgow G3 8SJ, UK
Tel: +44 141 201 0238; Fax: +44141 201 0837; E-mail: J.Y.Paton@clinmed.gla.ac.uk

Table 1 The Global Initiative for Asthma (GINA) recommended goals of asthma management and data from the Asthma Insights and Reality in Europe (AIRE results) study showing the results actually reported in 753 children

GINA recommendation	AIRE result	Symptoms in children (%)
Minimal chronic symptoms	Daytime symptoms once a week	38.2
	Sleep disturbances at least once a week	28.0
Minimal episodes	Reported episodes of coughing, wheezing, chest tightness or shortness of breath in the last month	51.5
No emergency visits	Unscheduled urgent care visits during last year	36.0
	Emergency visits during last year	18
Minimal need for ß2-agonists	Used as-required β_2-agonists during the last month	61.0
No limitations on activities	Limitation of activities	
	Sports	29.5
	Normal physical activity	19.1
	Choice of jobs/career	–
	Social activities	13.8
	Sleep	31.2
	Life-style	18.6
	Housekeeping chores	10.9
	School/work absence	42.7
Normal or near normal lung function	Never had a lung function test	60.5

Adapted from Rabe et al.[1]

morbidity associated with many other childhood illnesses has been decreasing. The most recent data suggest a slight decline in hospital admissions and deaths,[3] perhaps reflecting the effects of improved clinical care.

Prevalence rates vary substantially from country to country, tending to be highest in economically developed countries with a temperate climate, and being particularly high in English speaking countries and in Latin America.[4] There are also marked racial variations within countries that may reflect the impact of poverty and lack of access to health care.[3]

The causes of both the rising prevalence and the geographical variation in prevalence are not known. Differing exposures to as yet undefined environmental factors seem to be the most likely explanation. There have been hypothesised links to environmental changes associated with economic development, such as air pollution or changes in the indoor environment, as well as to changes in life-style and diet.

The increase in asthma over time seems to reflect a more general increase in the prevalence of allergic sensitisation and allergic disease. A more affluent life-style has many features that may be involved in the cause of asthma and allergy. One of the most striking observations about allergic sensitisation and, to a lesser extent, asthma is that it is less common in children with older siblings. It is nearly 15 years since David Strachan proposed 'the hygiene hypothesis' to explain this inverse association with family size.[5] Strachan suggested that the epidemiological observations could be explained 'if allergic diseases were prevented by infection in early childhood, transmitted by unhygienic contact with older siblings, or acquired prenatally'. Exposure to lower levels of infection might polarise the immune system towards an allergic phenotype and hence pose a greater risk of allergic disease. In general, an inverse association between infection and atopy has not been confirmed directly by epidemiological studies. The most consistent evidence of an inverse relationship between infection and allergic sensitisation has emerged from studies of hepatitis A. This and other studies have raised the interesting possibility that the intestinal flora may influence immunological maturation. Factors such as antibiotic therapy and diet in early childhood acting through gut flora perhaps may contribute to the variations in allergy within countries.

Whatever the causes for these variations, the current burden of childhood asthma is enormous.

SOME SIGNIFICANT PROBLEMS

PATTERNS OF ASTHMA AND WHEEZING IN EARLY CHILDHOOD

Over the last 15 years, longitudinal studies have made it clear that childhood asthma is not a single disease (Fig. 1). Rather, there are distinctive patterns of wheezing with different patterns of progression.

At one extreme, there is a large group of children (perhaps 20% of the population) who present in the first 3 years of life with recurrent wheezing during viral lower respiratory infections. Respiratory symptoms often disappear as the child grows, such that between 60–70% of babies who wheezed during the first 6 months of life have stopped wheezing by 3–6 years of age ('transient early wheezers'). These children usually do not have any of the important, particularly the allergic, risk factors associated with asthma in later childhood. Children of mothers who smoke during pregnancy are particularly at risk. In this group, Martinez et al.[6] showed that there is often reduced lung function, which can be detected before any wheezing illnesses develop. Taken altogether, the data suggest that it is the mechanical properties of the airways which play a dominant role in transient early wheezing.

At the opposite extreme is a the group of young children (10% of the population) who may also wheeze during viral infections, but who also have present the allergic risk factors associated with persistent asthma in later childhood. The onset of symptoms before age 3 years is associated with increased asthma severity and bronchial hyper-responsiveness as well as more significant loss in pulmonary function. In this group, early allergic sensitisation may be an important factor in the development of persistent asthma; specific factors such as increased exposure in early life to other children, pets, or farm animals, may protect against the development of asthma.

Unfortunately, there is often significant overlap between these groups. At the stage when a child first develops a wheezy illness, it is not yet possible to know with certainty whether they will merely experience transient symptoms or whether they will go on to develop persistent asthma. Since the adverse

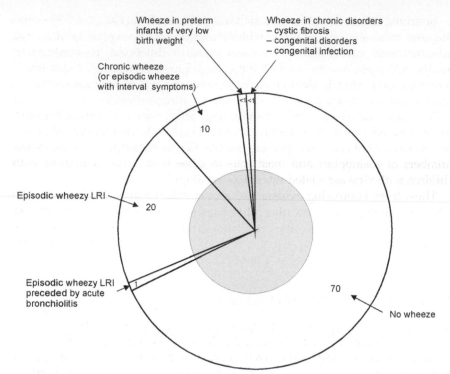

Wheeze in preterm
infants of very low
birth weight

Wheeze in chronic disorders
– cystic fibrosis
– congenital disorders
– congenital infection

Chronic wheeze
(or episodic wheeze
with interval symptoms)

<1 <1

10

Episodic wheezy LRI

20

Episodic wheezy LRI
preceded by acute
bronchiolitis

1

70

No wheeze

Fig. 1 Frequency of wheezing disorders in a UK population of infants. Figures are percentages. The central, grey-filled area represents the random distribution of the atopic genotype (about 30%) across all groups. From: *Childhood Asthma and Other Wheezing Disorders*, 2nd edn, edited by Prof. Michael Silverman, Arnold, with permission.

effects of asthma on lung function seem to occur before 5–6 years of age, distinguishing these different patterns types is likely to be very important in deciding the best approaches to asthma treatment and prevention.

This is a significant clinical problem because it has been estimated that, if all the children who presented with wheezing were treated with preventive asthma medication, something approaching half of all children would require treatment. The problem is made more difficult in young children, because a number of other often uncommon conditions, such as cystic fibrosis, can present with symptoms very similar to asthma.

IS CHILDHOOD ASTHMA AN INFLAMMATORY DISEASE?

It is well established that in adults asthma is a chronic inflammatory disease of the airways. Endoscopic biopsy studies have documented mucosal inflammation within the airways even in mild-to-moderate asthma. Air-flow limitation and bronchial hyper-responsiveness, the pathophysiological hallmarks of asthma, are thought to arise as consequences of persistent airway inflammation. In chronic asthma, the repair processes are also disturbed and remodelling of airway structures occurs. Although endoscopic airway biopsy has provided the gold standard test for diagnosing airway inflammation, it is neither technically nor ethically straightforward when applied to children.

In school children with atopic asthma, the limited data available indicate that the morphological picture with basement membrane thickening and inflammatory cell infiltration in the airways is similar to that encountered in adults, although not all studies have found eosinophilic inflammation.[7,8] Basement membrane thickening has been demonstrated even in children with mild/moderate asthma.[7]

In young children with different wheezing phenotypes, information is even more limited. Broncho-alveolar lavage studies have shown different inflammatory cell profiles depending on the allergic background, with greater numbers of eosinophils and mast cells in those with atopy compared with children with viral associated wheeze or no atopy.[9]

Thus, there is growing evidence of airway inflammation in children who wheeze. Whether and how the inflammatory processes in the airways of children with asthma and wheezing differ from those in adults, and how the inflammatory processes vary with age and stage of disease, as well as with atopic status, require further detailed research.

OUTCOMES – OLD AND NEW

In clinical work or for research purposes, asthma outcomes are usually based on measures such as changes in symptoms, pulmonary function, quality of life or economic costs. Despite the array of options, choosing outcome measures that are of value in making an accurate diagnosis or evaluating the benefits of treatment is often difficult in children. Standard symptom reports can be unreliable. For example, accurate reporting of nocturnal symptoms depends on the carer being awake to notice them. Lung function provides an objective measure, but is often impossible in young children. Validated quality of life instruments measure the impact of a disease on a patient's daily activities. However, there may be little correlation between the concerns of the child about his or her asthma, the effects on the family reported by the parent or the clinician's view of asthma control.[10]

Recently, there has been increasing interest in objective, non-invasive markers which might reflect directly the extent of airway inflammation. One of the most promising has been the measurement of nitric oxide exhaled breath (eNO). Increased eNO levels are thought to result from an increase in the expression in cells in the respiratory tract of an inducible nitric oxide synthase, induced by the action of pro-inflammatory cytokines. Exhaled NO levels (FENO) are increased in atopic asthmatics compared to non-atopic controls, increase during an exacerbation, decrease with anti-inflammatory therapy, and rise as the dose of inhaled corticosteroids is reduced.

This opens up the possibility that eNO could be a useful method of monitoring response to therapy,[11] and perhaps even of diagnosing asthma in some children.[12] The possibility is attractive as eNO is measured non-invasively, can be easily obtained, followed serially, and used in infants and young children too young to perform other lung function tests.

Other non-invasive markers of inflammation are being actively studied. Molecules such as hydrogen peroxide and leukotrienes have been found in condensates of exhaled air as well as markers of oxidative damage. Such non-invasive markers may help characterise patterns of lower airway inflammation.

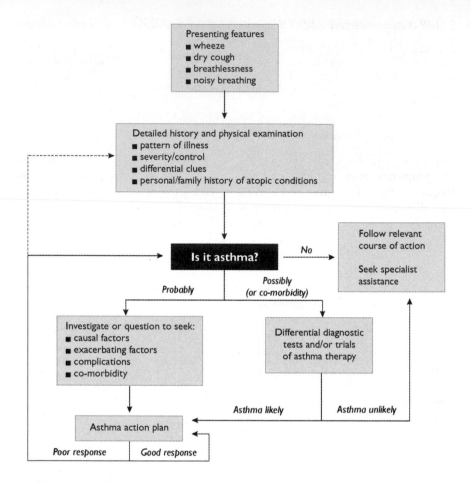

Fig. 2 Algorithm for the diagnosis of asthma in children (from British guideline on the management of asthma[2]).

THE DIFFICULTIES OF DIAGNOSIS

The most difficult step in managing childhood asthma is often making an accurate diagnosis. Parents expect that there will be a blood, skin or X-ray test which will give a definite diagnosis. Yet there is still no gold standard test, and the diagnosis of asthma remains clinical.[2] This is particularly true for pre-school children. Lung function tests may corroborate the diagnosis in older children; however, in those under 5 years of age, lung function testing is still largely a clinical research tool.

A PRACTICAL APPROACH TO DIAGNOSIS AND MANAGEMENT

The diagnosis of asthma in children is usually a process, rather than a single step (Fig. 2). The stages are: (i) recognising the presence of key clinical features; (ii) carefully considering alternative diagnoses; (iii) assessing the response to trials of treatment; and (iv) re-assessing the child over time and questioning the diagnosis if management is ineffective.

SYMPTOMS – WHAT ARE THE CLINICAL FEATURES?

Because of the lack of objective measurements, diagnosing childhood asthma is dependent on parental symptom reporting. The classic symptoms of asthma are the same at all ages – wheezing, difficulty breathing and dry cough. In asthma, these symptoms vary over time and improve after bronchodilator treatment. Increased wheezing with viral infections is particularly common in children.

Unfortunately, this typical picture conceals some major difficulties in children, highlighted by Cane and Mackenzie: some parents confuse respiratory sounds; night time symptoms are difficult to quantify; recollection of symptoms may change; parents' and children's reports of symptom frequency may not agree; and clinicians' and parents' words for symptoms may differ. In some languages, there is no word for 'wheeze' – a problem in an increasingly multicultural society. In more detailed studies, Cane and MacKenzie found that only about a third of mothers recognised their child was wheezy by 'sound' alone. Indeed, a quarter of mothers reported using only non-auditory clues to recognise whether their child was wheezy and two-thirds used difficulty in breathing and/or being unwell as the main way of knowing that their child was unwell.[13]

There is perhaps an even greater problem with isolated persistent cough. Very few children with a chronic non-productive cough without wheeze will turn out to have asthma.[14] Further, isolated cough does not respond well to asthma treatments. Paediatric respiratory specialists have been increasingly concerned that too many children whose only symptom is cough have been inappropriately diagnosed as having asthma and treated with asthma medications, including high dose inhaled corticosteroids.

More objective tests for diagnosing childhood asthma would clearly help. In the meantime, symptoms such as wheezing and cough should be viewed circumspectly. Silverman and Keeley[15] suggest the following approach: 'Let parents use their own words. Do not offer the word 'wheeze' but wait to see if the parents use it. If they do, clarify what it means.' For pre-school children, it may even be best to arrange to examine the child when parents think symptoms are present.

Because of these difficulties, it is important to look for other supporting clinical features. Evidence of atopy – either eczema or rhinitis, or from positive allergy tests – is the factor most clearly linked to asthma. A family history of asthma and rhinitis, particularly in the mother, predicts the presence of symptoms throughout childhood. It is also important to remember that many other conditions cause childhood wheezing. Clinical features such as wheezing that starts in early infancy, moist cough, the presence of finger clubbing, or poor growth, are not features of asthma and should point to other diagnoses.

PROGRESS WITH MANAGEMENT

At present, asthma cannot be cured, only controlled. The most effective available treatments are pharmacological. Most asthma guidelines recommend a stepwise approach to pharmacological treatment starting with β_2-agonists for mild inter-mittent symptoms through to daily oral corticosteroids for the most severe disease. The starting level of treatment should be based on an assessment of asthma severity.

A major issue for paediatricians is that the evidence base in children younger than 5 years is often thin, because of the small number of studies available. As a

Table 2 Age-specific recommendations for inhaled drug delivery devices

Age (years)	First choice	Second choice	Comments
0–2	MDI + spacer and face mask	Nebuliser	Ensure optimum spacer use Avoid 'open vent' nebulisers
3–6	MDI + spacer	Nebuliser	Very few children at this age can use dry powder inhalers adequately
6–12 (broncho-dilators	MDI + spacer, breath actuated or dry powder inhaler	–	If using breath actuated or dry powder inhaler, also prescribe MDI + spacer for acute exacerbations
6–12 (steroids)	MDI + spacer	Dry powder inhaler	May need to adjust dose if switching between inhalers Advise mouth rinsing or gargling
12+ (broncho-dilators)	Dry powder inhaler or breath actuated MDI	–	
12+ (steroids)	MDI + spacer	Dry powder inhaler or breath actuated MDI	May need to adjust dose if switching between inhalers Advise mouth rinsing or gargling
Acute asthma (all ages)	MDI + spacer	Nebuliser	Written instructions for what to do in acute asthma

MDI, meter dose inhaler.
From O'Callaghan and Barry.[42]

consequence, treatment recommendations are often based on extrapolation from studies of older children or adults.

INHALED OR ORAL?

Although administering inhaled drugs to children is often difficult, there are clear potential benefits. Direct delivery to the airways means beneficial effects can be achieved rapidly with much smaller doses, resulting in lower systemic drug concentrations and fewer adverse side effects. All these benefits would be likely to remain important even if oral drugs of similar effectiveness to inhaled drugs were to become available.

Even in 2003, incorrect inhaler use is still all too common, and large numbers of children are prescribed inhalers they cannot use. Age- and drug-specific recommendations have been made and are a useful starting point (Table 2). Clinicians should pick one or two of each type of device for use in their practice and become completely familiar with their use. If inhaled therapy is to be successful, then the device must be appropriate to a child's developmental skills, the child and their carers must be carefully taught and must be able to demonstrate satisfactory technique. Device use should be checked at each clinical review.

WHICH DRUG, WHEN?

Relievers

For asthma symptom relief and for the prevention of exercise-induced asthma, inhaled short-acting β_2-agonist bronchodilators remain the drugs of choice. A Cochrane Review has confirmed that there is no clear advantage in using β_2-agonists regularly, supporting guideline recommendations to use bronchodilators for symptom relief on an as-needed basis.[2]

The long debate on the effectiveness of bronchodilators in infants and young children continues. The evidence remains surprisingly limited. A meta-analysis, which included only 8 RCTs, found no clear benefit of using β_2-agonists in the management of recurrent wheeze in the first 2 years of life, although the evidence was conflicting.[16] The review highlights that problems in defining the precise phenotype and measuring suitable outcomes will need to be addressed before those young children with wheezing who might respond to bronchodilators can be confidently identified. Fortunately, the likelihood of a clinical bronchodilator response increases with age.

Preventers

Inhaled corticosteroids are now considered the mainstay of asthma treatment even in young children.[2] The exact threshold when prophylactic treatment should be started has never been definitely established. The latest UK guideline recommends starting inhaled corticosteroids when bronchodilator treatment is needed more than once a day, when there is nocturnal asthma or impaired lung function or after a recent exacerbation.[2] The most recent US guideline update places the threshold slightly lower and suggests intervention when symptoms occur twice a week, or nocturnal waking more than twice a month; for younger children, exacerbations more than 6 weekly or more than 3 episodes of sleep disturbing wheezing lasting more than 24 h in a year are also indications.[17]

The problem in young children is that many wheeze only with viral infections and have no interval symptoms. Clinical trials over many years have never shown any benefit of corticosteroids (oral or inhaled) in acute viral bronchiolitis. There is also no evidence that regular low-dose inhaled corticosteroids are effective in the prevention or management of episodic, mild, viral-induced wheeze.[18] If the child has no interval symptoms but only develops wheezing with triggers such as viral infections, bronchodilators are the treatment most likely to provide symptom relief. Current guidelines recommend that a short course of oral corticosteroids can be added for significant exacerbations. However, a very recent RCT found no clear benefit of parent-initiated oral prenisolone for viral wheeze in children aged 1–5 years, suggesting this stategy may need re-evaluation.[19]

Chronic ('interval') respiratory symptoms when the child has no obvious cold or other trigger mark out those children who will respond to prophylactic treatment. Rhinitis without colds may be another clinical marker of symptoms that will persist. In these children with chronic persistent symptoms, inhaled corticosteroids are the most effective regular anti-inflammatory drugs, even in infants and toddlers.

At what dose?

Probably the most important recent development in asthma management has been the realisation that most children with asthma require only a low dose of an

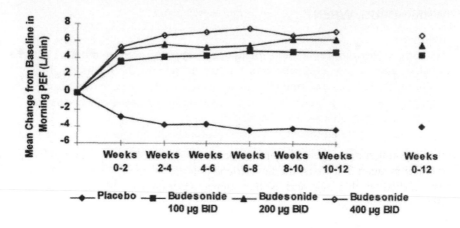

Fig. 3 Dose response curve for inhaled corticosteroids in children. Mean change from baseline in morning PEF for placebo- and budesonide-treated groups by treatment week and as average value throughout 12-week treatment period (weeks 0–12). Improvements in morning PEF observed in groups receiving 100, 200, and 400 µg of budesonide twice daily were statistically significant ($P < 0.001$), in comparison with placebo group. The difference between the budesonide groups receiving 100 and 400 µg twice daily was also statistically significant ($P < 0.05$). Statistically significant improvements in morning PEF were observed within 2 weeks of initiation of treatment of budesonide.[20]

inhaled corticosteroid for effective treatment. This is because the dose-response curve for inhaled corticosteroids reaches a plateau at relatively modest doses of between 100–200 µg/day beclomethasone dipropionate equivalent.[19] Increasing the dose beyond these levels rarely improves asthma control and by then the dose may be on the steep part of the side-effect curve. The result is that, as the steroid dose is increased, there may no clinical benefit but an increased risk of systemic side effects (Fig. 3). Most children can be managed with < 400 µg/day budesonide or equivalent. If control is inadequate, then it is usually better to add another drug rather than increase the inhaled corticosteroid dose. Such an approach maximises the chances of asthma control while minimising the risk of side effects.

How often?
Inhaled steroids have usually been given twice a day. Once satisfactory control is established, they can often be maintained giving the same daily dose only once per day.[2] There is substantial evidence to support this, especially for budesonide. Indeed, once-a-day inhaled corticosteroids may be all that is ever required for many children.[21] Whether the drug is given in the morning or evening does not seem to matter, at least for budesonide;[20] thus, administration can be adapted to family routine, hopefully improving long-term compliance.

WHEN SHOULD THERAPY BE INCREASED OR AUGMENTED AND, IF SO, WITH WHAT?

For those children, who are not controlled on a modest dose of inhaled corticosteroids (< 400 µg/day budesonide or equivalent) where next? Before any increase in therapy, it is always important to check that the child can use the prescribed device correctly, to investigate compliance and check whether continuing exposure to any asthma triggers may be preventing improvement.

For children over 5 years, the first choice for an add-on therapy is an inhaled long-acting β_2-agonist (salmeterol or formoterol twice daily). Both long-acting β_2-agonists are available in combination with an inhaled corticosteroids. While there is no difference in efficacy in giving the long-acting bronchodilator and inhaled corticosteroids in combination or separately, the combination may lead to better compliance. None of the add-on therapies have been adequately studied in children younger than 5 years, a gap that has been identified as a research priority. For children, aged 2–5 years, the leukotriene antagonist, monteleukast, has been most studied at this age and is the suggested drug to add on to inhaled corticosteroids at present.[2]

For those children with poor control on moderate doses of inhaled cortico-steroids and an add-on therapy, there is essentially no clinical evidence what to do next. The new British asthma guidelines suggest a sequential trial of: (i) increasing the inhaled corticosteroids to 800 µg/day; (ii) a leukotriene receptor antagonist; or (iii) oral theophylline. The treatment should be evaluated over 6–8 weeks. If it is ineffective, it should be stopped and the next choice tried.

There are still a very few children in whom all these treatments will fail and who may require continuous oral steroids, or more experimental therapies. These children are best evaluated using a systematic protocol in specialist centres experienced in the management of children with severe asthma.

Leukotriene modifier drugs

The leukotriene modifiers are the only new class of drugs to come on the market in the last two decades. These agents block the action or inhibit the synthesis of cysteinyl leukotrienes, mediators which cause bronchoconstriction, mucous secretion and increased vascular permeability. There are two pharmacological classes of drugs – 5-lipo-oygenase inhibitors (*e.g.* zileuton) and leukotriene receptor antagonists (*e.g.* monteleukast). Monteleukast has been the one most widely studied in children. It is approved for children older than 2 years, is given once daily and is available both as a liquid and a chewable tablet making it particularly useful in treating young children. It reduces the signs and symptoms of chronic asthma in children as young as 2 years.[22] Monteleukast also rapidly attenuates exercise-induced bronchoconstriction. However, there is not enough data yet to be clear about the best way to use monteleukast in the treatment of childhood asthma.

Is it important to start early?

An important question has been whether starting an inhaled corticosteroids early in the course of asthma can alter the natural history of the disease. Inhaled corticosteroids improve symptoms and the occurrence of exacerbations; however, when treatment is stopped, most patients relapse over days or weeks suggesting that drugs has only a suppressant effect on inflammation.[23] Pedersen and Agertoft reported better long-term lung function in children with mild/moderate persistent asthma if inhaled corticosteroids were started within 2 years of symptoms starting.[24] In one recent study, pre- and post-bronchodilator lung function was already reduced at study entry even though two-thirds of the subjects had had asthma for less than a year. Lung function continued to decrease in both groups, although at a slower rate in those treated with budesonide.[21] The large US CAMP study also found no benefit in terms of lung function for children given inhaled budesonide or nedocromil compared with therapy given as need for control of symptoms.[25] Inhaled corticosteroids are clearly effective at controlling symptoms and preventing exacerbations, but do not appear to prevent on-going reduction in lung function which seems most rapid early in the disease. Whether 'even earlier' intervention might prevent the development of permanent structural changes in the airways outcomes remains moot.

Reducing therapy

Just as the threshold for when to start inhaled corticosteroid is not clearly defined, there is little evidence about how to reduce treatment in children. Guidelines suggest halving the dose every 3 months if the patient remains symptom-free. In fact, in most cases, the parents or the child will have already experimented by reducing or even stopping completely if the symptoms have settled.

A TRIAL OF THERAPY

With the difficulties of diagnosis, it is hardly surprising that a trial of anti-asthma treatment is often an important step in managing childhood asthma.

In infants with frequent or prolonged wheeze, Cochrane proposed an 8-week trial of moderately high-dose inhaled steroid (800 µg/day beclomethasone dipropionate or equivalent) on the basis that a generous dose will increase the likelihood of a clear response if there is going to be one.[26] If there is an excellent response after 6–8 weeks, the dose should be 'stepped down' to the minimum required to control symptoms. If, on the other hand, there is no response, the drug should be stopped completely.

WHAT'S NEW IN SIDE EFFECTS

Systemic effects of inhaled corticosteroids

Inhaled corticosteroids have been in use for around 30 years, yet concerns about their side effects continue, especially as they are used earlier, in younger children and for longer periods and as new more potent steroids become available.

Inhaled corticosteroids cause systemic effects to the extent that they are absorbed from the gastrointestinal tract and the airways. The amount absorbed varies with the dose, with the site of deposition, with the metabolism of the particular drug and with the device. Newer inhaled steroids (fluticasone propionate, mometasone) are minimally absorbed from the gastrointestinal tract and/or undergo extensive first-pass liver metabolism so that only a small amount reaches the systemic circulation. However, significant amounts of inhaled steroids can be absorbed through the lungs where they escape first-pass metabolism in the liver and can cause systemic effects.

Adrenal insufficiency

Until 1999, published reports of acute adrenal insufficiency associated with inhaled corticosteroids were exceptionally rare. It came as a shock when cases of acute adrenal insufficiency attributed to inhaled corticosteroids were reported in the literature. In a subsequent national UK survey, Todd *et al.* identified 33 asthmatic patients (28 children, 5 adults) with acute adrenal crisis associated with inhaled corticosteroids.[27] Of the 28 children, 23 had symptoms of acute hypoglycaemia (13 decreased conscious level or coma; 9 with coma and convulsions; one with coma, convulsions and death).

The fact that the majority of these cases were receiving inhaled fluticasone propionate via meter dose inhaler ± spacer was unexpected. This may reflect the fact fluticasone propionate had become the preferred steroid for many patients requiring higher inhaled corticosteroids doses because of a perceived superior benefit/risk ratio. It may also reflect particular pharmacokinetic properties of fluticasone propionate such as its high potency and lipophilicity. Nevertheless, the reports of adrenal suppression with both budesonide and beclomethasone dipropionate suggest that the effect is at least, in part, a class effect of high-dose inhaled corticosteroids. Thus, while other steroids may be safer than fluticasone propionate, no steroid is completely safe. The results also emphasised the importance of having a secure diagnosis of asthma if potent inhaled corticosteroids were to be used at high doses. In the study, 8 children had persistent cough; of these, 3 did not have asthma; in 5, persistent cough unresponsive to inhaled corticosteroids may have led to increasing treatment.

Clinical adrenal insufficiency is simple to treat – if the condition is recognised. Clinicians should be particularly vigilant when children with asthma using inhaled corticosteroids present with disturbed consciousness, unusual behaviour or autonomic symptoms suggestive of hypoglycaemia.

Todd *et al.* suggested that adrenal function should be monitored in children receiving > 400 μg/day fluticasone propionate or equivalent for a year or more with a low dose ACTH test;[27] however, as yet, there is no overall consensus on the method or frequency of testing.

Growth

The other long-running concern has been the effects of inhaled corticosteroids on growth. It has been very difficult to separate out the growth effects of chronic asthma from the side effects of inhaled corticosteroids. Price *at al.*[28] identified 18 growth studies investigating the effects of inhaled corticosteroids that included a control group, measured height by stadiometry and lasted a year or longer; 17 were susceptible to one or more important confounding factors. Nevertheless, the findings were consistent. Budesonide and beclomethasone dipropionate impair growth velocity in comparison with placebo, non-steroidal therapy and fluticasone propionate during 1–2 years of treatment but have no impact on final height. Children treated with low-dose fluticasone propionate (< 200 μg/day) for 1 year grow similarly to those receiving placebo or non-steroidal therapy, but there are no data yet on fluticasone propionate's effect on final height.

The most important outcome is long-term growth as assessed by final adult height and compared with the predicted values for sex and mid-parental height. The only prospective study reported on 142 children treated with budesonide for a mean of 9.2 years (range, 3–13 years) at a mean daily dose 412 μg/day. They reached their target adult height to the same extent as their healthy siblings and children who had never received budesonide.[29] Agertoft and Pedersen noted that the growth during the first year of treatment was on average 1 cm less than during the run-in period, in keeping with the results from medium-term studies of budesonide; however, this initial reduction in growth rate did not persist, and adult height was not adversely affected.

Preventing side effects
It is quite clear that the safest way to use inhaled corticosteroids is to titrate to the lowest possible dose necessary to achieve satisfactory control of asthma. Higher dose inhaled corticosteroids should only be used when the diagnosis of asthma is secure, preferably supported by objective measurements, and under the careful supervision of a paediatrician experienced in managing asthma.

ALTERNATIVE THERAPIES

Concerns about drug side-effects are one of the factors that lead parents to try complementary and alternative medical therapies. Such treatments are surprisingly widely used in children. The range of therapies is extensive – one study identified 117 different therapies recommended as treatment for asthma. For most of the available asthma therapies, the evidence-based review undertaken for the latest British asthma guidelines[2] found the current evidence base to be inadequate in terms of the level, amount and quality of evidence available. Although some progress is being made in improving the evidence base, large gaps remain in our knowledge of such therapies.

Most alternative therapies are self-prescribed and are taken in addition to conventional drugs. However, only a minority of patients and families will discuss their use of, or reasons for using, alternative therapies with out prompting. Nevertheless, the wide-spread use of alternative therapies emphasises that there are important patient needs and concerns which current pharmacological therapy is not addressing. At present, the best advice is to question patients and families directly about their use of alternative therapies, to try to understand their motivations in using such therapies, and to explain dispassionately the known facts about any alternative therapy.

THE IMPORTANCE OF EDUCATION IN ASTHMA MANAGEMENT

The disparity between the wide availability of effective asthma treatments and poor asthma symptom control has led to the conclusion that there is an 'asthma knowledge gap' between clinicians' performance and patients' behaviours. Managing asthma is complex. For effective asthma control, parents and children must carry out a number of tasks such as using inhaler devices correctly, avoiding asthma trigger factors and self-managing most asthma exacerbations. The place of education in helping families develop the necessary knowledge, attitudes, beliefs and skills to manage asthma effectively has been increasingly recognised.[2] A recent systematic review of educational interventions in childhood asthma concluded that asthma self-management education programmes improved a wide range of outcomes, particularly in children with moderate-severe asthma.[30]

TREATING ACUTE ASTHMA – ANYTHING NEW?

In the UK, 14% of all acute paediatric hospital admissions are due to asthma attacks. Pre-school children have the highest rate for hospitalisation for diagnosed asthma of any age group.[31]

The mainstays of acute asthma treatment in children remain supplemental oxygen, if appropriate, high dose inhaled β_2-agonists and systemic corticosteroids.[2]

Oxygen saturation should be measured in all children with acute asthma. As well as allowing oxygen therapy to be targeted to those with low SpO_2 levels, low values after bronchodilator therapy (< 92%) identify those children with severe asthma who are likely to be admitted.

For children with mild-to-moderate exacerbations, a meter dose inhaler + spacer is the preferred delivery method for β_2-agonists. For reasons that remain unclear, children receiving β_2-agonists via spacers are less likely to have tachycardia and hypoxia than if given the same drug via nebuliser.[2] In school-aged children, bronchodilator via a dry powder inhaler may be as good as via a spacer.[32] In children with severe exacerbations, adding multiple doses of anticholinergics to β_2-agonists is safe, improves lung function and helps avoid hospital admission in 1 of 12 such treated patients.[2]

Early treatment with oral corticosteroids is highly effective and results in earlier discharge, shorter lengths of stay and less frequent relapse.[33] Prednisolone has the advantages of reliability, simplicity, convenience and cost and is the treatment of choice.

Only a few children will fail to respond to bronchodilators and steroids. For these children, the best evidence supports the addition of intravenous aminophylline,[34] which appears more effective then a single bolus dose of intravenous salbutamol.[35] UK data show that currently only about 5% of children admitted with acute asthma receive aminophylline.

For life-threatening asthma unresponsive to conventional therapies, treatment with intravenous magnesium sulphate has been used.[2] A very recent adult study reported that the using isotonic magnesium sulphate solution as an adjuvant to nebulised salbutamol resulted in clinically significant enhancement of bronchodilation in the treatment of severe asthma. Whether salbutamol nebuliser solution with adjuvant magnesium sulphate will have a role in the treatment of children with severe asthma awaits study.[36]

Any acute exacerbation provides an opportunity to review and educate parents about the management of future acute episodes. Studies of hospitalised children have shown that such education can significantly reduce subsequent asthma admissions.[37]

WHAT ABOUT ALLERGIES?

The idea that avoiding exposure to allergens within the environment might either prevent asthma or reduce the need for drug treatment is very appealing, both for patients and doctors. Primary prophylaxis is the term used for interventions applied before any evidence of disease is present with a view to preventing its occurrence. Secondary prevention applies to interventions made after the disease has developed to reduce its impact.

Unfortunately, despite considerable research, clear messages seem increasingly elusive. Sporik and Platts-Mills summarised the evidence as showing a proven association between allergen exposure and sensitisation and a strong association between allergen sensitisation and asthma. Despite strong evidence for a role of indoor allergens in asthma, there is still controversy about whether allergens play a *casual* role in the development of asthma.[38]

Doubt about the role of allergen exposure in the development of asthma has come about because it has not translated into simple therapies. Domestic avoidance measures are not easy to apply. They are often expensive and the results of controlled trials have not been consistent. Short-term trials of extreme allergen avoidance, for example at high altitude or in controlled environment such hospitals, have shown short-term benefit. But Sporik and Platts-Mills have pointed out that 20 years of research into mite avoidance measures (including pillow and mattress encasements, carpet removal, dehumidification, essential oil washes, steam cleaning, heat treatment, and improved vacuum cleaner filtration systems) have not provided simple and totally effective control measures.[38]

Things have become even more complicated because of increasing evidence of the phenomenon of high dose tolerance. For example, children raised in a household with a cat are less likely to become sensitized to cat allergen. The very high level of exposure to cat allergen induces a form of immunological tolerance.[39] In contrast, moderate exposure to cat allergen is sufficient to induce sensitisation in a large number of children who have never had a cat at home.

If avoidance of allergen is proving so complicated, is there a role for the induction of tolerance by immunotherapy? Paradoxically, there is actually quite good evidence of consistent benefit compared with placebo.[40] At present, the place of immunotherapy compared with pharmacotherapy and the relative risks and benefits need further study.

IS THERE ANYTHING THE PARENTS CAN DO?

SMOKING

For once, the message is clear. Children and young people, with, and without, asthma should not be exposed to environmental tobacco smoke so parents who smoke should stop. In very young children, banning smoking in the home was the only harm reduction strategy that reduced exposure to environmental tobacco smoke.[41] Newer smoking cessation interventions may offer a better framework to help parents give up smoking.

WHERE NEXT?

For children with asthma, highly effective evidence-based treatments are available that can make a substantial difference to their experience of asthma symptoms and the impact of these symptoms on their lives and families. Nevertheless, asthma control for many children remains suboptimal.

There are also many areas of childhood asthma management where evidence is deficient or even absent. This is particularly true for pre-school children where the main burden of childhood asthma rests; a better understanding of the wheezing phenotypes and their relation to airway inflammation, better diagnostic tests and a stronger evidence base for treatment are all required. Parents are right to be surprised that the diagnosis in particular is based on such shaky foundations.

Changes are afoot. Increasingly, large trials in well-defined groups of children with measurable asthma outcomes are being undertaken. New, non-invasive measures of inflammation are coming and there is a clear recognition of the need to close the gap between effective therapies and the fact that asthma control remains suboptimal for so many. The future will be different.

Key points for clinical practice

Asthma is amongst the commonest chronic diseases of childhood throughout the world.

- The prevalence in children has increased steadily over the last 30 years but is now stabilising.

- The cause for the increase in prevalence in not known but is most likely related to exposure to an as yet undefined environmental factor.

Childhood asthma is not a single disease.

- There are distinctive patterns of wheezing with different patterns of progression.

The diagnosis of asthma in children is clinical.

- Diagnosing asthma is usually a process rather than a single step.

- Symptoms such as wheezing and cough need careful evaluation.

- Isolated cough is rarely the sole manifestation of asthma.

Currently asthma can be controlled, not cured.

- As required, inhaled β_2-agonists are recommended for symptom relief.

- Inhaled corticosteroids are the mainstay of treatment for the control of persistent symptoms.

- Most children can be controlled with < 400 µg/day beclomethasone dipropionate equivalent.

- The preferred first choice add-on in school-aged children not controlled with low dose inhaled corticosteroids is a long-acting β_2-agonist.

- High-dose inhaled corticosteroids have been associated with adrenal insufficiency.

Education is an important part of asthma management and improves outcomes.

[continued on next page]

Key points for clinical practice (continued)

Supplemental oxygen, high-dose bronchodilators and oral steroids remain the main treatments for acute asthma.

- Meter dose inhaler + spacer is the preferred method for delivering β_2-agonists in children with mild to moderate exacerbations.

- Adding multiple doses of anticholinergics is effective in children with severe asthma.

- The evidence supports the addition of intravenous aminophylline for those that fail to respond.

Children and young people with (and without) asthma should not be exposed to environmental tobacco smoke.

Clear messages for patients and doctors about what to do about allergen avoidance, especially for dogs and cats, are currently elusive.

References

1. Rabe KF, Vermeire PA, Soriano JB, Maier WC. Clinical management of asthma in 1999: the Asthma Insights and Reality in Europe (AIRE) study. *Eur Respir J* 2000; **16**: 802–807.
2. Anon. British guideline on the management of asthma. *Thorax* 2003; **58 (Suppl 1)**: 1–94.
3. Akinbami LJ, Schoendorf KC. Trends in childhood asthma: prevalence, health care utilization and mortality. *Pediatrics* 2002; **110**: 315–322.
4. ISAAC. Worldwide variations in the prevalence of asthma symptoms: the International Study of Asthma and Allergies in Childhood (ISAAC). *Eur Respir J* 1998; **12**: 315–335.
5. Strachan DP. Family size, infection and atopy: the first decade of the 'hygiene hypothesis'. *Thorax* 2000; **55 (Suppl 1)**: S2–S10.
6. Martinez FD, Wright AL, Taussig LM, Holberg CJ, Halonen M, Morgan WJ. Asthma and wheezing in the first six years of life. The Group Health Medical Associates. *N Engl J Med* 1995; **332**: 133–138.
7. Barbato A, Turato G, Baraldo S *et al*. Airway inflammation in childhood asthma. *Am J Respir Crit Care Med* 2003; **168**: 798–803.
8. Cokugras H, Akcakaya N, Seckin I, Camcioglu Y, Sarimurat N, Aksoy F. Ultrastructural examination of bronchial biopsy specimens from children with moderate asthma. *Thorax* 2001; **56**: 25–29.
9. Stevenson EC, Turner G, Heaney LG *et al*. Bronchoalveolar lavage findings suggest two different forms of childhood asthma. *Clin Exp Allergy* 1997; **27**: 1027–1035.
10. Williams J, Williams K. Asthma-specific quality of life questionnaires in children: are they useful and feasible in routine clinical practice? *Pediatr Pulmonol* 2003; **35**: 114–118.
11. Covar RA, Szefler SJ, Martin RJ *et al*. Relations between exhaled nitric oxide and measures of disease activity among children with mild-to-moderate asthma. *J Pediatr* 2003; **142**: 469–475.
12. Malmberg LP, Pelkonen AS, Haahtela T, Turpeinen M. Exhaled nitric oxide rather than lung function distinguishes preschool children with probable asthma. *Thorax* 2003; **58**: 494–499.
13. Cane RS, Ranganathan SC, McKenzie SA. What do parents of wheezy children understand by 'wheeze'? *Arch Dis Child* 2000; **82**: 327–332.
14. Wright AL, Holberg CJ, Morgan WJ, Taussig LM, Halonen M, Martinez FD. Recurrent cough in childhood and its relation to asthma. *Am J Respir Crit Care Med* 1996; **153**:

1259–1265.

15. Keeley DJ, Silverman M. Issues at the interface between primary and secondary care in the management of common respiratory disease. 2: Are we too ready to diagnose asthma in children? *Thorax* 1999; **54**: 625–628.

16. Chavasse R, Seddon P, Bara A, McKean M. Short acting beta agonists for recurrent wheeze in children under two years of age (Cochrane Review). In: *The Cochrane Library, Issue 2 2003*. Oxford: Update Software 2003.

17. National Asthma Education and Prevention Program. Expert Panel Report: Guidelines for the diagnosis and management of asthma update on selected topics – 2002. *J Allergy Clin Immunol* 2002; **110 (Suppl 5)**: S141–S219.

18. McKean M, Ducharme F. Inhaled steroids for episodic viral wheeze of childhood. *Cochrane Database Syst Rev* 2000;(2): CD001107.

19. Oommen A, Lambert PC, Grigg J. Efficacy of a short course of parent-initiated oral prednisolone for viral wheeze in children aged 1–5 years; randomised controlled trial. *Lancet* 2003; **362**:1433–1438.

20. Szefler S, Pedersen S. Role of budesonide as maintenance therapy for children with asthma. *Pediatr Pulmonol* 2003; **36**: 13–21.

21. Pauwels RA, Pedersen S, Busse WW *et al*. Early intervention with budesonide in mild persistent asthma: a randomised, double-blind trial. *Lancet* 2003; **361**: 1071–1076.

22. Knorr B, Franchi LM, Bisgaard H *et al*. Monteleukast, a leukotriene receptor antagonist, for the treatment of persistent asthma in children aged 2 to 5 years. *Pediatrics* 2001; **108**: E48.

23. Waalkens HJ, Essen-Zandvliet EE, Hughes MD *et al*. Cessation of long-term treatment with inhaled corticosteroid (budesonide) in children with asthma results in deterioration. The Dutch CNSLD Study Group. *Am Rev Respir Dis* 1993; **148**: 1252–1257.

24. Agertoft L, Pedersen S. Effects of long-term treatment with an inhaled corticosteroid on growth and pulmonary function in asthmatic children. *Respir Med* 1994; **88**: 373–381.

25. The Childhood Asthma Management Program Research Group. Long-term effects of budesonide or nedocromil in children with asthma. *N Engl J Med* 2000; **343**: 1054–1063.

26. Cochran D. Diagnosing and treating chesty infants. A short trial of inhaled corticosteroid is probably the best approach. *BMJ* 1998; **316**: 1546–1547.

27. Todd GR, Acerini CL, Ross-Russell R, Zahra S, Warner JT, McCance D. Survey of adrenal crisis associated with inhaled corticosteroids in the United Kingdom. *Arch Dis Child* 2002; **87**: 457–461.

28. Price J, Hindmarsh P, Hughes S, Efthimiou J. Evaluating the effects of asthma therapy on childhood growth: what can be learnt from the published literature? *Eur Respir J* 2002; **19**: 1179–1193.

29. Agertoft L, Pedersen S. Effect of long-term treatment with inhaled budesonide on adult height in children with asthma. *N Engl J Med* 2000; **343**: 1064–1069.

30. Wolf FM, Guevara JP, Grum CM, Clark NM, Cates CJ. Educational interventions for asthma in children. *Cochrane Database Syst Rev* 2003;(1): CD000326.

31. National Asthma Campaign. Starting as we mean to go on. An audit of children's asthma in the UK. *Asthma J* 2002; **8**: S1–S11.

32. Drblik S, Lapierre G, Thivierge R *et al*. Comparative efficacy of terbutaline sulphate delivered by Turbuhaler dry powder inhaler or pressurised metered dose inhaler with Nebuhaler spacer in children during an acute asthmatic episode. *Arch Dis Child* 2003; **88**: 319–323.

33. Smith M, Iqbal S, Elliott TM, Everard M, Rowe BH. Corticosteroids for hospitalised children with acute asthma. *Cochrane Database Syst Rev* 2003; (2): CD002886.

34. Mitra A, Bassler D, Ducharme FM. Intravenous aminophylline for acute severe asthma in children over 2 years using inhaled bronchodilators. *Cochrane Database Syst Rev* 2001; (4): CD001276.

35. Roberts G, Newsom D, Gomez K *et al*. Intravenous salbutamol bolus compared with an aminophylline infusion in children with severe asthma: a randomised controlled trial. *Thorax* 2003; **58**: 306–310.

36. Hughes R, Goldkorn A, Masoli M, Weatherall M, Burgess C, Beasley R. Use of isotonic nebulised magnesium sulphate as an adjuvant to salbutamol in treatment of severe asthma in adults: randomised placebo-controlled trial. *Lancet* 2003; **361**: 2114–2117.

37. Madge P, McColl J, Paton J. Impact of a nurse-led home management training programme in children admitted to hospital with acute asthma: a randomised controlled study. *Thorax* 1997; **52**: 223–228.

38. Sporik R, Platts-Mills TA. Allergen exposure and the development of asthma. *Thorax* 2001; **56 (Suppl 2)**: ii58–ii63.

39. Platts-Mills T, Vaughan J, Squillace S, Woodfolk J, Sporik R. Sensitisation, asthma, and a modified Th2 response in children exposed to cat allergen: a population-based cross-sectional study. *Lancet* 2001; **357**: 752–756.

40. Abramson MJ, Puy RM, Weiner JM. Allergen immunotherapy for asthma. *Cochrane Database Syst Rev* 2000; (2): CD001186.

41. Blackburn C, Spencer N, Bonas S, Coe C, Dolan A, Moy R. Effect of strategies to reduce exposure of infants to environmental tobacco smoke in the home: cross sectional survey. *BMJ* 2003; **327**: 257.

42. O'Callaghan C, Barry PW. How to choose delivery devices for asthma. *Arch Dis Child* 2000; **82**: 185–187.

43. Oommen A, Lambert PC, Grigg J. Efficacy of a short course of parent-initiated oral prednisolone for viral wheeze in children aged 1-5 years; randomised controlled trial. *Lancet* 2003; **362**:1433–1438

Harry Baumer

3

Advances in diabetes mellitus

When I started looking after children with diabetes about 25 years ago, I could not have known how things would change, although I had supposed that their care would improve with time. I certainly did not predict that the annual incidence of type 1 diabetes would rise by a factor of 2 or 3 over my professional life-time, nor that we would be faced with the appearance of type 2 diabetes in obese children. It is ironic to be writing of recent advances in the light of these changes.

Insulin is now identical to human insulin thanks to genetic engineering techniques, and is being complemented with insulin analogues with improved properties. The needles and syringes are now disposable, with tiny gauge 28–31 needles, and we now have insulin pen injector devices some of which will deliver insulin in 0.5 unit increments. Routine urine testing has long ago been completely replaced by home blood glucose monitoring, with meters that can store many results with dates and times (facilitating early awareness of falsified results).

Glycated haemoglobin tests give important information about medium-term diabetes control, and we now know that improved glycaemic control reduces the risk of microvascular complications. Sadly, we do not know what impact these changes in the last 25 years have had on the overall control of diabetes, although few would believe that the prospects for diabetes control today are unchanged. However, the average child with diabetes in the UK at the start of the 21st century still has poor control of their diabetes. In spite of the emergence of diabetes specialist nurses and the multiprofessional team, the service for children with diabetes in many hospitals remains woefully deficient. Much of our current management is unsupported by good quality research-evidence in children. We have a long way to go.

Harry Baumer MBChB, FRCP, FRCPCH
Consultant Paediatrician, Women & Children's Health Division, Level 12, Derriford Hospital, Plymouth PL6 8DH, UK. Tel: +44 1752 763450; E-mail: harry.baumer@phnt.swest.nhs.uk

Why has the incidence of newly diagnosed diabetes in children increased? The short answer is that we still do not know. Childhood type 1 diabetes is now recognised as being of multifactorial aetiology, an autoimmune condition with a strong genetic basis and unknown environmental triggers. A large number of susceptibility loci are known to be associated with an increased risk of diabetes in children. A Finnish twin study showed that 13% of monozygotic twins both had type 1 diabetes, suggesting a major role for genetic factors. The search for further responsible genes is continuing. The underlying genetic causes of a number of rare forms of diabetes, including maturity onset diabetes of youth, have already been clarified. Over the last few decades, the improved obstetric outcomes for women with diabetes has increased the proportion of children with susceptible genes. The rate of increase of diabetes in the population seems too rapid for this to be the only explanation.

The social circumstances of children with diabetes exactly mirror those of the rest of the population, which suggests that such factors as the decline in breast-feeding rates (which has a strong social class bias) are unlikely to be important.[1] It has been suggested that as children are getting more overweight this is accelerating their development of diabetes so that it is occurring at a younger age.[2] This is certainly responsible for the appearance of type 2 diabetes in children, and the distinction between the two types is not always clear.

I intend to focus on advances that already have a direct impact on diabetes management in children with type 1 diabetes.

DIABETES CONTROL

The landmark Diabetes Control and Complications Trial (DCCT) demonstrated that intensified treatment improved glycaemic control, and delayed the onset and slowed the progression of microvascular complications.[3] The study was on adults, but included 195 adolescents recruited between the ages of 13 and 17 years, who were also described separately.[4] Adolescents randomised to intensive treatment experienced a reduction of similar magnitude to adults in glycated haemoglobin levels, risk of retinopathy and microalbuminuria, but with higher average glycated haemoglobins in both conventional (9.76% versus 9.02%) and intensive treatment (8.06% versus 7.12%) arms. Those adolescents in the intensive treatment group also experienced a 3-fold increased risk of severe hypoglycaemia compared to those on conventional treatment. This was a very similar increase in risk of hypoglycaemia as that seen overall in the adults.

The trial reported the observed association between average glycated haemoglobin and rate of progression of retinopathy and risk of severe hypoglycaemia. These figures, reproduced in Figure 1, suggest that irrespective of the current glycated haemoglobin level, reduction will reduce the risk of microvascular complications and increase the risk of severe hypoglycaemia.

How did the trial intensify treatment? Conventional treatment included once or twice daily mixed insulin, once daily monitoring of blood or urine glucose levels, with education on diet and exercise, and 3-monthly clinic visits to a multiprofessional team. Frequent adjustment of insulin was discouraged; although glycated haemoglobin was tested at 3-monthly intervals, the results were only divulged to the patients and diabetes team if they were above 13%. Some aspects, such as urine glucose testing, once daily insulin injections and

A   B

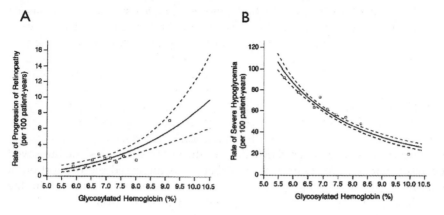

Fig. 1 Risk of sustained progression of retinopathy (A) and rate of severe hypoglycaemia (B) in the patients receiving intensive therapy, according to their mean glycosylated haemoglobin values during the trial. (A) The glycosylated haemoglobin values used were the mean of the values obtained every 6 months. (B) The mean of the monthly values was used. Squares indicate the crude rates within deciles of the mean glycosylated haemoglobin values during the trial; each square corresponds to more than 400 patient-years. The solid lines are regression lines estimated as a function of the log of the mean glycosylated haemoglobin value in (A) and the log of the glycosylated haemoglobin value in (B); the dashed lines are 95% confidence intervals. Reproduced with permission. Copyright© 1993 Massachusetts Medical Society. All rights reserved.

managing diabetes without access to regular glycated haemoglobin results would not now be considered best practice in the UK.

Intensive treatment included 3 or more insulin injections daily or an insulin pump (patients chose which they preferred and could swap) with frequent adjustment of dose, at least four blood tests each day with specific blood glucose targets, monthly review by clinic staff and telephone contact in between, and target glycated haemoglobin of 6% or less.

The study presents an important challenge to improve diabetes control, especially in adolescents. It does not in itself identify which aspects of these interventions were important in improving diabetes control. The balance between the increased risks resulting from severe hypoglycaemic episodes and the benefits in terms of improved control is likely to differ in pre-adolescent children.

We are beginning to get comparable information on diabetes control in UK children. A Scottish study of 18 centres within the last 5 years used a single method for glycated haemoglobin performed at one reference laboratory, which allowed direct comparisons between centres. The average glycated haemoglobin in children of all ages was 9.1%, and was 9.5% in those aged 10–15 years.[5] There was a highly significant variation in performance between centres after taking into account factors associated with poor control.

Although there are many different test methods for glycated haemoglobin, and no simple method for comparing results between them, in the UK many laboratories now report glycated haemoglobins as 'DCCT-aligned'. The results from different DCCT-aligned methods are increasingly comparable, and have been pooled in two national audits of paediatric diabetes covering England, Wales and Northern Ireland. The second of these, in 2001, involved 111 centres, and the overall glycated haemoglobin was 9.1%. As seen in Figure 2, there

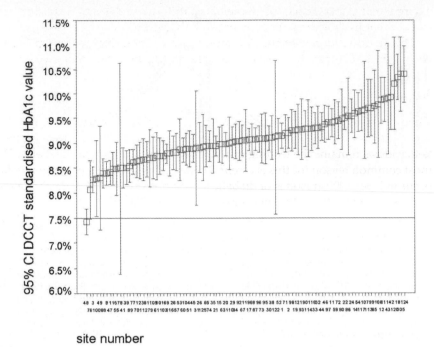

site number

Fig. 2 Pooled DCCT-aligned data for overall glycated haemoglobin from 111 centres in England, Wales and Northern Ireland.

were large variations in mean glycated haemoglobin between individual centres, as was seen in Scotland. Centres with lower mean results tended to report lower rates of severe hypoglycaemia.

HYPOGLYCAEMIA AND ITS SEQUELAE

The consequences of severe hypoglycaemia have to be considered alongside the benefits from improved control. Parents who have witnessed a hypoglycaemic fit may worry about their child dying or being brain damaged in future episodes. Unless this is addressed, their efforts may continue to be focused on this at the expense of satisfactory diabetes control. A recent UK study found that death is in fact an extremely rare consequence of hypoglycaemia, most deaths being from diabetic ketoacidosis even among those dying unexpectedly at home.[6]

There is concern that severe hypoglycaemia in children may cause neurodevelopmental sequelae. A 7-year prospective longitudinal study of 16 children, 9 of whom had previous hypoglycaemic seizures, found significant decline in verbal, but not visuospatial, ability, particularly in those with seizures.[7] Similar findings have not been seen in adult onset diabetes.

Asymptomatic nocturnal hypoglycaemia is common in children, especially when attempting to optimise glycaemic control. One study found evidence of depressed mood, but not disturbed cognitive function, the day following profound nocturnal hypoglycaemia.[8] It is unclear whether recurrent asymptomatic nocturnal hypoglycaemia contributes to the long-term cognitive impairment in children with early onset of diabetes.

This does not argue against the importance of achieving optimal glycaemic control, but underlines the importance of close blood glucose monitoring in children.

DIABETIC KETOACIDOSIS

Children with diabetes have an overall risk of dying that is just over twice that for all children, but in the 1–4-year-olds this risk is increased 9 times. Diabetic ketoacidosis remains the leading cause of death in children with diabetes. The most common reason for this is cerebral oedema,[6] which has been estimated to occur in 7 per 1000 episodes of diabetic ketoacidosis, with a quarter dying and with severe neurological sequelae in over a third of survivors.[9]

The pathogenesis of cerebral oedema remains uncertain. It has been suggested as being due to fluid shifts to the intracellular space with rapid rehydration. However, a recent case control study from the US found that severe hypocarbia and high blood urea were the only two independent associations with the development of cerebral oedema. This suggests that the pathogenesis may be brain ischaemia secondary to impaired cerebral circulation either due to the hypocarbia or due to extreme dehydration.[10]

The optimum management of diabetic ketoacidosis in minimising cerebral oedema therefore remains controversial.[11,12] Early recognition of cerebral oedema and rapid administration of intravenous mannitol, as well as rapid restoration of circulating blood volume, appear important. However, as half the children with cerebral oedema present with respiratory arrest, presumably secondary to cerebral herniation and with a high mortality, prevention is important. In the 2001 national audit, the rate of diabetic ketoacidosis (excluding those admitted at first presentation) varied from 0% in about 1 in 5 centres to over 30% in the centre with the highest rate. This must be interpreted with caution, but suggests that there may be scope for preventing diabetic ketoacidosis in some centres.

DELIVERING DIABETES CARE

THE DIABETES TEAM

Professional opinion, enshrined in the National Service Framework for diabetes,[13] is that a multidisciplinary team should provide the care of diabetes in children in separate diabetic clinics. Paediatric specialist diabetes nurses play a vital part in improving diabetes care in children and young people, and the team should include a consultant paediatrician with specialist expertise in children's diabetes care, a paediatric dietician with expertise in diabetes, and a senior paediatric ward nurse with expertise in children's diabetes. There should also be easy access to psychology, podiatry and ophthalmology. Paediatricians caring for children should have an adequate caseload so as to avoid occasional practice. Paediatric specialist diabetes nurses should not have an excessive caseload above 100 children.[14]

Observational evidence supporting the need for paediatricians having a reasonable caseload of children with diabetes came from a regional audit in the

South West in 1994.[15] Children under the care of paediatricians with a caseload of more than 40 children were less likely to be admitted to hospital with hypoglycaemia or for all diabetes problems, had lower glycated haemoglobin results, were more likely to be screened for microalbuminuria, and were more likely to attend clinic appointments.

FREQUENCY OF CONTACT

The Diabetes Control and Complications Trial included monthly review by clinic staff and telephone contact in between. The characteristics of care in the best performing centre in the Scottish study[5] were 'a policy of frequent contact (both medical and nursing), with at least monthly formal advice (more if required), together with a rapid 'troubleshooting' service and frequent change in insulin regimen with no fixed 'favourite' and the aim of a near-normal target for HbA1c (glycated haemoglobin) concentration (< 7.5%)'. Clearly, this would have considerable resource implications. However, in my view, this is likely to be important if improved diabetes control is to be achieved.

PSYCHOSOCIAL SUPPORT

A recent systematic review of educational and psychological interventions for adolescents with diabetes[16] identified 25 relevant randomised controlled trials, principally from the US. Nine of the 14 randomised controlled trials with glycated haemoglobin as an outcome and involving a face-to-face psychology based intervention (including 443 of the 544 adolescents in the 14 trials) reported significant reductions in glycated haemoglobin compared to the control group.

The largest effect was over 2% improvement in average glycated haemoglobin compared to the control group. In this study,[17] teenagers with diabetes taught their parents how to inject themselves (with saline!), perform blood tests and urine tests, recording a meal and exercise plan, and continue this for a week. Parents then discussed the experience in a small group.

A second study, a particularly well-conducted randomised controlled trial from the US, involved role play in small groups of 2 or 3 young people with a trainer, using scenarios that confronted difficult situations such as making appropriate food choices when with friends. Sessions lasted 60–90 min, weekly for 6 weeks and then monthly over 12 months. Control adolescents received intensification support from the diabetes team without the coping strategy training. This approach led to improvements in a number of measures including a 1% mean lower glycated haemoglobin than in the control group at 1 year.[18]

Factors contributing to psychological problems include low socio-economic status, family conflict and communication difficulties, maternal depression, and too much responsibility falling to the emotionally immature child. Screening for specific psychological problems, particularly maladaptive coping strategies (coping in ways that do not actively try to solve the difficulty) and eating disorders, is recommended in a recent evidence-based guideline.[19] Maintaining parental involvement and communication, with targeted psychological support are recommended.

A cross-sectional observational study also demonstrated the association between family stress and poor glycated haemoglobin, with stress accounting for approximately 25% of the variance in glycated haemoglobin.[20] Two UK studies have shown an association between the absence of one parent and poor diabetes control.[5,15] Children with diabetes have high rates of depression. One study found clinical depression in one in 5 children two years after diagnosis.[21]

Attention to the psychosocial circumstances and ensuring that support is available for children with diabetes is, therefore, crucial if diabetes control is to be improved. In my view, there exists a sufficiently strong body of evidence to warrant routine psychology input in children's diabetes clinics.

The 1989 Children Act, section 17, includes legislation regarding children in need. The more recent Department of Health publication[22] *Framework for the Assessment of Children in Need and their Families* sets out the mechanism for initiating a multi-agency assessment of such children. However, many diabetes services experience great difficulty in obtaining social work support for families with a child in need.

Unfortunately, children's diabetes teams continue to be inadequately resourced. We demonstrated this in the South West region in 1998 despite improvements in practice following a regional audit,[23] and the latest national UK survey demonstrated wide-spread continuing deficiencies.[24] Some unacceptable practices continue, including: (i) children being managed in general paediatric clinics; (ii) lack of regular monitoring of glycated haemoglobin; (iii) paediatricians caring for very small numbers of children with diabetes; (iv) lack of paediatric dietetic support in clinic; and (v) lack of easy access to psychology support.

It is to be hoped that the Diabetes National Service Framework will bring the standards of children's services up to a more acceptable norm.

INSULIN TREATMENT

INSULIN ANALOGUES

Insulin lispro and aspart

Human insulin has been available for around 20 years. Unfortunately, it consists of a mixture of monomers and hexamers, only the former of which are absorbed into the circulation. The timing of its onset, peak and duration of action are too slow to match the speed of glucose absorption following a meal.

Insulin lispro differs from soluble insulin in having two amino acids in the B-chain reversed, with lysine at B-28 and proline at B-29. This inhibits its tendency to form hexamers; therefore, it enters the blood stream more rapidly. A second analogue, insulin aspart, has aspartic acid at position B-28 instead of proline, with almost identical effects to insulin lispro. These analogues have a peak blood level by 60 min and a return to baseline by 4 h, instead of a peak at 2–3 h with return to baseline at 6–8 h as in soluble insulin.

These insulin analogues have shown no increased risk of adverse events or allergic reactions to date. Insulin lispro is structurally similar to insulin growth factor-1, which raises theoretical concerns about possible adverse properties including accelerated progression of retinopathy. There are no relevant data available regarding longer-term risks, and their long-term safety does need to be monitored.

Improvements in glycated haemoglobin have not been seen in the randomised trials of these analogues to date. Their main advantage is in providing improved post-prandial glycaemic control with reduction of overnight hypoglycaemia, when compared to soluble insulin. Care is needed to ensure that this is not accompanied by hyperglycaemia before the next meal or in the early part of the night, and adjustment to the longer-acting insulin may be needed.

A practical benefit to families is that insulin is given immediately before meals, rather than 15–30 min in advance as with soluble insulin. In one study in toddlers,[25] similar post-prandial blood glucose levels were seen when the insulin was given immediately after the meal. This has great advantages in young children whose eating pattern is unpredictable. I now use insulin aspart routinely in preference to soluble insulin.

Insulin glargine

This is a long-acting insulin analogue in which two additional arginine molecules have been added to the NH_2-terminal end of the B-chain, and glycine substituted for asparagine at position 21 of the A-chain. Glargine is soluble at pH 4, but precipitates at a neutral pH when injected subcutaneously, producing delayed absorption. It has a slow onset and prolonged (> 24 h) duration of action without a peak at 4–6 h as is found with isophane (Neutral Protamine Hagedorn) insulin. A steady state is reached 2–4 days after the first dose.

Glargine cannot be mixed with other insulins. It is currently available either for use with a pen or needle and syringe, to be used once daily before bed. It is now recommended in the UK as an option for patients with type 1 diabetes, with a product licence for children down to the age of 6 years.

A large multicentre randomised controlled trial compared glargine with isophane insulin in children and adolescents aged 5–16 years on at least 3 insulin injections each day.[26] This study showed no improvement in glycated haemo-globin results over a 6-month period despite significantly lower fasting blood glucose levels. There was also a statistically non-significant reduction in severe hypoglycaemias. This is not dissimilar to adult studies, where no reduction in glycated haemoglobin was found, but fewer nocturnal hypoglycaemias were seen. A more detailed investigation of children in one centre contributing to this study found less variation in blood glucose levels overnight with glargine.[27]

It seems reasonable to use insulin glargine in children who have problems with nocturnal hypoglycaemia. Further studies are needed to clarify its place in treating children under 6 years, the very group where prevention of severe overnight hypoglycaemia might be of greatest benefit.

INSULIN REGIMENS

How many injections each day should children be having? There is a lack of good evidence to support an answer to this question. There are few advocates for a single injection each day. In prepubertal children, it can sometimes provide good control. However, it can then be difficult for a child to have to face up to the need for twice or even three-times a day injections as they enter adolescence. This argument is probably the most convincing for avoiding the routine use of once daily regimens in prepubertal children. The most common regimen remains twice daily injections of a mixture of quick acting and intermediate acting insulin.

There are children for whom a three times a day insulin regimen is beneficial. The morning injection continues to be a mixture of quick acting and intermediate acting insulin. The tea-time injection is split so that the child has only quick acting insulin, with the longer acting component being given before bed. A number of studies suggest that this reduces the frequency of nocturnal hypoglycaemia.[5] However, other approaches may also be helpful in reducing nocturnal hypoglycaemia, including reducing the tea-time dose of quick-acting insulin or changing to a tea-time, rapidly acting insulin analogue.

Another alternative is the basal bolus system of injections, using an insulin pen device. This involves a single dose of longer-acting insulin at bed-time, with three injections of quick acting insulin before each main meal. There is no evidence that this regimen in itself improves control, although improved glycaemic control is seen in some individuals. The main problem is that children forget their lunch-time injection.

INSULIN DELIVERY

Pen devices are increasingly used to deliver subcutaneous insulin. Many children prefer them to the needle and syringe method for a number of reasons including their ease of use. With pre-mixed insulins, one cannot adjust one insulin at a time without swapping to a different mixture, which means either being inflexible or wasteful. It can be difficult for children with smaller hands to do the injection. It is easier for a child to conceal the fact that they have not given all the insulin from a watching attendant than when using a needle and syringe.

Some pens are now designed to deliver doses in increments down to 0.5 U. Small doses of insulin are difficult to deliver accurately, especially since insulin was standardised to 100 U/ml. Reproducibility is important as it will determine the amount of unintended day-to-day variation in delivered dose. One study[28] found that pen devices delivered insulin doses closer to the intended dose than even 30 U insulin syringes, but that the reproducibility did not differ between pens and syringes. I have not been able to find any published information on the accuracy of delivery of newer pen devices.

Optimum needle length is important: too deep, and intramuscular injection increases the risk of hypoglycaemia with exercise – too superficial and insulin may leak from the injection site. A recent study used ultrasound to measure depth of subcutaneous fat and injection delivery site in a group of older, lean children with diabetes.[29] Injections were performed by a nurse perpendicularly to a two finger skinfold pinch. Compared with 12.7 mm needles, 8 mm needles reduced the rate of intramuscular injections from 88% to 48% of injections into the arm and from 84% to 28% of those in the thigh. The effects of a 45° angle of injection and of 5 mm needles need to be studied in children of different ages. I routinely recommend 8 mm needles, and encourage a 45° angle of injection. In slim children, I consider 5 mm needles acceptable unless insulin leakage is seen (which it commonly is).

INSULIN PUMPS

Continuous subcutaneous insulin infusion via an insulin pump is not new, but improvements in the pump technology and experience obtained largely in adults in the UK makes it a choice for a minority of children and adolescents.

In Sweden, however, pump therapy for children is common-place. Insulin pumps were used by some of the teenagers in the diabetes control and complications trial (chosen in preference to a multiple injection regime). The infusion set is changed every 2–3 days, and a rapid-acting insulin analogue is infused at basal and bolus rates that can be adjusted according to blood glucose results.

Those contemplating starting children on insulin pump therapy need to consider a number of factors. The diabetes team must be trained to enable them to provide education and support. Which children are likely to benefit?

The following seem reasonable indications to try insulin pump therapy:

1. Well motivated, well supported and no significant psychosocial problems.

2. Can demonstrate ability to maintain at least 4 blood tests each day.

3. Capable of managing an insulin pump with available education and support.

4. Poor control (NICE guidance suggests glycated haemoglobin above 7.5% despite the use of multiple injections) or frequent hypoglycaemia despite alternative treatments including insulin analogues, or clear patient preference.

Despite the relatively few children who would fit the criteria above, it is an important option to have available for those who could benefit.

The insulin regimen does need to be individualised to each child's needs and, if possible, wishes. Factors such as their age, preference for a pen device and how they feel about injections need to be taken into consideration. I always try to find out how each child feels about their injections. A question such as 'what do you think is the worst thing about having diabetes?' provokes very varied and sometimes unexpected answers. A child who says that the worst thing is their injections is unlikely to feel positive about a suggestion to increase the number of injections each day. Children with diabetes have only limited control over decisions about diabetes management, so it is important to give choice to children about their diabetes management wherever possible.

DIET

A 'healthy eating' approach to diet advises a reduction in sugar and low-fat diet, with increased soluble non-starch polysaccharide fibre intake. It has replaced carbohydrate counting which did not result in improved glycaemic control and may have contributed to the higher rate of eating disorders in children with diabetes.[30] The glycaemic index is a method for quantifying the post-prandial glycaemic response to different foods. This has not been formally evaluated in children.

SURVEILLANCE FOR MICROVASCULAR COMPLICATIONS

Microvascular complications are commonly seen in early adulthood. Should routine surveillance be undertaken in children and adolescents?

NEPHROPATHY

The development of microalbuminuria precedes the development of overt diabetic nephropathy. It is also said to be a marker of other microvascular complications, including proliferative retinopathy, and macrovascular complications including coronary heart disease.[31] Improving diabetic control can potentially modify its progression. In adults with diabetes and microalbuminuria, angiotensin converting enzyme inhibitors have been shown to reduce urinary albumin excretion rates by lowering renal vascular resistance and, thereby, lowering glomerular capillary pressure. One randomised cross-over study of captopril in 12 normotensive adolescents with diabetes and microalbuminuria aged 12–17 years showed a significant reduction in microalbuminuria over 3 months compared to placebo.[32]

A large cross-sectional study in UK children aged 10 years or more demonstrated a prevalence of 9.7% of abnormal urinary albumin creatinine ratio[33] in at least 2 of 3 samples.[34] The development of microalbuminuria was associated with poorer glycaemic control and longer duration of diabetes. However, the average duration of diabetes in those with microalbuminuria was less than 8 years, and the shortest duration was less than 2 years. It was much commoner in girls, and occurred in a small proportion of prepubertal children. Less than 1 in 5 children with microalbuminuria were hypertensive. However, one study failed to demonstrate progression over 3 years in 8 of 9 children with microalbuminuria.[35]

The Oxford Regional Prospective Study followed a large cohort of children from diagnosis of diabetes between 1986 and 1996 and defined the natural history of microalbuminuria.[36] They found 13% of children developed microalbuminuria within a median of 5 years from diagnosis: this regressed in half of the children. The risk of developing microalbuminuria was doubled in girls, trebled after the age of 11 years, and rose by 36% for every 1% rise in mean glycated haemoglobin. Some 18% of children had developed persistent microalbuminuria by 11 years from diagnosis.

The purpose of surveillance for microalbuminuria is 2-fold. First, to provide further motivation to the child, family and diabetes team to improve glycaemic control. Second, to allow early intervention with angiotensin converting enzyme inhibitors when persistent microalbuminuria with or without persistent hypertension occurs. The case for routine surveillance for micro-albuminuria is strong, but when should this start?

The Oxford study found microalbuminuria 2 years from diagnosis in approximately 5% of children diagnosed after the age of 11 years, whereas in children diagnosed up to the age of 11 years, this risk of microalbuminuria was present 5 years from diagnosis. Surveillance should be undertaken annually using an albumin creatinine ratio on an early morning urine. Those with abnormal results (albumin creatinine ratio above 3.5 mg/mmol) should have timed overnight urine albumin excretion (and a urine culture) checked. Those with abnormal albumin excretion (> 35 µg/min on two of three consecutive timed overnight urine samples) should have efforts made to improve their diabetes control, and the test repeated after an appropriate interval.

The Oxford study found a rise in blood pressure with the onset of microalbuminuria, though very few had overt hypertension.[37] An annual blood pressure measurement should be checked. Reference charts for systolic and diastolic blood pressure, including 91st, 98th and 99.6th centiles are now available from Harlow Printing Ltd derived from three UK studies using an oscillometric method.

RETINOPATHY

A recent cohort study of children with diabetes from one centre in Germany found a 50% risk of developing mild non-proliferative retinopathy by the time they had had diabetes for 16.6 years.[39]

It has been suggested that children are protected from developing retinopathy before puberty. In children with prepubertal onset of diabetes, retinopathy occurred after a median pubertal duration of 10.9 years compared with 15.1 years in children with pubertal onset of diabetes. There is, therefore, at least some contribution of prepubertal diabetes, and good diabetes control before puberty is important for avoiding retinopathy. Although the risk of retinopathy was low in the first 5 years, the shortest duration of diabetes at onset of retinopathy was 2.2 years, and the youngest child developing retinopathy was 5.5 years.

The Scottish Intercollegiate Guideline Network[19] recommends annual surveillance for retinopathy 3 years from diagnosis after the onset of puberty, and from the age of 12 years with prepubertal onset. Laser photocoagulation is effective for sight threatening, moderate proliferative or more severe retinopathy. This should be stabilised before rapid improvement in diabetes control is attempted, as this may lead to short term worsening of retinopathy.

SCREENING FOR OTHER CONDITIONS

THYROID DYSFUNCTION

Thyroid antibodies are found in between a quarter and a third of children with type 1 diabetes, and thyroid dysfunction, more commonly hypothyroidism, with a prevalence of around 4%, is more common than in the general population. Clinical signs may be difficult to identify during routine care; therefore, it seems beneficial to screen children for thyroid problems. I check thyroid antibodies at 5-year intervals, and supplement these with annual thyroid function tests in those with raised antibodies.

COELIAC DISEASE

A recent review[40] estimates that about 4.5% of children with diabetes will develop co-existent coeliac disease. In about 1 in 10 of these, coeliac disease will precede the diabetes. Serological screening can be undertaken with a variety of antibodies including anti-gliadin, anti-endomyseal, anti-reticulin and anti-tissue transglutaminase. The latter two tests have the best sensitivity and specificity. However, a single screening test at or soon after diagnosis will not pick up all affected children; in order to do so, repeated serological surveillance is needed, perhaps at 5-year intervals (how long this surveillance should continue after diagnosis is unclear). It must be emphasised that the diagnosis can only be made following a jejunal biopsy. Even when the specificity of the screening test is as high as 99%, assuming the prevalence quoted above and a highly sensitive test, only approximately 80% of those with positive screening test results will have the condition. Overall, the rate of positive jejunal biopsies in the published series to date is below 70%, suggesting a lower test specificity of nearer 97%.

Many children identified in this way either have no symptoms, or symptoms that are unrecognised by the family. The case for a gluten-free diet is convincing for professionals (improved diabetes control, reduced hypoglycaemia, and reduced longer-term risks including lymphoma), but unfortunately less convincing for some children and their families.

My own experience with coeliac screening has been less than satisfactory, with some deciding against a jejunal biopsy or being unable to sustain a gluten-free diet even when the biopsy is abnormal. There is no point in undertaking a jejunal biopsy if the child and parents would not consider a gluten-free diet even with an abnormal result. I would still argue for antibody surveillance, with very careful assessment and counselling of the individual child and their family before proceeding to a jejunal biopsy. Where adherence to a gluten-free diet appears unlikely, I watch the child carefully for early clinical or laboratory evidence of the condition, with a view to discussing the matter again.

Key points for clinical practice

- Improved glycaemic control markedly reduces long-term risks of microvascular complications and remains an important goal, recognising the increased risk of severe hypoglycaemia, with consequences for cognitive function.

- Most children in the UK with diabetes have sub-optimal glycaemic control, with marked variation between centres.

- Many children's diabetes services in the UK are understaffed, particularly with suitably trained diabetes specialist nurses, dieticians and psychological support. This hampers efforts to improve diabetes control.

- The main risk from diabetic ketoacidosis is the complication of cerebral oedema. The pathogenesis remains unclear; therefore, the optimum management of diabetic ketoacidosis is uncertain, but prevention and early recognition are important.

- The insulin analogues, lispro and aspart, improve post-prandial glycaemic control compared to human insulin. They are given immediately before meals and in very young children with unpredictable eating patterns may be given immediately afterwards. They probably reduce the risk of nocturnal hypoglycaemia.

Key points for clinical practice (continued)

- Administering isophane insulin alone before bed, or substituting insulin glargine, probably reduce nocturnal hypoglycaemia.

- Insulin pump therapy can be an alternative for well-motivated children who are unable to achieve good diabetes control with other available regimens.

- Correct needle length is important; 8 mm needles are preferable to 12.7 mm needles.

- Nephropathy surveillance should start no later than 5 years from diagnosis. This should include microalbuminuria and blood pressure measurement.

- Annual retinopathy surveillance should start 3 years from diagnosis or from the 12th birthday, whichever comes later.

- Thyroid surveillance should be undertaken, with regular thyroid function tests in those with raised antibodies.

- Coeliac antibody surveillance should be undertaken, with jejunal biopsy where it seems likely that the child will adhere to a gluten-free diet, and close watching otherwise.

References

1. Baumer JH, Hunt LP, Shield JPH. Social disadvantage, family composition, and diabetes mellitus: prevalence and outcome. *Arch Dis Child* 1998; **79**: 427–430.
2. Wilkin TJ. The accelerator hypothesis: weight gain as the missing link between type I and type II diabetes. *Diabetologia* 2001; **44**: 914–922.
3. The Diabetes Control and Complications Trial Research Group. The effect of intensive treatment of diabetes on the development and progression of long-term complications in insulin-dependent diabetes mellitus. *N Engl J Med* 1993; **329**: 977–986.
4. Diabetes Control and Complications Trial Research Group. Effect of intensive diabetes treatment on the development and progression of long-term complications in adolescents with insulin-dependent diabetes mellitus: Diabetes Control and Complications Trial. *J Pediatr* 1994; **125**: 177–188.
5. Scottish Study Group for the Care of the Young Diabetic. Factors influencing glycaemic control in young people with type 1 diabetes in Scotland: a population-based study (DIABAUD2). *Diabetes Care* 2001; **24**: 239–244.
6. Edge JA, Ford-Adams ME, Dunger DB. Causes of death in children with insulin dependent diabetes 1990–96. *Arch Dis Child* 1999; **81**: 318–323.
7. Rovet JF, Ehrlich RM. The effect of hypoglycaemic seizure on cognitive function in children with diabetes: a 7 year prospective study. *J Pediatr* 1999; **134**: 503–506.
8. Matyka KA, Wigg L, Pramming S, Stores G, Dunger DB. Cognitive function and mood after profound nocturnal hypoglycaemia in prepubertal children with conventional treatment for diabetes. *Arch Dis Child* 1999; **81**: 138–142.
9. Edge JA, Hawkins MH, Winter DL, Dunger DB. The risk and outcome of cerebral oedema developing during diabetic ketoacidosis. *Arch Dis Child* 2001; **85**: 16–22.
10. Glaser N, Barnett P, McCaslin I *et al*. Risk factors for cerebral edema in children with diabetic ketoacidosis. *N Engl J Med* 2001; **344**: 264–269.
11. Inward CD, Chambers TL. Fluid management in diabetic ketoacidosis: have we got it right yet? *Arch Dis Child* 2002; **86**: 443–444.
12. Harris GD, Fiordalisi I. Physiologic management of DKA. *Arch Dis Child* 2002; **87**: 451–452.

13. Diabetes National Service Framework. Standards. <http//www.doh.gov.uk/nsf/diabetes>.
14. Royal College of Nursing. Paediatric Diabetes Specialist Interest Group. *The role and qualifications of the nurse specialising in paediatric diabetes.* London: Royal College of Nursing, 1993.
15. Baumer JH, Hunt LP, Shield JPH. Audit of diabetes care by caseload. *Arch Dis Child* 1997; **77**: 102–108.
16. Hampson SE, Skinner TC, Hart J *et al.* Effects of educational and psychosocial interventions for adolescents with diabetes mellitus: a systematic review. *Health Technol Assess* 2001; **5**: 1–79.
17. Satin W, La Greca AM, Zigo MA, Skyler JS. Diabetes in adolescence: effects of multifamily group intervention and parent simulation of diabetes. *J Pediatr Psychol* 1989; **14**: 259–275.
18. Grey M, Boland EA, Davidson M, Li J, Tamborlane V. Coping skills training for youth with diabetes mellitus has long-lasting effects on metabolic control and quality of life. *J Pediatr* 2000; **137**: 107–113.
19. Scottish Intercollegiate Guidelines Network. *Management of Diabetes.* SIGN Executive, RCP Edinburgh 2001 ISBN 1 899893 82 2
20. Viner R, McGrath M, Trudinger P. Family stress and metabolic control on diabetes. *Arch Dis Child* 1996; **74**: 418–421.
21. Grey M, Cameron ME, Lipman TH, Thurber FW. Psychosocial status of children with diabetes in the first 2 years after diagnosis. *Diabetes Care* 1995; **18**: 1330–1336.
22. Department of Health. *Framework for the assessment of children in need and their families.* London: Stationery Office, 2000.
23. Drake AJ, Baumer JH. Improved clinical practice but continuing service deficiencies following a regional audit of childhood diabetes mellitus. *Arch Dis Child* 2000; **82**: 302–304.
24. Jefferson IG, Swift PGF, Skinner TC, Hood GK. Diabetes services in the UK: third national survey confirms continuing deficiencies. *Arch Dis Child* 2003; **88**: 53–56.
25. Rutledge KS, Chase HP, Klingensmith GJ, Walravens PA, Slover RH, Garg SK. Effectiveness of postprandial Humalog in toddlers with diabetes. *Pediatrics* 1997; **100**: 968–972.
26. Schober E, Schoenle E, Van Dyk J, Wernicke-Panten K, Pediatric Study Group of Insulin Glargine. Comparative trial between insulin glargine and NPH insulin in children and adolescents with type 1 diabetes mellitus. *J Pediatr Endocrinol Metab* 2002; **15**: 369–376.
27. Mohn A, Strang S, Wernicke-Panten K, Lang AM, Edge JA, Dunger DB. Nocturnal glucose control and free insulin levels in children with type 1 diabetes by use of the long-acting insulin HOE 901 as part of a three-injection regimen. *Diabetes Care* 2000; **23**: 557–559.
28. Gnanalingham MG, Newland P, Smith CP. Accuracy and reproducibility of low dose insulin administration using pen-injectors and syringes. *Arch Dis Child* 1998; **79**: 59–62.
29. Tubiana-Rufi N, Belarbi N, du Pasquier-Fediaevsky L *et al.* Short needles (8 mm) reduce the risk of intramuscular injections in children with type 1 diabetes. *Diabetes Care* 1999; **22**: 1621–1625.
30. Jones JM, Lawson ML, Daneman D, Olmsted MP, Rodin G. Eating disorders in adolescent females with and without type 1 diabetes: cross-sectional study. *BMJ* 2000; **320**: 1563–1566.
31. Deckert T, Kofoed-Envoldsen A, Norgaard K, Borch-Johnsen K, Feldt-Rasmussen B, Jensen T. Microalbuminuria. Implications for micro- and macrovascular disease. *Diabetes Care* 1992; **15**: 1181–1191.
32. Cook J, Daneman D, Spino M *et al.* Angiotensin converting enzyme inhibition therapy to decrease microalbuminuria in normotensive children with insulin-dependent diabetes mellitus. *J Pediatr* 1990; **117**: 39–44.
33. Shield JPH, Hunt LP, Baum JD, Pennock CA. Screening for microalbuminuria in routine clinical care: which method? *Arch Dis Child* 1995; **72**: 524–525.
34. Moore THM, Shield JPH. Prevalence of abnormal urinary albumin excretion in adolescents and children with insulin dependent diabetes: the MIDAC study. *Arch Dis Child* 2000; **83**: 239–243.
35. Shield JPH, Hunt LP, Karachaliou F, Karavanaki K, Baum JD. Is microalbuminuria

progressive? *Arch Dis Child* 1995; **73**: 512–514.

36. Schultz CJ, Konopelska-Bahu T, Dalton RN *et al*. Microalbuminuria prevalence varies with age, sex, and puberty in children with type 1 diabetes followed from diagnosis in a longitudinal study. *Diabetes Care* 1999; **22**: 495–502.

37. Schultz, CJ, Neil HA, Dalron RN *et al*. Blood pressure does not rise before the onset of microalbuminuria in children followed from diagnosis of type 1 diabetes. *Diabetes Care* 2001; **24**: 555–560.

38. Jackson LV, Thalange NKS, Cole TJ. Blood pressure centiles for children and young people aged 4–24 years in Great Britain. *Arch Dis Child* 2003; **88 (Suppl 1)**: A68.

39. Holl RW, Lang GE, Grabert M *et al*. Diabetic retinopathy in pediatric patients with type-1 diabetes: effect of diabetes duration, prepubertal and pubertal onset of diabetes, and metabolic control. *J Pediatr* 1998; **132**: 790–794.

40. Holmes GKT. Screening for coeliac disease in type 1 diabetes. *Arch Dis Child* 2002; **87**: 495–499.

Helen P. Roper

4

Muscular dystrophy

Before the mid-19th century, muscle weakness was considered secondary to skeletal abnormalities or diseases of the nerves or brain. Meryon[1] suggested muscle as a primary site of disease, citing cases of what he termed 'paralysis from granular degeneration of muscles'. He described a third affected brother who by age 5 years had difficulty climbing stairs, by 9 years could scarcely stand unsupported, and who died of pneumonia at age 14 years. At autopsy, there were abnormalities only in the voluntary muscles and Meryon inferred that this was 'a form of paralysis in which the nervous centres or conducting nerves were not implicated'. He described the process as 'a breaking up of the sarcolemma of the elementary primitive fibres'.

Meryon placed this emphasis on the diagnosis of primary muscle disease apparently in reply to suggestions made by Duchenne in 1861 that the site of this disease was the brain. By 1868, when Duchenne wrote his series of astute observations[2] of 'la paralysie musculaire pseudo-hypertrophique ou paralysie myo-sclerosique', he had drawn different conclusions. Duchenne recounted that he noted the association with delayed speech and impaired intellect and first inferred it was a disease of brain, but having studied muscle biopsies from his patients and autopsies in which no central nervous system abnormality was found, he abandoned this hypothesis.

Careful clinical description has remained very important in this field. Whilst Duchenne muscular dystrophy is the most common from of muscular dystrophy in most populations, the recognition of different phenotypes, followed by the delineation of specific molecular genetic and protein defects, has allowed the categorisation of the different subtypes of muscular dystrophy.

Helen P. Roper MD, FRCPCH, FRCP
Consultant Paediatrician, Department of Child Health, Birmingham Heartlands Hospital, Bordesley Green East, Birmingham B9 5SS, UK
Tel: +44 121 424 3687; Fax: +44 121 773 6458; E-mail: helen.roper@heartsol.wmids.nhs.uk

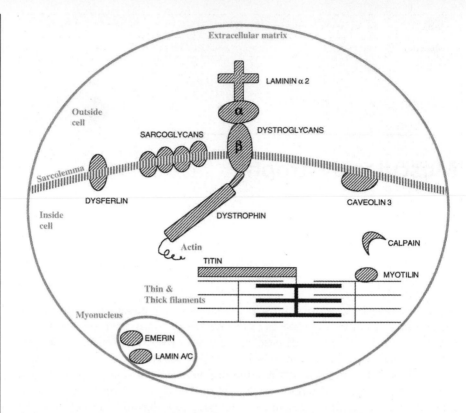

Fig. 1 Representation of the localisation of muscle proteins involved in the muscle dystrophies.

Muscular dystrophies are defined as genetically determined disorders producing progressive muscle weakness. In many of the muscular dystrophies, the primary defect has been identified as an abnormality of a specific protein which contributes to the integrity of the sarcolemma or those structures linking through the sarcolemma to the extra-cellular matrix (Fig. 1). Thus, Duchenne and Becker muscular dystrophy arise as a result of defects of dystrophin, limb girdle muscular dystrophies as abnormalities for instance of the sarcoglycans or dysferlin, congenital muscular dystrophies often defects of components linking sarcolemmal spanning proteins with components of the extra-cellular matrix. This concept that the pathogenesis of the muscular dystrophies relates to membrane defects jeopardising sarcolemmal integrity has been expanded as specific abnormalities have been found in other forms of muscular dystrophy involving the contractile apparatus and myonuclear proteins. Table 1 lists the known protein defects in the muscular dystrophies.

DUCHENNE MUSCULAR DYSTROPHY

CLINICAL PRESENTATION

Duchenne muscular dystrophy (DMD) is an X-linked recessive disorder occurring in around 1 in 3500 boys in all populations. Its natural history is of

Table 1 Protein defects in the muscular dystrophies

Muscular dystrophy	Protein defect
Duchenne muscular dystrophy	Dystrophin
Becker muscular dystrophy	Dystrophin
Limb girdle muscular dystrophies	
LGMD1A	Myotilin
LGMD1B	Lamin A/C
LGMD1C	Caveolin-3
LGMD1D	Unknown
LGMD1E	Unknown
LGMD 2A	Calpain
LGMD 2B	Dysferlin
LGMD 2C	γ-Sarcoglycan
LGMD 2D	α-Sarcoglycan
LGMD 2E	β-Sarcoglycan
LGMD 2F	δ-Sarcoglycan
LGMD 2G	Telethonin
LGMD 2H	TRIM32
LGMD 2I	Fukutin-related protein
LGMD 2J	Titin
Emery-Dreifuss muscular dystrophy	
X-linked	Emerin
Autosomal dominant	Lamin A/C
Congenital muscular dystrophies	
Merosin-deficient	Laminin α2
MDC 1B	Unknown
MDC 1C	FRKP
Ullrich syndrome	Collagen 6 α2 chain
Fukuyama	Fukutin
Muscle eye brain disease	O-Linked-mannose-acetylglucosaminyl-transferase
Walker-Warburg syndrome	O-Mannosyltransferase 1

progressive weakness becoming evident at 3–6 years, with loss of walking at 6–12 years, and death, usually from respiratory failure, in the late teens. There is a high rate of new mutations, arising in around one-third of cases, with suggestions that the disorder is more common in deprived populations.[3] Although the clinical features of the disorder are well known, we often do not make a timely diagnosis.[4]

Motor problems

Most boys will present with motor difficulties, but for some this will be part of global delay and their motor problems are not necessarily disproportionate to other developmental difficulties. Boys with DMD usually start to walk at a later age than their unaffected siblings and often beyond the 18-month point at which screening has been advocated.[5] They can never run properly (their running gait resembles that of a racing walker, or someone walking through water), cannot jump with both feet off the ground nor climb stairs with one foot per stair. Most boys will need to use a Gowers' manoeuvre to get up from the floor by the time of diagnosis.

Global developmental delay

Boys with DMD have non-progressive learning difficulties. The IQ distribution is shifted 1 SD lower than the normal population. 30% have an IQ of < 70 and the mean IQ is 85.[6] This is skewed, with the verbal IQ being lower than the performance IQ. Many boys with DMD will have speech delay, often identified before muscle weakness is recognised.

Isoforms of dystrophin are usually present in the brain, and are absent from the cerebrum and cerebellum of boys with DMD and intellectual impairment. Absence of brain dystrophin is not associated with macroscopic morphological abnormalities but there are abnormalities of dendrites and loss of those neurones that normally express dystrophin.[6]

Failure to recognise this presentation is often associated with late diagnosis and the risk of a second or third affected brother being born before the parents have an opportunity of genetic counselling.

Failure to thrive and spurious 'liver disease'

Boys with DMD often follow a specific growth pattern and may present with failure to thrive.[7] They are of normal birth weight and length but from 1–3 years of age fall across the centiles for both height and weight. They then return to normal growth velocities but do not regain their original centiles. This may relate to excess energy consumption associated with intense muscle necrosis.

Investigation of boys in this setting has led to inappropriate diagnoses of liver disease and on occasion their being subjected to serial liver biopsies. This is because transaminases are found to be raised when 'liver function tests' are requested, although all other measures of liver function are normal. These transaminases leak from damaged muscle cells just as does creatine kinase (CK). Any boy with unexplained isolated raised transaminase levels should have his CK measured.

Anaesthetic problems

Boys with DMD or Becker muscular dystrophy (BMD) may be vulnerable to acute rhabdomyolysis under general anaesthesia, producing a malignant hyperthermia-like crisis. Occasionally, this may be the presenting feature, either leading to sudden cardiac arrest secondary to hyperkalaemia, or in milder cases to myoglobinuria after a general anaesthetic. This is most likely if suxamethonium or volatile anaesthetic agents are used in a previously undiagnosed child.[8]

Screening

DMD does not fulfil the usual criteria for a disease appropriate for neonatal screening, as there is no available early intervention to modify its course. However, one could argue that an intervention (*i.e.* genetic counselling) might modify the course for the family (*i.e.* potentially avoiding further affected children).

The Welsh programme includes creatine kinase in neonatal blood screening taken on day 6 or 7, with a 92% uptake of the test. Of positive results, 50% represent transient high CK. Most parents whose sons were confirmed as having DMD were in favour of the screening programme, though a minority regretted knowing the diagnosis so early: 80% changed their reproductive plans, usually by delaying a further pregnancy.[9]

DIAGNOSIS OF DUCHENNE MUSCULAR DYSTROPHY

Duchenne muscular dystrophy is caused by lack of dystrophin. Measurement of serum CK is used as an initial investigation to confirm the presence of significant muscle disease involving muscle cell damage, but is not specific. CK is always very high, except in the end stages of the disease when there is little remaining muscle, usually of the order of 50–100 times the upper limit of the laboratory normal range. A normal or mildly raised CK in a young child excludes the diagnosis of DMD.

The specific investigations are the identification of a mutation in the dystrophin gene and the study of dystrophin expression in muscle.

The dystrophin gene

Until recently, dystrophin remained the largest human gene to be identified. It has now been superseded by another muscle protein gene, that coding for titin. The dystrophin gene is 2.5 Mb in length, consisting of 79 exons, coding for a very large protein with a molecular weight of 427 kDa, comprising 3685 amino acids in skeletal muscle. Despite the protein's size, only 0.6% of the gene contributes to the coding areas.

Dystrophin is a rod-shaped protein, which links between the dystroglycan complex in the sarcolemma and cytoskeletal actin. Absence of dystrophin may make the sarcolemma vulnerable to damage during repeated cycles of contraction and relaxation of the muscle fibre. Dystrophin exists in a number of different isoforms; there are three full-length isoforms present in skeletal muscle, cardiac muscle and brain, and at least five shorter isoforms expressed in different brain areas.

When Becker muscular dystrophy was recognised as allelic to DMD,[10] it was at first expected that patients with DMD would have a large gene deletion and those with BMD a smaller deletion. There is, in fact, no relationship between deletion extent and disease severity. The reading frame hypothesis provides an explanation for this[11] and applies in > 90% of cases. Mutations which disrupt the reading frame of the triplet codons ('out-frame' or 'frame shift' mutations) lead to the production of no dystrophin and hence the DMD phenotype, whilst those that maintain the reading frame ('in-frame') lead to the production of a semi-functional protein and hence the milder BMD phenotype (Fig. 2).

In 70% of affected boys, deletions of the dystrophin gene are detected by techniques used routinely in genetic laboratories. The remaining 30% have point mutations or duplications, which are more difficult to detect and these investigations are available in only a small number of centres. Thus, a report that a deletion has not been detected does not exclude a diagnosis of DMD or BMD.

Confirmation of the diagnosis

If one sees a boy with apparently typical clinical features of DMD and a CK of 10,000 U/l, how should the diagnosis be confirmed?

(A) Frame shift deletion:

A small deletion – here of G in the first codon – disrupts the reading frame.
The gene code cannot be read appropriately and no protein is produced

<u>TTG CAG CCT TAA CTG CGG CTC ATA</u>   **Parent gene**

<u>TTC AGC CTT AAC TGC GGC TCA TA</u>   **Small frame shift mutation**
                                                → nonsense → no protein

(B) In frame deletion

There is a large deletion but it involves complete triplet codons so the reading frame is maintained
and a truncated semi-functional protein is produced

<u>TTG CAG CCT TAA CTG CGG CTC ATA</u>   **Parent gene**

                          <u>CGG CTC ATA</u>   **Large in-frame deletion**
                                                → reading frame maintained → semi-functional protein

Fig. 2 Representation of the reading frame hypothesis.

It is important to confirm the diagnosis definitively to allow accurate genetic counselling and discussion of the prognosis. If the boy has a mutation in the dystrophin gene, then he must have either DMD or BMD. If the clinical features are clearly those of DMD (for instance a boy of 5 or 6 years who is unable to run or jump at presentation), one could argue that performing a muscle biopsy does not add further information. Certainly, a biopsy to look at dystrophin expression must be undertaken in the 30% of boys in whom no gene deletion is demonstrated. It is important also to biopsy those boys in whom the phenotype appears mild. It is possible to be misled by those small numbers of boys with BMD with severe learning difficulties who may present with motor delay but later have a milder clinical course. A biopsy is likely to be mandatory if future specific therapy becomes available, to follow progress before and after treatment. Some argue that the diagnosis should always be confirmed by muscle biopsy,[12] while others feel that the greater availability of more sensitive DNA techniques will allow the recognition of frame shift mutations in an increasing proportion of patients.[13]

Electromyography has no role in confirming the specific diagnosis of DMD. It will confirm only that there is an underlying myopathy and is likely to be uncomfortable for a child.

MANAGEMENT OF DUCHENNE MUSCULAR DYSTROPHY

Exercise

Some have extrapolated from animal studies that exercise may accelerate muscle damage. This is, after all, the model for disease pathogenesis. In the mdx mouse (a dystrophin-deficient animal) this applies particularly to eccentric exercise,[14] where the muscle must be put into action whilst stretched (*e.g.* the quadriceps muscle in downhill running). In these animals, endurance exercise did no harm and possibly was beneficial. There are few studies of boys with DMD. It seems appropriate to encourage non-eccentric exercise, such as swimming, which may enhance general fitness.[15] There is no evidence to support or refute the role of stretching or passive exercises in non-ambulant boys.

Orthoses

There is evidence to support the use of night splints to control Achilles tendon (TA) contractures.[16] Boys with DMD develop TA contractures as they tend to toe walk to compensate for hip extensor weakness by adopting a hyperlordotic stance. Parents are usually taught passive stretching exercises to control the evolution of TA tightness. Hyde *et al.*[16] demonstrated in a prospective randomised study that contractures developed less rapidly in boys who used stretches and night splints than in those who used stretching alone. This is important, as impaired ankle dorsiflexion is a predictor of loss of ambulation, together with impairment of hip extension.[17]

Boys should not wear splints during the day as they prevent their using a lordotic stance and make walking harder.

Long leg splints (also known as knee-ankle foot orthoses or KAFOs) can prolong assisted walking[18] and their use may lead to later better control of contractures. Successful use is dependent on a good fit, often associated with the need for TA release surgery, a motivated child, and active rehabilitation. Some boys are fearful of falling in them even if well supported.

Early multiple release of lower limb contractures in ambulant boys does not confer long-term benefit.[19]

Weight control

Many boys with DMD begin to gain weight rapidly as they approach loss of ambulation. The evidence that this has negative implications for respiratory function is lacking. For those boys who become very obese, there are practical difficulties with daily care and in finding appropriate wheelchairs. At 7 years of age, boys' weight for height is similar to the normal population. Thereafter, the prevalence of overweight increases until by 13 years 54% of boys have a weight for age > 90th centile.[20] Many boys with DMD are short because of the early period of poor growth velocity and median height stabilises at –1.5 SD.[21] Whilst a small number of boys remain very obese, many lose weight as teenagers and by 17 years, 45% of boys have a weight for age < 10th centile.

Weight loss and poor appetite are often a sign of impending respiratory failure.[22] Late weight loss also reflects loss of muscle bulk, and appropriate weight is often difficult to assess, without using specific charts.[20]

Dietary advice and calorie requirement calculations, for either the overweight or underweight child, should not be based on standard requirements for an ambulant child.

Steroids

The use of steroids to slow progression in DMD was suggested some years ago.[23] There are now more long-term studies demonstrating their efficacy in prolonging independent ambulation with a clearer assessment of the likely side effects.

Steroids do not effect a cure. How they exert an effect is not known; theories include a reduction in the rate of muscle breakdown, reduction of focal inflammation and necrosis, or stimulation of muscle regeneration.

Some groups have used prednisone or prednisolone and others deflazacort.[24] The early studies remain difficult to interpret, as boys of widely differing age and disease stage were included with no clear end-point. More recent studies have started steroids in younger boys and used age at loss of independent walking as an outcome measure. Long-term studies of the use of daily steroids, initially at a dose of 0.75 mg/kg/day[23] demonstrated that continuing use of this dose was unsustainable because of side effects, with > 50% of subjects reducing the dose or stopping altogether. The long-term outcome of daily steroid use in some of this original cohort was to prolong walking by 4 years.[25] Similar results in prolonging ambulation have been reported for the use of deflazacort.[24]

Intermittent dose regimens were introduced to reduce the high incidence of side effects. A regimen of prednisolone given at 0.75 mg/kg/day for the first 10 days of the month produced early benefits in strength which were not maintained and this was modified to a regimen of 10 days on and 10 days off. There are fewer side effects in boys taking this regimen but it may be less effective.[26]

A study of weekly high-dose prednisone showed improvements in strength with fewer side effects but this regimen has not yet been used for long enough to demonstrate an effect on age at loss of walking.[27]

There has been no long-term randomised control trial of steroid use. Many studies compare outcome against historical controls and most are open studies.

The most common side effect is weight gain, seen in boys taking prednisone or deflazacort, although perhaps less common in the latter.[28] More than 50% of boys taking steroids for some time have height velocity slowing. Cataracts occur in 30–40% of boys taking deflazacort[24] though most are not visually significant. Parents report behaviour changes with irritability or excitability. There is a significant risk of immunosuppression, particularly for those boys taking a continuous regimen. Before steroids are started, the boy's zoster immunity should be determined and vaccination given if necessary.

Ambulant boys with DMD have decreased bone density compared with age-matched controls.[29] Fractures are common in boys with DMD and probably increase after steroid use, whether prednisolone or deflazacort, with more than 50% sustaining long bone or vertebral fractures. In one report, 75% had vertebral fractures after 100 months of prednisone use.[30] There are no data on the use of bisphosphonates, calcium or vitamin supplementation in this situation.

Most regimens stop steroids at loss of independent ambulation. The effects of continued steroids on later respiratory function or the development of cardiomyopathy are not yet documented although there are some suggestions of a positive effect.[25]

Steroids are now widely used in Europe and North America. It is probably appropriate to suggest a trial of steroids in an ambulant boy at the plateau of his motor ability. There should be regular assessments of muscle strength and functional ability using validated techniques. It is important to monitor for side effects with weight and blood pressure measurement, and eye screening and bone density scanning if steroids are continued beyond 12 months. If there is no benefit of steroids after 6 months they should be stopped.

Scoliosis

Boys never develop a scoliosis whist still walking as the lordotic stance is protective, but more than 90% will develop a scoliosis after losing independent ambulation. This is usually a thoraco-lumbar curve with pelvic obliquity. The scoliosis produces problems with comfortable sitting, particularly because of the pelvic tilt, and may exacerbate the decline in respiratory function.

There is no evidence that spinal bracing prevents progression of the curve. Surgical management, using various methods of segmental wiring derived from the Luque technique, is widely used. There is no clear evidence that spinal surgery improves survival, nor slows the decline in respiratory function. Most boys will have some loss of vital capacity postoperatively.

Nevertheless, > 90% of boys are glad they have had spinal surgery and experience improvements in quality of life.[31] Seating is more comfortable and boys feel taller and happier with their appearance. There are practical problems that should be discussed pre-operatively – some will lose head control and may be unable to feed themselves; they may also lose the ability to stand in KAFOs if they are still so doing.

There are different approaches to the timing of surgery, with some centres operating earlier at a lesser curve, but better residual respiratory function. It is clear that surgery is not feasible if respiratory function is less than 30% predicted or if there is a significant cardiomyopathy.

Cardiac involvement

Most boys with DMD will develop a cardiomyopathy but usually this becomes symptomatic only late in the course of the disease. Symptoms are less likely to manifest because of their immobility. In a few boys, a cardiomyopathy develops early and leads to death before there is established respiratory failure.

ECG changes may be seen in young boys with DMD, usually as tall R waves and $R/S > 1$ in the right praecordial leads, and are not helpful in predicting those who will develop symptomatic involvement. Sinus tachycardia is present in most from the age of 5 years and precedes left ventricular dysfunction. It is usual practice to perform echocardiography once boys have lost ambulation to look for the development of the hypertrophic cardiomyopathy which later progresses to dilated cardiomyopathy. As the myocardium is replaced by fibrous tissue, left ventricular function diminishes and in later stages arrhythmias may occur.

If cardio-active therapy is started once cardiac failure is apparent, there is little impact on outcome. It is not known whether pre-symptomatic treatment of left ventricular dysfunction delays the onset of cardiac failure and improves prognosis.

There is undoubtedly a risk of cardiac involvement in obligate carriers, although the incidence of clinically significant problems varies widely in studies from 41%[32] to < 10%.[33] The risk increases with age and does not correlate with the presence of skeletal muscle weakness. It is suggested that carriers should be screened with echocardiography at 5-yearly intervals.

Respiratory function and non-invasive ventilation

Respiratory failure is the usual cause of death in DMD, muscle weakness producing a restrictive ventilatory defect exacerbated by scoliosis.

Relative hypoventilation in sleep is ubiquitous and is exaggerated when there is muscle weakness. Night-time alveolar hypoventilation leads to carbon dioxide retention and periods of hypoxia. Thus patients with DMD are vulnerable to night-time respiratory failure before day-time respiratory failure. It is inappropriate to treat this with oxygen as this diminishes the respiratory drive further, worsening hypercapnia and risking the acceleration of respiratory failure and death. The classical symptoms of nocturnal hypoventilation are day-time sleepiness and headaches, but earlier symptoms may be recognised including weight loss, poor appetite and increased frequency of night-time waking.[22]

The recognition of this phenomenon has led to the development of programmes of non-invasive ventilatory support. The aim is to anticipate incipient nocturnal respiratory failure by monitoring respiratory function regularly and performing sleep studies once the vital capacity falls to 20% of predicted and certainly if the boy is symptomatic. It has been demonstrated that such support improves well being, is associated with longer survival, and that most who use night support will not need daytime support for at least 5 years.

Non-invasive ventilation (NIV) is usually delivered by face-mask and with air. Oxygen may be needed during respiratory infections. The machines are pre-set and easy to manage at home.

The mean age at onset of need for night time NIV in one study was 20 years,[34] with a 1-year survival after starting NIV of 85% and 5-year survival of 73%. Eagle compared life expectancy in those ventilated in this way and those not, and demonstrated an increase in survival of at least 5 years in the ventilated cohort.[22] A minority died of symptomatic cardiac disease, but most remained stable on night support alone with a good quality of life.

All boys should have regular influenza and pneumococcal vaccination once there is a decline in respiratory function.

Specific therapy for Duchenne muscular dystrophy

No specific treatment is yet available for DMD. Challenges to effective gene therapy include those common to other disorders – including the T-cell immune response to the viral vector and the humoral antibody response to the new foreign protein thus produced – and those specific to the disorder – including the fact that dystrophin gene is larger than the vector, and the difficulties of repeated therapy delivery to multiple muscle sites. Recent work has focused on 'exon-skipping' – a process whereby an oligonucleotide sequence is inserted to convert an out-frame deletion to an in-frame deletion (*i.e.* potentially converting the phenotype from DMD to BMD).

Myoblast transfer involves the injection of myogenic cells from an immune-compatible donor into specific muscle sites. This technique has failed to produce functional effects. Most injected myoblasts do not survive because of the immune response they generate, and those that do usually fail to migrate from the injection site.

Gentamicin has been used to restore dystrophin expression in the mdx mouse,[35] but it works only where the gene mutation is a point mutation inserting a premature stop codon. This is the usual mutation in the mdx mouse but is unusual in human DMD. One would be concerned about the long-term risks of aminoglycoside toxicity.

CLINICAL PRESENTATION OF BECKER MUSCULAR DYSTROPHY

The incidence of Becker muscular dystrophy (BMD) is one-third that of DMD. The age at onset of symptoms varies from < 5–60 years although most develop symptomatic weakness in the second decade. The rate of progression of BMD is also very variable. Young men with BMD will be ambulant until at least 16 years.

The distribution of weakness is the same as that seen in DMD. Most will present with motor difficulties, but an important clinical feature is that of cramps, particularly in the calves, on exertion. In teenagers, this symptom is often more disabling than weakness. Affected boys may experience myoglobinuria after strenuous exercise. There may be early cardiac involvement disproportionate to the degree of skeletal muscle weakness and, occasionally, this is the presenting feature.

The degree of learning difficulty is usually milder than in boys with DMD, but can occasionally be severe and this may present difficulties in the diagnosis if the boy presents early with global delay.

LIMB GIRDLE MUSCULAR DYSTROPHY

It is only in the last few years that the different limb girdle muscular dystrophies (LGMDs) have been clearly delineated by phenotype, by the protein involved and by gene location. Previously, all limb girdle syndromes had been lumped together and indeed at one time the existence of limb girdle muscular dystrophy as a separate entity had been questioned, with the suggestion that such weakness was predominantly due to anterior horn cell disease or inflammatory myopathies.

The LGMDs differ from Duchenne and Becker muscular dystrophy in that the different subtypes vary in incidence in different populations. The first to be described and identified were what are now known as the sarcoglycanopathies. These conditions are relatively common in people of North African origin but rare in white northern Europeans. Conversely, the recently described LGMD2I, with a defect in fukutin-related protein, is relatively common in the UK.

The nosology of LGMD divides the different forms into those which are autosomal dominant, termed type 1, and those which are autosomal recessive, termed type 2. A separate letter denotes each disorder. Table 1 lists the specific protein defects. It is important to make a precise diagnosis to allow accurate genetic counselling and to screen appropriately for associated problems. Some LGMDs have a high risk of cardiac involvement (*e.g.* LGMD1B, LGMD2I) while others do not (LGMD2A).

The diagnosis is based on the clinical phenotype, variable rise in CK, a muscle biopsy to demonstrate a dystrophic histology and immunocytochemical studies to identify the specific protein defect. In some forms, it is not possible to identify the protein defect on biopsy; however, other forms can be excluded and then specific gene mutation screening undertaken on the basis of the clinical picture. It is not feasible to approach initial diagnosis of LGMDs by gene screening alone as so many potential genes are involved.

Why different gene disorders produce specific distributions of muscle weakness remains unanswered. One might expect all muscles to be similarly affected if the gene is expressed in all skeletal muscle. Yet it is this variation that is the key to precise diagnosis.

SALIENT CLINICAL FEATURES OF SOME LIMB GIRDLE MUSCULAR DYSTROPHIES

Sarcoglycanopathies (LGMD2C, LGMD2D, LGMD2E, LGMD2F)

These conditions present a similar clinical picture to DMD or BMD. They are autosomal recessive disorders, usually presenting with motor difficulties in childhood. There is often calf hypertrophy. In contrast to boys with DMD, these children have no intellectual impairment. There maybe associated cardiac involvement.

Calpainopathy (LGMD2A)

This arises as a result of a defect of calpain, a muscle specific calcium-dependent protease enzyme. There is no muscle hypertrophy and affected children have a characteristic broad-based stance, as there is relatively greater weakness of the hip adductors compared with abductors. There is early wasting and weakness of the posterior thigh muscles and scapular winging. Most will present in the early teenage years and the average age of loss of independent walking is 17 years. There are no reports of cardiac involvement.

Dysferlinopathy (LGMD2B)

Lack of dysferlin protein may produce two different phenotypes even within the same family. Children tend to present with proximal lower limb weakness in their teens and develop upper limb weakness after an interval of some years. Early motor abilities are completely normal, in contrast to other muscular dystrophies where there is often a history of poor agility even before overt weakness. Other family members may present with distal lower limb weakness, initially involving gastrocnemius (termed Myoshi myopathy). The risk of cardiac involvement is low. CK is very high, even in those who are pre-symptomatic.

LGMD2I

This is probably the commonest form of LGMD in the UK. Patients may have striking hypertrophy of the calves and thighs although the shape of the hypertrophy seems subjectively different to that seen in DMD or BMD. As in BMD, affected individuals may have episodes of myoglobinuria. The age at onset is very variable and there is a significant risk of development of cardiomyopathy.[36]

Laminopathies

Defects of the lamina A/C nuclear envelope protein have been found in a number of distinct disorders (LGMD1B, autosomal dominant Emery-Dreifuss muscular dystrophy, autosomal recessive Charcot Marie Tooth disease type 2A, familial partial lipodystrophy, autosomal dominant dilated cardiomyopathy with AV block and, most recently, progeria[37]).

The LGMD1B phenotype presents as limb girdle weakness at 4–35 years of age, with a high risk of cardiac conduction defects and cardiomyopathy developing in early adulthood.

In the autosomal dominant Emery-Dreifuss form, there is a similar pattern of weakness and contractures to the X-linked form of Emery-Dreifuss muscular dystrophy. The age at onset is variable and may be earlier than EDMD. Contractures may not be evident at first presentation but evolve over time, comprising flexion contractures of the elbows and fingers, with increasing neck and spinal rigidity. Although this is a dominant disorder, 75% of cases are new mutations.[38] There is a high risk of cardiac disease at any time from the teens onwards.

OTHER MUSCULAR DYSTROPHIES PRESENTING IN CHILDHOOD

Emery-Dreifuss muscular dystrophy

This X-linked recessive muscular dystrophy produces a specific pattern of weakness, with proximal weakness in the upper limbs and distal peroneal weakness in the lower limbs. This is associated with contractures particularly at the elbows and Achilles tendons, usually present at presentation in the teens, with later evolution of neck and spinal rigidity. Many patients develop cardiac conduction defects, usually after the age of 20 years. The disorder is due to a lack of emerin,[39] a nuclear envelope protein.

Facioscapulohumeral muscular dystrophy

Facioscapulohumeral muscular dystrophy (FSHD) is the most common autosomal dominant from of muscular dystrophy. The classical presentation is in adolescence or early adulthood with facial and shoulder girdle weakness, but there is considerable intrafamilial variation. Affected individuals may present with pelvic girdle weakness and little facial involvement, or in infancy with severe facial weakness.[40] These children are often misdiagnosed as having Moebius syndrome, although there is no associated 6th nerve palsy. There is an association with high-tone deafness, retinal problems and learning difficulties in these severely affected children.

FSHD is associated with deletion of units of a DNA repeat sequence on chromosome 4. The molecular genetics is complex but such investigations confirm the diagnosis and provide an explanation for the severity of early onset cases.

CONGENITAL MUSCULAR DYSTROPHY

Just as the LGMDs have proven to be a group of many different disorders with different phenotypes, pathogenesis and prognosis, so too have the congenital muscular dystrophies. Children with congenital muscular dystrophy present with hypotonia, weakness and wasting at birth or within the first few months.

A number of the congenital muscular dystrophies are associated with progressive contracture formation and have been shown to arise as a result of defects of proteins linking the muscle cell to the extracellular matrix (*e.g.* merosin, collagen 6). Severely affected infants may present with arthrogryposis and this should be considered in arthrogrypotic infants with a persistently high CK beyond the first week of life.

The different disorders may be divided into those in which there is intellectual impairment and those without. The former often have structural brain abnormalities reflecting abnormal neuronal migration.

Those without intellectual impairment include merosin-deficient congenital muscular dystrophy, Ullrich syndrome and fukutin-related protein deficiency.

Merosin-deficient congenital muscular dystrophy

This was the first specific defect to be identified in congenital muscular dystrophy. Lack of merosin (the α2 chain of laminin), produces a specific phenotype comprising generalised weakness, a tendency to develop contractures, and the presence of white matter brain changes, which are not associated with intellectual impairment,[41] but confer a significant risk of epilepsy. Affected children do not achieve independent ambulation and are prone to develop nocturnal hypoventilation in the first or second decade.

Ullrich syndrome

Ullrich syndrome is an example of a recessive disorder producing severe disease where a milder form of muscle disease (in this case Bethlem myopathy) is produced by different autosomal dominant mutation of the same gene. The defect is in collagen 6 formation.[42] Children usually attain independent walking but have contractures from birth, spinal rigidity often associated with a severe scoliosis, and develop respiratory failure often during childhood.

Fukutin-related protein deficient congenital muscular dystrophy

A form of congenital muscular dystrophy presenting with hypotonia, early calf hypertrophy and macroglossia is allelic to LGMD2I and is also caused by a defect of fukutin-related protein.[43]

Those associated with intellectual impairment include Fukuyama congenital muscular dystrophy, which is virtually exclusively to those of Japanese ethnic origin; muscle-eye-brain disease and Walker-Warburg syndrome, where there are abnormalities of retinal development with or without glaucoma or cataract.

All are due to defects in genes involved in protein glycosylation.

CONCLUSIONS

Over last 20 years, advances in molecular biology have hugely enhanced the understanding of the muscular dystrophies. No specific therapy is yet available although there are now opportunities for more precise diagnosis and there is an evidence base for management of the disorders, which may enhance and perhaps prolong life.

Key points for clinical practice

- Boys with Duchenne muscular dystrophy often present with global delay, with their motor problems not disproportionate to other developmental difficulties.

- Boys with Duchenne muscular dystrophy may fail to thrive in the first 3 years of life, and although they later resume normal growth velocities, they do not regain their original centiles.

- Where a child has raised transaminases with no other abnormalities of liver function, it is likely to be a reflection of muscle rather than liver disease and creatine kinase should be measured.

- Boys with Duchenne or Becker muscular dystrophy may experience rhabdomyolysis during general anaesthesia, leading to myoglobinuria or unexpected cardiac arrest.

- The diagnosis of Duchenne muscular dystrophy is confirmed with a combination of muscle biopsy and molecular genetic tests. EMG is not specific and should be avoided.

- Night splints help control the development of Achilles tendon contractures in Duchenne muscular dystrophy. Boys should not wear day splints as they make walking harder.

- The use of steroids in Duchenne muscular dystrophy prolongs independent ambulation by several years, but there is a significant risk of side effects.

- Carriers of dystrophin gene mutations are at risk for the development of a cardiomyopathy.

- Non-invasive night ventilation prolongs life in Duchenne muscular dystrophy and is associated with an improved quality of life.

- Boys with Becker muscular dystrophy often present with cramps, sometimes in association with myoglobinuria. The cramps may be more disabling than weakness at presentation.

- The limb girdle muscular dystrophies may be differentiated by clinical phenotype. It is important to make a precise diagnosis to screen appropriately for associated problems, including cardiac or respiratory involvement.

- Facioscapulohumeral dystrophy may present with severe facial weakness in infancy.

References

1. Meryon E. *Practical and Pathological Researches on the Various Forms of Paralysis.* London: Churchill, 1864; 200–215.
2. Duchenne GB. Recherches sur la paralysie musculaire pseudohypertrophique, ou paralysie myosclerosique. *Arch Gen Med* 1868; **11**: 5–25, 179–209, 305–321, 421–443, 552–558.
3. Bushby K, Raybould S, O'Donnell S, Steele JG. Social deprivation in Duchenne muscular dystrophy: population based study. *BMJ* 2001; **323**: 1035–1036.
4. Bushby KMD, Hill A, Steele JG. Failure of early diagnosis in symptomatic Duchenne muscular dystrophy. *Lancet* 1999; **353**: 557–558.
5. Gardner Medwin D. Recognising and preventing Duchenne muscular dystrophy. *BMJ* 1983; **287**: 1083–1084.
6. Anderson JL, Head SI, Rae C, Morley JW. Brain function in Duchenne muscular dystrophy. *Brain* 2002; **125**: 4–13.
7. Call G, Ziter FA. Failure to thrive in Duchenne muscular dystrophy. *J Pediatr* 1985; **106**: 939–941.
8. Breucking E, Reimnitz P, Schara U, Mortier W. The incidence of severe anaesthetic complications in patients and families with progressive muscular dystrophy of the Duchenne and Becker types. *Anaesthesist* 2000; **49**: 187–195.
9. Parsons EP, Clarke AJ, Hood K, Lycett E, Bradley DM. Newborn screening for Duchenne muscular dystrophy: a psychological study. *Arch Dis Child Fetal Neonatal Edn* 2002; **86**: F91–F95.
10. Kingston HM, Thomas NS, Pearson PL, Sarfrazi M, Harper PS. Genetic linkage between Becker muscular dystrophy and a polymorphic DNA sequence on the short arm of the X chromosome. *J Med Genet* 1983; **20**: 255–258.
11. Monaco AP, Bertelson CJ, Liechti-Gallati S, Moser H, Kunkel LM. An explanation for the phenotypic differences between patients bearing partial deletions of the DMD locus. *Genomics* 1988; **2**: 90–95.

12. Muntoni F. Is a muscle biopsy in Duchenne dystrophy really necessary? *Neurology* 2001; **57**: 574–575.
13. Mendell JR, Buzin CH, Feng J *et al*. Diagnosis of Duchenne muscular dystrophy by enhanced detection of small mutations. *Neurology* 2001; **57**: 645–650.
14. Petrof BJ. The molecular basis of activity-induced muscle injury in Duchenne muscular dystrophy. *Mol Cell Biochem* 1998; **179**: 111–123.
15. Eagle M. Report on the Muscular Dystrophy Campaign workshop: exercise in neuromuscular diseases. *Neuromusc Disorders* 2002; **12**: 975–983.
16. Hyde SA, Floytrup I, Glent S *et al*. A randomized comparative study of two methods for controlling Tendo Achilles contracture in Duchenne muscular dystrophy. *Neuromusc Disorders* 2000; **10**: 257–263.
17. Bakker JPJ, de Groot IJM, Beelen A, Lankhorst GJ. Predictive factors of cessation of ambulation in patients with Duchenne muscular dystrophy. *Am J Phys Med Rehabil* 2002; **81**: 906–912.
18. Bakker JP, de Groot IJ, Beckerman H, de Jong BA, Lankhorst GJ. The effects of knee-ankle-foot orthoses in the treatment of Duchenne muscular dystrophy: review of the literature. *Clin Rehabil* 2000; **14**: 343–359.
19. Manzur AY, Hyde SA, Rodillo E, Heckmatt JZ, Bentley G, Dubowitz V. A randomized controlled trial of early surgery in Duchenne muscular dystrophy. *Neuromusc Disorders* 1992; **2**: 379–387.
20. Willig T-N, Carlier L, Legrand M, Riviere H, Navarro J. Nutritional assessment in Duchenne muscular dystrophy. *Dev Med Child Neurol* 1993; **35**: 1074–1082.
21. Eiholzer U, Bolthauser E, Frey D, Molinari L, Zachmann M. Short stature: a common feature in Duchenne muscular dystrophy. *Eur J Pediatr* 1988; **147**: 602–605.
22. Eagle M, Baudouin SV, Chandler C, Giddings DR, Bullock R, Bushby K. Survival in Duchenne muscular dystrophy: improvements in life expectancy since 1967 and the impact of home nocturnal ventilation. *Neuromusc Disorders* 2002; **12**: 926–929.
23. Mendell JR, Moxley RT, Griggs RC *et al*. Randomized, double-blind six-month trial of prednisone in Duchenne's muscular dystrophy. *N Engl J Med* 1989; **320**: 1592–1597.
24. Biggar WD, Gingras M, Fehlings DL, Harris VA, Steele CA. Deflazacort treatment of Duchenne muscular dystrophy. *J Pediatr* 2001; **138**: 45–50.
25. Pandya S, Myers G, Moxley RT. Effect of daily prednisone on independent ambulation in patients with Duchenne muscular dystrophy treated for up to 15 years. World Muscle Society Congress, Salt Lake City, Utah, 5–8th Sept, abstract. *Neuromusc Disorders* 2001; **11**: 630.
26. Sansome A, Royston P, Dubowitz V. Steroids in Duchenne muscular dystrophy; pilot study of a new low-dosage schedule. *Neuromusc Disorders* 1993; **3**: 567–569.
27. Connolly AM, Schierbecker JM, Renna R, Florence J. High dose weekly oral prednisone improves strength in boys with Duchenne muscular dystrophy. *Neuromusc Disorders* 2002; **12**: 917–925.
28. Bonifati MD, Ruzza G, Bonometto P *et al*. A multicenter, double-blind, randomized trial of deflazacort versus prednisone in Duchenne muscular dystrophy. *Muscle Nerve* 2000; **23**: 1344–1347.
29. Larson CM, Henderson RC. Bone mineral density and fractures in boys with Duchenne muscular dystrophy. *J Pediatr Orthop* 2000; **20**: 71–74.
30. Bothwell JE, Gordon KE, Dooley JM, MacSween J, Cummings EA, Salisbury S. Vertebral fractures in boys with Duchenne muscular dystrophy. *Clin Pediatr* 2003; **42**: 353–356.
31. Granata C, Merlini L, Cervellati S *et al*. Long-term results of spine surgery in Duchenne muscular dystrophy. *Neuromusc Disorders* 1996; **6**: 61–68.
32. Politano L, Nigro V, Nigro G *et al*. Development of cardiomyopathy in female carriers of Duchenne and Becker muscular dystrophies. *JAMA* 1996; **275**: 1335–1338.
33. Grain L, Cortina-Borja M, Forfar C, Hilton-Jones D, Hopkin J, Burch M. Cardiac abnormalities and skeletal weakness in carriers of Duchenne and Becker muscular dystrophies and controls. *Neuromusc Disorders* 2001; **11**: 186–191.
34. Simonds AK, Muntoni F, Heather S, Fielding S. Impact of nasal ventilation on survival in hypercapnic Duchenne muscular dystrophy. *Thorax* 1998; **53**: 949–952.
35. Barton-Davies ER, Cordier L, Shoturma DI, Leland SE, Sweeney HL. Aminoglycoside antibiotics restore dystrophin function to skeletal muscles of mdx mice. *J Clin Invest* 1999; **104**: 375–381.

36. Poppe M, Cree L, Bourke J *et al*. The phenotype of limb-girdle muscular dystrophy type 2I. *Neurology* 2003; **60**: 1246–1251.
37. Eriksson M, Brown WT, Gordon LB *et al*. Recurrent *de novo* point mutations in lamin A cause Hutchinson-Gilford progeria syndrome. *Nature* 2003; April 25 (epub ahead of print).
38. Bonne G, Mercuri E, Muchir A *et al*. Clinical and molecular genetic spectrum of autosomal dominant Emery-Dreifuss muscular dystrophy due to mutations of the lamin A/C gene. *Ann Neurol* 2000; **48**: 170–180.
39. Bione S, Maestrini E, Rivella S *et al*. Identification of a novel X-linked gene responsible for Emery-Dreifuss muscular dystrophy. *Nat Genet* 1994; **8**: 323–327.
40. Jardine PE, Koch MC, Lunt PW *et al*. *De novo* facioscapulohumeral muscular dystrophy defined by DNA probe p13E-11 (D4F104S1). *Arch Dis Child* 1994; **71**: 221–227.
41. Tome FM, Evangelista T, Leclerc A *et al*. Congenital muscular dystrophy with merosin deficiency. *C R Acad Sci III* 1994; **317**: 351–357.
42. Camacho Vanegas O, Bertini E, Zhang R-Z *et al*. Ullrich scleroatonic muscular dystrophy is caused by recessive mutations in collagen type VI. *Proc Natl Acad Sci USA* 2001; **98**: 7516–7521.
43. Brockington M, Blake DJ, Prandini P *et al*. Mutations in the Fukutin-related protein gene (FKRP) cause a form of congenital muscular dystrophy with secondary laminin α2 deficiency and abnormal glycosylation of α–dystroglycan. *Am J Hum Genet* 2001; **69**: 1198–1209.

Paula H.B. Bolton-Maggs

5

Childhood idiopathic thrombocytopaenic purpura

Idiopathic thrombocytopaenic purpura (ITP) in children is an uncommon condition with a dramatic presentation. It is usually self-limiting, presenting most commonly with a short history of purpura and bruising in children of either sex at any age, but usually between 2–10 years of age. The aetiology is not fully understood, but the disorder is caused by immune dysregulation, and may be triggered by a viral infection or immunisation. Platelet autoantibodies are produced leading to removal of antibody-coated platelets from the circulation and a consequent fall in count. Antibody-mediated platelet destruction can also occur in association with other disorders (secondary immune thrombocytopaenic purpura). Primary or idiopathic thrombocytopaenic purpura is a diagnosis of exclusion, and occasionally a more sinister diagnosis emerges over a period of days, weeks, or rarely, years. Fortunately, most children with ITP do not have serious bleeding problems and can be watched with sensible advice to the parents without giving pharmacological therapy to raise the platelet count. The treatments are mostly more unpleasant than the disease. The rare child with significant bleeding warrants therapy and options are discussed below.

PATHOPHYSIOLOGY

Idiopathic thrombocytopaenia is caused by immune mechanisms. Harrington infused plasma from affected patients into volunteers and demonstrated a fall in platelet count occurring within 3 h and lasting for 5 days.[1] The immune system produces antibodies reactive against platelet surface molecules. This may be triggered by viral infections or immunisations in some children, but in others no definite trigger can be identified. The antibodies are generally IgG,

Paula H.B. Bolton-Maggs FRCPCH FRCP FRCPath
Manchester Haemophilia Comprehensive Care Centre, Department of Clinical Haematology,
Manchester Royal Infirmary, Oxford Road, Manchester M13 9WL, UK
Tel +44 161 276 4811; Fax +44 161 276 4814; E-mail: paula.bolton-maggs@cmmc.nhs.uk

and usually target specific surface molecules, most commonly glycoprotein (Gp) IIb/IIIa, the complex with the largest number of molecules on the platelet surface. Gp IIb/IIIa is the receptor for fibrinogen and Gp 1b the receptor for von Willebrand factor. In some instances, antibodies against these antigens may produce platelet dysfunction, which may be associated with a more severe bleeding diathesis.[2,3] After varicella, the antibodies most commonly express activity against Gp V.[4] The sensitised platelets are cleared from the circulation by macrophages – most commonly, but not exclusively, in the spleen. The macrophages have surface receptors for the Fc portion of the immunoglobulin molecules. More recently, evidence has emerged that antibodies may target megakaryocytes as well as mature platelets;[5] thus, the peripheral thrombocytopaenia may result from both reduced production and increased peripheral destruction.

DIAGNOSIS

The diagnosis of ITP is a clinical one, made in the well child with profound thrombocytopaenia. Despite the dramatic skin appearances, the child with ITP usually has no other symptoms. This helps to differentiate the purpura from that associated with infection, particularly meningococcal disease. A clear history of acute onset together with careful examination of child and blood film is essential to exclude other diagnoses.

HISTORY

The history is typically short with an abrupt onset of cutaneous symptoms over 1–2 days, but history taking should include careful enquiry for evidence of life-long bleeding or a more chronic onset (which may indicate a congenital thrombocytopaenia), and whether other family members have either thrombocytopaenia or other types of immune disease. ITP is a disorder of immune regulation and there may be an increased frequency of other autoimmune diseases in the family. In some families, X-linked thrombocytopaenia has been mistaken for ITP.

EXAMINATION

Examination is normal apart from signs related to the low platelet count. Extensive purpura and bruising are common. There may be mucosal lesions in the mouth. The fundi should be examined if possible, but retinal haemorrhages are very rare in typical ITP. Lymphadenopathy and splenomegaly are not usual and should alert the clinician to additional infection (e.g. ITP in association with Epstein Barr virus or cytomegalovirus) or to an alternative diagnosis. Congenital abnormalities may indicate an associated congenital thrombocytopaenia. Other diagnostic considerations are given below.

WHAT INVESTIGATIONS?

The full blood count is typically normal apart from the very low platelet count, usually less than $20 \times 10^9/l$. Film examination shows a reduced number of platelets which are usually larger than normal. Iron deficiency is common in this age group, so there may be features to suggest this, such as microcytosis and hypochromia with or without anaemia. It is sensible to examine the urine for blood both macroscopically and by bed-side testing. Occasional children have significant haematuria, and its presence precludes the use of antifibrinolytic drugs for other mucous membrane bleeding because of the risk of inducing clot colic. Further investigations are not indicated unless other disorders need to be excluded. A coagulation screen is unnecessary and does not contribute to the differential diagnosis of purpura. Rarely, von Willebrand's disease may be associated with thrombocytopaenia (some less common subtypes) and present in infancy – this will be associated with a life-long bleeding history, and other members of the family are also likely to have symptoms,[6] particularly menorrhagia in adult affected women. A von Willebrand profile will confirm the diagnosis (factor VIIIC assay, von Willebrand factor antigen and activity assays) but the coagulation screen may well be normal and is not useful for excluding von Willebrand's disease, and such children should be investigated in association with a haemophilia specialist.

There has been recent interest in *Helicobacter pylori* infection as a trigger for ITP. In some adults, detection and eradication of this organism has resulted in remission from ITP,[7,8] but there are no data for childhood ITP. It may be worth screening for this in the child with chronic ITP and gastrointestinal symptoms.

Anti-platelet antibodies can usually be detected in patients with ITP but this is not a discriminating investigation, being both non-specific and not usually available in sufficient time. Other specialist tests are under development but are not yet generally available to assist in diagnosis, and are not recommended.[9] For example, in ITP the bone marrow increases platelet output from megakaryocytes; these young (reticulated) platelets can be labelled and counted, and measurements in thrombocytopaenic children correlate well with the cause of thrombocytopaenia.[10] Thrombopoietin levels in children with ITP are typically normal, compared to the raised levels found in disorders with reduced platelet production.[11,12]

Bone marrow examination is not usually indicated. Acute leukaemia rarely presents with a low platelet count alone, but aplastic anaemia may. Any atypical clinical or laboratory features should, therefore, prompt bone marrow examination. This is not necessary in most children with the typical clinical presentation and blood count, and in whom no treatment is contemplated. Children with Down syndrome need special consideration. Acute megakaryoblastic leukaemia may present in infancy in these children with a prodromal thrombocytopaenia.[13] Congenital thrombocytopaenias may be missed because they are very rare indeed, and are forgotten.[14] In Bernard Soulier syndrome (deficiency of the Gp 1b complex) the bleeding is usually more dramatic than the platelet count would suggest (*e.g.* significant bleeding with a platelet count of $30 \times 10^9/l$). Parents of these children are often related (autosomal recessive inheritance), and it is thus more common in communities where cousin marriages are frequent. Diagnosis requires demonstration of absent or reduced Gp 1b on the platelets. In Wiskott Aldrich syndrome (X-linked inheritance) the characteristic immune deficiency and eczema may not be prominent in the early years of life, but the platelets are characteristically smaller than normal in contrast to the larger than normal platelets seen in ITP.

Wiskott Aldrich syndrome is caused by mutations in the *WASP* gene (X11p), which codes for a protein expressed in lymphocytes and megakaryocytes. This protein plays a role in signal transduction and formation of the cytoskeleton. Forms of X-linked thrombocytopaenia occur due to mutations in the *WASP* gene, but without the other features of the full syndrome.[15] There are several other rare causes of inherited thrombocytopaenia, therefore an alternative diagnosis should be considered particularly in the child with thrombo-cytopaenia where the time of onset of symptoms was not clear, where the thrombocytopaenia persists and if there is no rise in platelet count if the child is treated with immune modulation (see below). The presence of other affected family members is an important pointer, as familial ITP is very rare indeed. The child should be carefully examined to exclude congenital abnormalities, such as abnormalities of the digits, which would suggest that the isolated thrombocytopaenia might be the first clue to Fanconi's anaemia. Other congenital abnormalities, such as deafness, can be associated with familial thrombocytopaenias.[14]

ASSOCIATED DISORDERS

ITP in association with varicella is well-recognised, and these children should be reviewed carefully because their course may be complicated by other auto-antibody-induced problems, particularly the rare association with acquired protein S deficiency and microvascular thrombosis.

Immune thrombocytopaenia may be associated with other autoimmune diseases (secondary ITP) such as autoimmune haemolysis (Evans' syndrome), SLE or antiphospholipid syndrome. These disorders are uncommon, and may present before the thrombocytopaenia, concurrently, or several months or years later. They are probably more common in older children, particularly girls, and usually in association with chronic ITP. Immune thrombocytopaenia may complicate the course of HIV infection in children but is rarely the presenting feature.

MANAGEMENT

In typical childhood ITP, most children remit spontaneously within 6–8 weeks and have only cutaneous or mild bleeding symptoms, so that treatment to raise the platelet count, even when it is very low or unmeasureable ($< 10 \times 10^9/l$), is not always required.[9,16] The few platelets function more efficiently and automated machines are inaccurate at these very low levels.[17] Pooled data from two UK centres demonstrated that more than 50% of 108 untreated children had achieved a platelet count of more than $50 \times 10^9/l$ within 2 weeks (Fig. 1).[18]

EXPECTANT MANAGEMENT

It is important to explain carefully to the parents and child the nature of the disease, the rarity of serious bleeding and the good outcome.[18] Unfortunately, it is impossible to predict at diagnosis how rapidly a child will remit, although a longer history is associated with a longer course. Parents should have access to advice and admission as necessary should more serious bleeding occur. It is

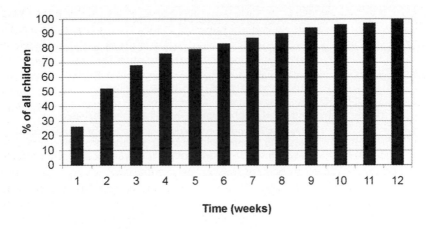

Fig. 1 Time to reach a platelet count of > 50 x 10⁹/l in 108 children with acute ITP.[18]

important that the family learn how to manage their life with the low count, and to carry on with all normal activities as far as possible. The number of platelets should not dominate family life. Quality of life for a child or adolescent will be impaired by unnecessary restriction of activity, particularly when this continues for months or years. Counts at very low levels are not accurate, and a difference between say, $5 \times 10^9/l$ and $15 \times 10^9/l$ is not significant. The child should not be excluded from school or nursery; a patient group, the ITP Support Association (view at <www.itpsupport.org.uk>), produces good leaflets for schools and family. Restrictions of activity should be minimal and confined to avoiding sports in which contact is a deliberate part of the activity, such as rugby, boxing and some of the martial arts. Swimming, cycling and other non-contact sports should continue. There is no evidence that travel by air is likely to precipitate bleeding in ITP so that holidays abroad may be taken with appropriate advice; a letter about the condition is often helpful. Parents need advice about when hospital review is necessary (*e.g.* after injury). It is helpful to discuss what treatment might be given if indicated, and the reasons for reserving this for more significant bleeding. There is no benefit in admission to hospital of children with acute ITP and cutaneous manifestations alone. Parents will usually be guided by the advice they are given. Most have no knowledge of low platelet counts until given advice by a doctor (words and body language). Sensible advice (avoidance of contact sports, attendance at hospital in the face of accidents) and a contact name and number are usually sufficient - such as those used for other patients with bleeding disorder (haemophiliacs). The count should perhaps be repeated within the first 10 days to exclude other emerging marrow disorders such as aplastic anaemia, but generally there is no need to do repeated counts while the child has purpura as such symptoms indicate a low count, and the absolute level should not determine treatment. It is more interesting to reserve repeat counts for when the child becomes asymptomatic when remission may be occurring.

There has been a tendency to focus on the platelet count rather than the child and his or her symptoms. When intravenous immunoglobulin (IVIG) became available for treatment, a group of UK paediatric haematologists became concerned that this invasive treatment was being used unnecessarily,

Table 1 Clinical assessment of children with acute ITP – UK studies[16]

Asymptomatic	A low platelet count was discovered by chance when the child was having a blood test for other reasons
Mild symptoms	Bruising and petechiae; occasional minor epistaxis, very little or no interference with daily living
Moderate	More severe skin manifestations with some mucosal lesions and more troublesome epistaxis and menorrhagia
Severe	Bleeding episodes (epistaxis, melaena and/or menorrhagia) requiring hospital admissions and/or blood transfusions – symptoms seriously interfering with quality of life

and produced guidelines.[19] A national review of the management of acute childhood ITP in the UK was undertaken in 1995–1996 against these guidelines. An important feature of this analysis was the definition of clinical severity as mild, moderate or severe (Table 1). Over a 14-month period, data were collected for 427 children. Although 82% had platelet counts < 20 x 10^9/l, the majority were classified as clinically mild by their physicians (73% of children with counts < 10 x 10^9/l; Fig. 2).[16] Only 13 (3%) children had severe bleeding manifestations (usually epistaxis or gastrointestinal haemorrhage); there were no intracranial bleeds or deaths. The audit confirmed that acute ITP is a benign condition in most children, but showed that many children (61%) are treated on the basis of a low count with steroids or intravenous immunoglobulin (IVIG).[16] After publication of the results and dissemination of this information, the audit was repeated in 2000. A similar population of children was reviewed, with almost identical characteristics in relation to count, clinical severity and outcome. This second audit demonstrated that there had been a reduction in the number of children treated with drugs; there

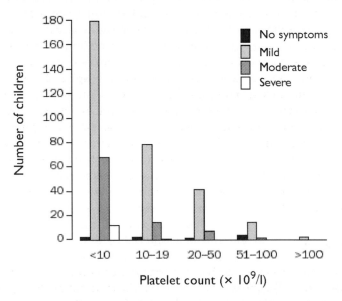

Fig. 2 Clinical classification of children with acute ITP in relation to platelet count; data from first UK national audit.[16]

was also a reduction in the number of children having bone marrow examinations presumably related to this.[20]

Many haematologists and paediatricians, therefore, consider that most children with acute ITP do not need active treatment, which is in contrast to practice in the US where guidelines published in 1996 did not countenance a 'no treatment' option.[21] These two contrasting sets of 'guidelines' were produced from the same evidence-base. There are insufficient trials of good quality upon which to base decisions, in particular, most trials of treatment (steroids versus IVIG or anti-D) have focused on the platelet count alone, and not the bleeding symptoms. The tendency to treat the low count arises from the assumption that a low count increases the risk of serious bleeding complications, in particular, intracranial haemorrhage. It is clear that clinical definitions are required in addition to laboratory parameters and a further useful clinical grading system has been published (Table 2).[22] This needs to be validated in larger studies. The Intercontinental ITP Study Group (ICIS) have an on-going international study of bleeding symptoms in children with acute ITP, which may help to inform future practice (for details see <www.unibas.ch/itpbasel/>)

Intracranial haemorrhage in children with ITP is very uncommon. Although many text books quote an incidence of 1–3%, it is much rarer than this. Careful examination of the literature and a recent survey in the UK led to an overall incidence of 0.1% in acute ITP, but the relative risk increases in those rare children who persist for more than 6 months (chronic ITP) with a very low count of less than $10 \times 10^9/l$, because there are fewer of them.[23,24] Unfortunately, at present, ICH cannot be predicted; it is not more common close to the time of diagnosis and is not predicted by whether or not the child has 'wet' purpura (*i.e.* mucosal bleeding). ICH can occur many months into the disorder, in children who have clinically mild disease, and without any warning. Some children have an underlying risk factor such as recent head injury or an arterio-venous malformation as a contributory factor. An important observation is that these children can do very well if this serious complication is recognised early and treated energetically. The two children with ICH reported to the second national audit were both more than 10 years of age, and both made almost a complete recovery. These considerations also emphasise the importance of education – it is important that children with ITP who sustain head injuries attend hospital promptly and are treated to raise the count in addition to whatever other measures are necessary. It is an interesting observation that, although the incidence of ICH in severe haemophilia in the early neonatal period is much higher (estimated at about 1–4%[25]), there has not been the same pressure to give these affected infants prophylaxis at birth or thereafter to avoid this complication which is much more common than ICH in ITP which seems to drive the need to treat children who are otherwise minimally symptomatic.

ACTIVE THERAPY

So when is treatment required? Fortunately, serious bleeding in ITP is not common. Although 20% may have nose bleeds in addition to cutaneous bleeding, these are usually not severe. More serious bleeding occurs in 4–5%. These figures are similar to those found in a survey in Germany.[26] The most

Table 2 Grading of haemorrhage in children with ITP[22]

OVERALL BLEEDING SEVERITY

0	None	Definitely no new haemorrhage of any kind
1	Minor	Few petechiae ($\leq$ 100 total) and/or $\leq$ 5 small bruises ($\leq$ 3 cm diameter); no mucosal bleeding
2	Mild	Many petechiae (> 100 total) and/or > 5 large bruises (> 3 cm diameter); no mucosal bleeding
3	Moderate	Overt mucosal bleeding (epistaxis, gum bleeding, oropharyngeal blood blisters, menorrhagia, gastrointestinal bleeding, *etc.*) that does not require immediate medical attention or intervention
4	Severe	Mucosal bleeding or suspected internal haemorrhage (in the brain, lung, muscle, joint, *etc.*) that requires immediate medical attention or intervention
5	Life-threatening or fatal	Documented intracranial haemorrhage or life-threatening or fatal haemorrhage in any site

GRADES OF EPISTAXIS

0	None	
1	Minor	Spotting on sheet or pillow and/or blood noted in nares, no active bleeding or need to apply pressure
2	Mild	Active bleeding on one or more occasions with need to apply pressure for less than 15 min
3	Moderate	Active bleeding on one or more occasions with need to apply pressure for at least 15 min
4	Severe	Repeated, continuous and/or profuse bleeding

GRADES OF ORAL BLEEDING

0	None	
1	Minor	Petechiae on palate or buccal mucosa
2	Mild	One or more buccal blood blisters (haemorrhagic bullae or infiltrates) with or without petechiae, no active bleeding
3	Moderate	Intermittent active bleeding from gums, lips, buccal mucosa or posterior oropharynx
4	Severe	Continuous bleeding from gums, lips, buccal mucosa, or posterior oropharynx

GRADES OF SKIN BLEEDING

0	None	No new cutaneous bleeding
1	Minor	Possibly a few new petechiae ($\leq$ 100 total)
2	Mild	Definitely a few new petechiae ($\leq$ 100 total) and/or $\leq$ 5 small bruises (< 3 cm diameter)
3	Moderate	Numerous new petechiae (> 100 total) and/or > 5 large bruises (> 3 cm diameter)
4	Severe	Extensive (hundreds of) petechiae and > 5 large bruises (> 3 cm diameter)

common serious bleeding in ITP is epistaxis. When torrential, this causes anaemia and may need red cell transfusion. Guidance is not generally available as to what constitutes a severe nose bleed, but those which persist over 30 min and are difficult to stop usually indicate severe bleeding. Less troublesome nose bleeds can sometimes be controlled with oral antifibrinolytic agents given for short courses (*e.g.* 5 days). Haematemesis and melaena are most likely to occur from epistaxis, rather than due to primary gastrointestinal haemorrhage. Other sites of serious bleeding are the genito-urinary tract (gross haematuria or menorrhagia) and the nervous system.

WHEN THERAPY IS NEEDED, WHAT SHOULD BE USED?

Clearly, treatment can produce a rise in the platelet count, but at a cost to the child. Unfortunately, there is no currently available treatment which is not associated with significant side-effects in some or all children. Children given high dose steroids (1–2 mg/kg) usually suffer behaviour disturbances and insomnia, which can be hard to manage. Recent evidence suggests a very high dose of prednisolone of 4 mg/kg for 4 days will raise the count rapidly and may be sufficient. The lower doses should not be given for more than 14 days. If steroids have been started for a low count alone, it is difficult to continue their withdrawal in the face of a falling platelet count. Current recommendations are to use steroids as first-line therapy, in high doses but for limited periods.[9] IVIG is usually effective in raising the count, often within 24–36 h, but has a significant morbidity (75% of children had side-effects in one trial[27]) – and most children would rather not have a drip. The platelet count will rise more rapidly than the lower doses of oral steroids considered above. A single dose of 0.8 g/kg is often adequate, but high doses may carry a greater risk of side-effects.[9] If this dose does not produce an adequate response, it may be repeated and/or increased (another regimen is 1 g/kg daily for 2 days). Other treatments are available but should be supervised by a haematologist, preferably with a particular interest in ITP. There has been particular interest in the use of anti-D given as a single infusion (to D-positive individuals only). The theory is that antibody-coated D-positive cells are removed by the spleen, sparing the platelets coated with antibody. This treatment can be given as a short infusion as an out-patient; data are available for adults but there is less information about action in childhood ITP. It has not been available in the UK until recently. It has the disadvantage of being a pooled blood product as is IVIG. Serious side-effects may occur; there is commonly a reduction in the haemoglobin level (in 80% children in one study[28]), and some patients develop severe haemolysis requiring transfusion; renal failure has also occurred in children treated with this agent.[29] It is currently regarded as second-line therapy in adult ITP.[9] More information is required before this can be recommended for children; an early trial suggested that it would not be an appropriate agent for first-line therapy.[30] Numerous other drugs have been tried, but the experience is anecdotal. Azathioprine is probably the least toxic long-term therapy, but may not produce a response for several weeks, so a trial of 2–3 months' therapy is required. The guidelines list the other available agents that have been tried with varying success in adult ITP. There are some very interesting preliminary studies with monoclonal antibody treatment against components of the immune system; rituximab, an antibody directed against CD20, a surface molecule on B lymphocytes, has proved a useful agent in some adults, with relatively few side-effects[31] but there is very little experience with this in children.

Table 3 Recommendations for 'safe' platelet counts in adults[9]

Dentistry	$\geq 10 \times 10^9/l$
Extractions	$\geq 30 \times 10^9/l$
Regional dental block	$\geq 30 \times 10^9/l$
Minor surgery	$\geq 50 \times 10^9/l$
Major surgery	$\geq 80 \times 10^9/l$

Menorrhagia can be managed with oral antifibrinolytic agents (tranexamic acid) taken for the first few days of the period, or with hormonal control. These measures are generally more effective and less toxic than using measures to raise the platelet count.

Splenectomy is rarely indicated in children with ITP. It should only be considered in the child with severe (*i.e.* significant on-going bleeding) and more than 6 months from diagnosis (*i.e.* chronic ITP). Splenectomy must be preceded by vaccination against *Pneumococcus* spp., *Haemophilus influenzae* type b and *Meningococcus* type c, and followed by penicillin prophylaxis.[32] Children with severe bleeding and chronic ITP should be referred to a paediatric haematologist with an interest in chronic ITP. These children are very rare indeed.[24]

Is a bone marrow examination necessary prior to treatment? The first national audit suggested that clinicians feel comfortable giving IVIG, but are more cautious in using steroids without marrow examination. Some argue that leukaemia never presents with thrombocytopaenia alone, but not all hospitals have the benefit of familiarity with paediatric films; a number of respondents to the audit had seen children – at least in the past – with acute leukaemia who had received steroids for 'ITP' before the correct diagnosis was made, this single agent treatment perhaps jeopardising their long-term survival. It may be difficult to arrange a general anaesthetic for the procedure. If a bone marrow examination is not done before starting steroids, it must be recognised that very occasionally the diagnosis will be incorrect, with aplastic anaemia the most likely to be missed. Life-threatening or serious bleeding is fortunately rare, but should be treated promptly with IVIG, steroids and platelet transfusions in larger than normal doses. Apart from this, platelet transfusions are not indicated in ITP, which is a consumptive platelet disorder. It was disappointing in both national audits to find platelets being transfused for clinically mild, acute ITP (sometime on the advice of haematologists).

WHEN IS TREATMENT NEEDED PRIOR TO SURGERY?

The platelets in children with ITP function better than normal, and a lower count is acceptable for a given procedure than in children with marrow suppression. There is no good evidence in the literature as to what constitutes a safe cut-off, but guidelines for adults are reproduced in Table 3.[9] Adoption of these should reduce unnecessary therapy, but these limits need to be tested.

MANAGEMENT OF CHRONIC ITP

About 10–20% of children will fail to remit over 6 months (chronic ITP). This is more likely in older children, especially adolescent girls. Underlying diseases may be present (*e.g.* SLE). Many of these children do not run into significant bleeding problems and require no regular therapy. Splenectomy should be reserved for those who have chronic ITP and who have significant bleeding problems – up to 30% may relapse after splenectomy. Such children with clinically severe and chronic ITP are very rare. Some evidence suggests that response to splenectomy may be predicted by indium labelling of platelets and scanning.[33] Those patients whose labelled platelets are taken up mainly by the spleen have a high probability of remission after splenectomy (96%) compared with those whose platelets are consumed in the liver or mixed liver and spleen. This technique is cumbersome and currently not easily available. Splenectomy must be preceded by appropriate vaccinations, especially against *Pneumococcus* spp., and followed by long-term antibiotic prophylaxis.[32,34] Long-term follow-up of children with chronic ITP has shown that remissions continue to occur over a prolonged period even 10 years after diagnosis (predicted spontaneous remission rate 61% after 15 years).[35] Many individuals who do not remit nevertheless run a chronic course with moderate rather than severe thrombocytopaenia (by platelet count) and no significant symptoms. Adolescent girls may be more likely to develop other autoimmune phenomena and can be screened for the development of antinuclear and other antibodies, particularly against phospholipids. While the finding of these in the absence of symptoms does not affect the management, it may warn that there is trouble ahead. A recent study showed that the persistent finding of antiphospholipid antibodies, particularly the lupus anticoagulant, in adults with ITP carried an increased risk of the development of thrombosis.[36] Viral infections in children can produce transient antiphospholipid antibodies; it is the persistence for more than 6 months, particularly in older children, who may be more worrying, but there are no comparative data in a childhood population with ITP.

Key points for clinical practice

- .Childhood ITP is an uncommon disorder so that general practitioners will not be familiar with its management.

- ITP is a clinical diagnosis and there are no defining tests. An open mind needs to be maintained in case the diagnosis is wrong.

- Most children with acute ITP will remit very quickly or at least have a rise in platelet count to more than $50 \times 10^9/l$ within 2 weeks.

- Most children with ITP do not have serious bleeding symptoms and remain in very good health. However low the platelet count, these children do not necessarily require any treatment to raise the platelet count.

- There should not be unnecessary restriction on the child's activities. This is likely to cause psychological distress.

- Currently available treatments to raise the platelet count do not alter the underlying pathology, and the toxicity of treatment is usually worse than the disease.

(continued next page)

Key points for clinical practice (continued)

- Children whose ITP continues beyond 6 months are arbitrarily labelled as 'chronic', but the probability of remission remains high.

- The commonest bleeding problems (other than in the skin) in children with ITP are epistaxis and menorrhagia in adolescent girls. Oral tranexamic acid is useful for both of these manifestations.

- Splenectomy is very rarely indicated for the treatment of childhood ITP and should only be considered in the child with serious bleeding problems preferably more than 3–6 months from diagnosis. Such children should be referred to a specialist paediatric haematologist.

References

1. Harrington WJ, Minnich V, Hollingsworth JW, Moore CV. Demonstration of a thrombocytopenic factor in the blood of patients with thrombocytopenic purpura. *J Lab Clin Med* 1951; **38**: 1–10.
2. Yanabu M, Suzuki M, Soga T *et al*. Influences of antiplatelet autoantibodies on platelet function in immune thrombocytopenic purpura. *Eur J Haematol* 1991; **46**: 101–106.
3. Nomura S, Yanabu M, Soga T *et al*. Analysis of idiopathic thrombocytopenic purpura patients with antiglycoprotein IIb/IIIa or Ib autoantibodies. *Acta Haematol* 1991; **86**: 25–30.
4. Parker R. Immune-mediated platelet and coagulation disorders. In: Rich RR. (ed) *Clinical Immunology Principles and Practice*, vol. 2. St Louis, MO: Mosby-Year Book, 1996; 1301–1315.
5. Chang M, Makagawa PA, Williams SA, Schwartz MR, Infield KL, Nugent DJ. Immune thrombocytopenic purpura (ITP) plasma and purified ITP monoclonal antibodies inhibit megakaryocytopoiesis *in vitro*. *Blood* 2003; **102**: 887–895.
6. Donner M, Holmberg L, Nilsson I. Type IIB von Willebrand's disease with probable autosomal recessive inheritance and presenting as thrombocytopenia in infancy. *Br J Haematol* 1987; **66**: 349–354.
7. Gasbarrini A, Franceschi F, Tartaglione R, Landolfi R, Pola P, Gasbarrini G. Regression of autoimmune thrombocytopenia after eradication of *Helicobacter pylori*. *Lancet* 1998; **352**: 878.
8. Emilia G, Longo G, Luppi M *et al*. *Helicobacter pylori* eradication can induce platelet recovery in idiopathic thrombocytopenic purpura. *Blood* 2001; **97**: 812–814.
9. British Committee for Standards in Haematology. Guidelines for the investigation and management of idiopathic thrombocytopenic purpura in adults, children and in pregnancy. *Br J Haematol* 2003; **120**: 574–596.
10. Saxon BR, Blanchette VS, Butchart S, Lim-Yin J, Poon AO. Reticulated platelet counts in the diagnosis of acute immune thrombocytopenic purpura. *J Pediatr Hematol Oncol* 1998; **20**: 44–48.
11. Porcelijn L, Folman CC, Bossers B *et al*. The diagnostic value of thrombopoietin level measurements in thrombocytopenia. *Thromb Haemost* 1998; **79**: 1101–1105.
12. Kosugi S, Kurata Y, Tomiyama Y *et al*. Circulating thrombopoietin level in chronic immune thrombocytopenic purpura. *Br J Haematol* 1996; **93**: 704–706.
13. Craze JL, Harrison G, Wheatley K, Hann IM, Chessells JM. Improved outcome of acute myeloid leukaemia in Down's syndrome. *Arch Dis Child* 1999; **81**: 32–37.
14. Smith OP. Inherited and congenital thrombocytopenia. In: Lilleyman JS, Hann IM, Blanchette V. (eds) *Pediatric Hematology*. London: Churchill Livingstone, 1999; 419–435.

15. Nurden AT, Nurden P. Inherited defects of platelet function. *Rev Clin Exp Hematol* 2001; **5**: 314–334.
16. Bolton-Maggs PH, Moon I. Assessment of UK practice for management of acute childhood idiopathic thrombocytopenic purpura against published guidelines. *Lancet* 1997; **350**: 620–623.
17. Sutor AH, Grohmann A, Kaufmehl K, Wundisch T. Problems with platelet counting in thrombocytopenia. A rapid manual method to measure low platelet counts. *Semin Thromb Hemost* 2001; **27**: 237–243.
18. Bolton-Maggs PH, Dickerhoff R, Vora AJ. The nontreatment of childhood ITP (or 'the art of medicine consists of amusing the patient until nature cures the disease'). *Semin Thromb Hemost* 2001; **27**: 269–275.
19. Eden OB, Lilleyman JS. Guidelines for management of idiopathic thrombocytopenic purpura. The British Paediatric Haematology Group. *Arch Dis Child* 1992; **67**: 1056–1058.
20. Bolton-Maggs PHB, Moon I. National audit of the Management of Childhood Idiopathic Thrombocytopenic Purpura against UK Guidelines: closing the loop – education and re-audit demonstrate a change in practice. *Blood* 2001; **98**: 58b.
21. George JN, Woolf SH, Raskob GE *et al*. Idiopathic thrombocytopenic purpura: a practice guideline developed by explicit methods for the American Society of Hematology . *Blood* 1996; **88**: 3–40.
22. Buchanan GR, Adix L. Grading of hemorrhage in children with idiopathic thrombocytopenic purpura. *J Pediatr* 2002; **141**: 683–688.
23. Lilleyman JS. Intracranial haemorrhage in idiopathic thrombocytopenic purpura. Paediatric Haematology Forum of the British Society for Haematology. *Arch Dis Child* 1994; **71**: 251–253.
24. Lilleyman JS. Management of childhood idiopathic thrombocytopenic purpura. *Br J Haematol* 1999; **105**: 871–875.
25. Kulkarni R, Lusher J. Perinatal management of newborns with haemophilia. *Br J Haematol* 2001; **112**: 264–274.
26. Sutor AH, Harms A, Kaufmehl K. Acute immune thrombocytopenia (ITP) in childhood: retrospective and prospective survey in Germany. *Semin Thromb Hemost* 2001; **27**: 253–267.
27. Blanchette VS, Luke B, Andrew M *et al*. A prospective, randomized trial of high-dose intravenous immune globulin G therapy, oral prednisone therapy, and no therapy in childhood acute immune thrombocytopenic purpura. *J Pediatr* 1993; **123**: 989–995.
28. Moser AM, Shalev H, Kapelushnik J. Anti-D exerts a very early response in childhood acute idiopathic thrombocytopenic purpura. *Pediatr Hematol Oncol* 2002; **19**: 407–411.
29. Kees-Folts D, Abt AB, Domen RE, Freiberg AS. Renal failure after anti-D globulin treatment of idiopathic thrombocytopenic purpura. *Pediatr Nephrol* 2002; **17**: 91–96.
30. Blanchette V, Imbach P, Andrew M *et al*. Randomised trial of intravenous immunoglobulin G, intravenous anti-D, and oral prednisone in childhood acute immune thrombocytopenic purpura [see comments]. *Lancet* 1994; **344**: 703–707.
31. Saleh MN, Gutheil J, Moore M *et al*. A pilot study of the anti-CD20 monoclonal antibody rituximab in patients with refractory immune thrombocytopenia. *Semin Oncol* 2000; **27**: 99–103.
32. British Committee for Standards in Haematology. Guidelines for the prevention and treatment of infection in patients with an absent or dysfunctional spleen: Working party of the BCSH Clinical Haematology Task Force. *BMJ* 1996; **312**: 430–434.
33. Najean Y, Rain JD, Billotey C. The site of destruction of autologous ^{111}In-labelled platelets and the efficiency of splenectomy in children and adults with idiopathic thrombocytopenic purpura: a study of 578 patients with 268 splenectomies. *Br J Haematol* 1997; **97**: 547–550.
34. Davies JM, Barnes R, Milligan D. Update of guidelines for the prevention and treatment of infection in patients with an absent or dysfunctional spleen. *Clin Med* 2002; **2**: 440–443.
35. Reid MM. Chronic idiopathic thrombocytopenic purpura: incidence, treatment, and outcome. *Arch Dis Child* 1995; **72**: 125–128.
36. Diz-Kucukkaya R, Hacihanefioglu A, Yenerel M *et al*. Antiphospholipid antibodies and antiphospholipid syndrome in patients presenting with immune thrombocytopenic purpura: a prospective cohort study. *Blood* 2001; **98**: 1760–1764.

Nicholas Shaw Melanie Kershaw

6

Vitamin D deficiency in children

Although the impact of severe vitamin D deficiency has been recognised for over a century and is preventable, it continues to be a significant problem in the early years of the 21st century. It is now recognised that vitamin D has important biological actions other than its role in mineral metabolism. The receptor for 1,25-dihydroxyvitamin D is widely distributed in the body and 1,25-dihydroxyvitamin D is a potent inhibitor of cellular proliferation and inducer of cell maturation. There are important epidemiological associations between the risk of dying of colon, breast, prostrate and ovarian cancer and living at higher latitudes. One study[1] has reported that circulating concentrations of 25-hydroxyvitamin D greater than 20 ng/ml are associated with a 200% reduction in risk of dying from colon cancer. It is argued that the production of 1,25-dihydroxyvitamin D locally in cells may be important for maintaining normal cell growth and possible prevention of carcinogenesis.

Vitamin D deficiency has also been implicated as a risk factor for diabetes, ischaemic heart disease[2] and tuberculosis[3] in Asian subjects. There is experimental evidence that vitamin D deficiency reduces insulin secretion and that vitamin D supplementation can improve glycaemic control and reduce blood pressure. There is also evidence in teenage girls that longitudinal change in bone density is impaired in those with low vitamin D status which if it impacts on peak bone mass will increase the risk of adult osteoporosis.[4] Vitamin D deficiency has been shown to impair immune function in animals

Nicholas Shaw
Consultant Paediatric Endocrinologist, Department of Endocrinology, Birmingham Children's Hospital. Birmingham B4 6NH, UK
Tel: +44 121 333 9999; Fax: +44 121 333 8191; E-mail: nick.shaw@bch.nhs.uk (for correspondence)

Melanie Kershaw
Specialist Registrar in Paediatrics, Department of Endocrinology, Birmingham Children's Hospital. Birmingham B4 6NH, UK

and there is a strong association in children between pneumonia and vitamin D deficiency rickets.[5] Thus, the potential importance of maintaining adequate vitamin D status extends far beyond the prevention of rickets and osteomalacia.

There has been considerable debate in recent years as to what is regarded as an acceptable level of 25-hydroxyvitamin D for health. It is widely accepted that concentrations less than 20–25 nmol/l (8–10 ng/ml) indicate severe vitamin D deficiency and are associated with rickets and osteomalacia and laboratories will often quote such levels as the lower limit of normal. More recent work has argued that a normal concentration of 25-hydroxyvitamin D is much higher. A study of the relationship between 25-hydroxyvitamin D and serum PTH concentrations in healthy adults showed that those with 25-hydroxyvitamin D levels greater than 50 nmol/l (20 ng/ml) had no significant change in serum PTH when oral vitamin D was given.[6] Other studies in the elderly have shown that 25-hydroxyvitamin D levels of 100 nmol/l (40 ng/ml) are required to minimise serum PTH. However, such levels in the elderly may relate to factors such as a decline in renal function, the impact of oestrogen deficiency on bone turnover, and renal tubular re-absorption of calcium. Recent work in healthy male French adolescents showed that a 25-hydroxyvitamin D level less than 83 nmol/l was associated with a rise in serum PTH.[7] Thus, it has been argued that levels of 50–80 nmol/l (20–32 ng/ml) should be regarded as those associated with vitamin D sufficiency. In a recent review article,[8] it was argued that there are probably two levels to define vitamin D deficiency: (i) below 50 nmol/l (20 ng/ml) which puts an individual at risk of developing secondary hyperparathyroidism and precipitating osteoporosis or causing rickets or osteomalacia; and (ii) a higher level of 75 nmol/l (30 ng/ml) which is required to maximise cellular health. Such levels would indicate that in a country of Northern latitude such as the UK, vitamin D insufficiency is endemic and would require vitamin D supplementation for most ethnic and age groups during the winter months.

EPIDEMIOLOGY

A survey undertaken of paediatricians in the West Midlands region in 2000/2001 identified 24 cases of symptomatic vitamin D deficiency in children under the age of 5 years in one year (incidence 6.8 per 100,000), 15 of whom were of South-East Asian ethnic origin and 6 Black African or Caribbean.[9] An opportunistic survey of children aged 6–36 months (77% of whom were of South-East Asian ethnic origin) attending a child health clinic in Manchester identified 3 children as having active rickets giving a prevalence of 1.6%.[10] At the same time, a resurgence of rickets has been documented in the US particularly in black breast-fed infants who were not receiving vitamin D supplements.[11]

In addition to symptomatic vitamin D deficiency, there is considerable evidence of sub-clinical vitamin D deficiency in a variety of populations. A survey of 25-hydroxyvitamin D levels in South-East Asian 2-year-old children in England identified 20–34% of the children as having levels less than 25 nmol/l (< 10 ng/ml).[12] In Cardiff, 54% of pregnant Asian women had evidence of vitamin D deficiency with levels less than 8 ng/ml.[13] A study of 25-hydroxyvitamin D levels in the resident non-pregnant adult population in the catchment area of one Birmingham hospital showed that, in winter, 85% of Asians, compared to 3.3% of non-Asians, had vitamin D levels less than

Table 1 Aetiological factors for vitamin D deficiency

Vitamin D synthesis	
	Latitude
	Atmospheric pollution
	Clothing
	Melanin pigmentation
	Sunlight exposure
Vitamin D intake	
	Breast feeding
	Maternal vitamin D deficiency
	Unusual diets
Vitamin D metabolism	
	Low calcium intake
	Intestinal calcium absorption
	? Genetic variation

8 ng/ml. Furthermore, during summer, 38% of the Asians still had vitamin D levels less than 10 ng/ml (unpublished). A study[14] of other family members of index cases who had presented with clinical manifestations of vitamin D deficiency identified a 67% prevalence of severe vitamin D deficiency with levels less than 5 ng/ml. Vitamin D insufficiency is not confined to ethnic minority populations. A survey of French adolescent boys aged 13–16 years demonstrated that 72% had 25-hydroxyvitamin D levels of less than 10 ng/ml during the winter months.[15]

AETIOLOGY

The aetiology of vitamin D deficiency rickets is usually due to one or more of the factors listed in Table 1 with different factors being more significant in different situations. It is now rare to see it occurring in Caucasian children in the absence of gastrointestinal or liver disease or extreme restriction of sunlight exposure. An example is a report of a white infant in Toronto with rickets which appeared to be entirely due to the use of a potent sunscreen.[16] The majority of reports world-wide occur in dark-skinned infants and children. It is well known that increased melanin pigmentation reduces cutaneous vitamin D synthesis,[17] but this factor alone is unlikely to explain the occurrence of rickets in such children, particularly in countries with plentiful sunlight. The absence of any significant cutaneous vitamin D synthesis during the winter months in countries with latitudes above and below 35° is a contributory factor with dark-skinned children being more susceptible. This will partly account for the resurgence of rickets being seen in South-East Asian children in the UK and Norway and black children in the US, particularly so in breast-fed infants who are not receiving oral vitamin D to supplement the minimal vitamin D content of breast milk (~12–60 IU/l). An additional factor in many of these populations will be maternal vitamin D deficiency which has been demonstrated in pregnant and breast-feeding women. Thus, the infants will be born with depleted vitamin D stores which are not subsequently replenished because of inadequate cutaneous vitamin D synthesis, the absence of vitamin D in breast milk and no oral vitamin D supplementation.

Less commonly, diets of abnormal composition for infants are responsible which include prolonged exclusive breast feeding, macrobiotic and vegan diets without any vitamin D supplements. Again, these are more often reported in dark-skinned infants in countries where cutaneous vitamin D synthesis is compromised for a significant part of the year.

As previously mentioned, there are many reports of rickets occurring in countries with plenty of sunlight throughout the year such as Saudi Arabia, India and Australia. Here, limited sunlight exposure may be due to cultural practices such as clothing and veiling in Muslim women and spending a lot of time indoors at home. Certainly, reports of rickets from Australia are almost exclusively from ethnic minority groups with such cultural practices. In addition, overcrowding may limit sunlight exposure in some countries. The effect of atmospheric pollution in countries undergoing rapid industrialisation may also limit vitamin D synthesis. A recent report from Delhi showed a clear difference in vitamin D status between children in rural areas and those living in the polluted urban areas of the city.[18]

The role of calcium intake influencing vitamin D metabolism has also attracted attention in the past decade. Animal studies have shown that a low calcium intake enhances the catabolism of 25-hydroxyvitamin D. This is due to the effect of increased 1,25-dihydroxyvitamin D synthesis as a consequence of increased parathyroid hormone secretion. The elevated 1,25-dihydroxyvitamin D then acts on the liver to enhance the metabolic destruction of 25-hydroxyvitamin D.[19] This effect is seen in humans in other situations where 1,25-dihydroxyvitamin D concentrations are raised such as in primary hyperparathyroidism and chronic gastrointestinal disease. Thus, the same populations who are more susceptible to the impact of vitamin D deficiency often have a diet that is low in calcium. Alternatively, intestinal calcium absorption may be impaired as was speculated to contribute to vitamin D deficiency in South-East Asians in the UK due to the phytate content of chapatti flour.

Finally, a potential contributory element may be genetic factors influencing vitamin D metabolism. One study has suggested that Asian subjects living in the US have enhanced catabolism of 25-hydroxyvitamin D due to increased 25-OHD,24-hydroxylase activity.[20] As yet, this work has not been confirmed by other studies.

CLINICAL PRESENTATION

The presenting features of symptomatic vitamin D deficiency vary depending on the age of the affected child. In the survey undertaken in the West Midlands region of children presenting under the age of 5 years, there were three different modes of presentation.[9] One group presented under the age of 6 months with symptomatic hypocalcaemia, usually convulsions; another group presented with signs of rickets particularly bowed legs from the age of 1 year; and the third group presented with delayed walking with evidence of hypotonia and a proximal myopathy beyond the age of 18 months. This latter group were all black children of African/Caribbean ethnic origin in whom breast feeding was prolonged. Cardiomyopathy or stridor as a consequence of hypocalcaemia are other recognised modes of presentation in infancy (Table 2).

Table 2 Clinical presentation of vitamin D deficiency

Convulsions
Stridor
Tetany
Cardiomyopathy
Bowed legs/knock knees
Delayed walking
Fracture
Co-incidental X-ray finding
Hypercalcaemia due to tertiary hyperparathyroidism

FEATURES IN INFANCY

Some infants may present in the neonatal period with hypocalcaemia and evidence of rickets due to severe maternal vitamin D deficiency which has been termed 'congenital rickets'. On occasions, rickets may be identified as a co-incidental finding on an X-ray taken in a child presenting with another illness. The occurrence of a fracture in the osteopenic bones of a child with rickets is another potential mode of presentation (Fig. 1).

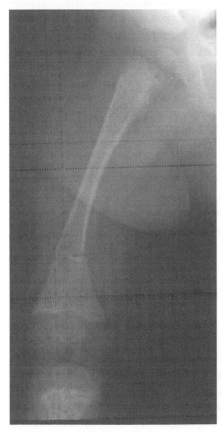

Fig. 1 Distal Femoral shaft fracture in a child with rickets.

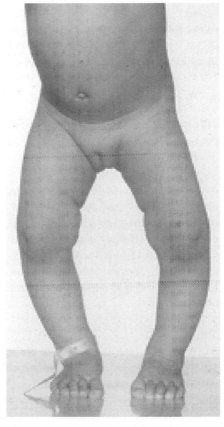

Fig. 2 Genu varum in toddler with rickets.

In the first year of life, the predominant clinical signs are palpable and visible enlargement of the extremities of the long bones, particularly wrists and ankles and costochondral junctions in the thorax ('rachitic rosary'). There may be a Harrison's sulcus due to the inward pull of the diaphragm on softened lower ribs. Examination of the skull will often show signs of poor mineralisation with softening of the occipital area ('craniotabes'), enlarged sutures, and delayed closure of the fontanelles. After the first year of life, the effects of weight bearing become evident in the legs resulting in genu varum (bow legs, Fig. 2) or genu valgum (knock knees). A large study of children in Nigeria aged 18 months or older who presented with leg deformity or inability to walk compared clinical features with radiographic evidence of rickets.[21] This identified wrist and costochondral enlargement as being the most predictive for active rickets.

TEETH

Development of the teeth is frequently impaired in vitamin D deficiency with delayed eruption and enamel hypoplasia. This is a useful distinguishing feature from hypophosphataemic rickets where early tooth development is normal. Evidence of an associated iron deficiency anaemia is often seen in infants. There is a recognised association between co-incidental illness particularly gastrointestinal and symptomatic hypocalcaemia in infants with vitamin D deficiency. There is also evidence of an increased risk of pneumonia in children with vitamin D deficiency.

ADOLESCENTS

The other age group where symptomatic vitamin D deficiency presents is during adolescence. In one study from Saudi Arabia, its prevalence is reported as 68 per 100,000 children aged 10–15 years.[22] Such individuals, who are often in early or mid puberty, usually present with hypocalcaemia either as convulsions or tetany. Other reported symptoms include diffuse limb pains and generalised weakness. There are often no clinical or radiological features of rickets in this age group. There is a striking female predominance when presenting at this age, and they are often consuming a diet low in calcium and vitamin D and have limited sunlight exposure. A rare presentation in this age group is with hypercalcaemia due to tertiary hyperparathyroidism secondary to prolonged parathyroid gland stimulation from severe vitamin D deficiency.

BIOCHEMICAL FEATURES

As a consequence of vitamin D deficiency, there is reduced intestinal calcium absorption, decreased extracellular calcium leading to defective mineralisation, and secondary hyperparathyroidism (Fig. 3). Biochemical findings are usually low or normal serum calcium and high serum parathyroid hormone levels leading to decreased tubular re-absorption of phosphate, aminoaciduria and low serum phosphate. There is evidence of increased bone turnover with high levels of alkaline phosphatase which are much higher than seen in hypophosphataemic

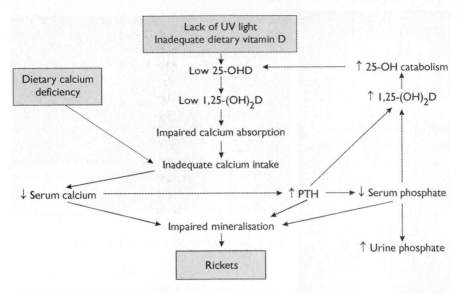

Fig. 3 Biochemical features of vitamin D deficiency.

rickets. Serum levels of 25-hydroxyvitamin D are usually low (< 8 ng/ml), but may be within the normal range if there has been recent exposure to vitamin D. 1,25-Dihydroxyvitamin D levels are usually within the normal or low-normal range, but have also been reported to be elevated though inappropriately low for the degree of hyperparathyroidism. Occasionally, elevated levels of serum phosphate can be seen in the face of secondary hyperparathyroidism giving a biochemical profile similar to that seen in pseudohypoparathyroidism. This entity which appears to occur more often in infants and adolescents who present with hypocalcaemia has also been termed 'partial hypoparathyroidism' and has been interpreted as a defective renal responsiveness to PTH.[23]

RADIOLOGICAL FEATURES

Radiological features predominantly appear at the growth plate and usually X-rays of the knee or wrist are the most useful for detecting early changes. The distal ulna is the best site to show early changes of rickets, particularly in young children, whereas in older children the knees are more useful. There is widening of the radiolucent space between the metaphyses and epiphyses as a consequence of the accumulation of uncalcified cartilage. With increasing severity of rickets the metaphyses show fraying and cupping or lateral spreading forming cortical spurs (Fig.4). The shafts of the long bones usually show reduced density with thin cortices and may show deformity, particularly bowing of the tibiae and femurs. On a chest X-ray, similar cupping at the costochondral junctions is seen corresponding to the palpable rachitic rosary. When rickets occurs during adolescence, typical changes may not be seen at the wrists and knees due to the narrowing and fusion of the epiphyseal growth plates. Here, radiographs of the pelvis may be useful as the centres of secondary ossification in the ischium and ilium may be abnormally wide. The appearance at the knees in an infant with rickets in conjunction with

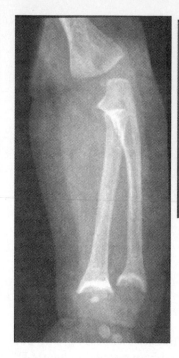

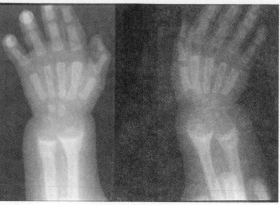

Fig. 4 (above) X-ray changes of florid vitamin D deficiency.

Fig. 5 (left) X-ray changes of healing rickets with band of provisional calcification.

disproportionate short stature has on occasion been thought to be that of a metaphyseal dysplasia. The first signs of healing rickets is the appearance of a zone of provisional calcification at the ends of the metaphyses which is usually seen within 3–4 weeks (Fig. 5).

TREATMENT

The most effective and physiological treatment for an infant with symptomatic hypocalcaemia, or rickets due to vitamin D deficiency, is either ergocalciferol (vitamin D_2) or cholecalciferol (vitamin D_3). This is the fastest means to replenish the depleted 25-hydroxyvitamin D levels, improve intestinal calcium absorption, and suppress the effect of secondary hyperparathyroidism. Alfacalcidol or calcitriol are not appropriate treatments; children treated with these preparations initially are often resistant to their effect. Currently, in the UK, preparations of ergocalciferol or cholecalciferol are not readily available and a liquid preparation suitable for infants is not listed in the British National Formulary (BNF). A calciferol solution containing 3000 U/ml is available from Martindale Pharmaceuticals (Bampton Road, Harold Hill, Romford, Essex RM3 8UG, UK). A dose of 3000 units daily for infants less than 6 months and 6000 units daily for those older than 6 months for 6 weeks to 4 months is usually adequate to replenish depleted vitamin D stores, correct biochemical abnormalities, and heal rickets. Normalisation of calcium and phosphate levels will occur within 3 weeks although alkaline phosphatase may remain elevated for several months. Measurement of serum PTH on treatment is also useful as it should normalise when the vitamin D deficiency has resolved. 1,25-Dihydroxyvitamin D concentrations rise rapidly with treatment and remain elevated for up to 10 weeks. Oral calcium supplements are also usually required initially if the child is hypocalcaemic and/or dietary intake is poor. One study from Nigeria in children with rickets and a low calcium intake indicated more rapid healing when calcium supplements were given alone or in combination with vitamin D than vitamin D alone.[24] Although they primarily had calcium deficiency as the cause of the rickets, one-third had additional evidence of vitamin D deficiency suggesting that calcium supplements should be routinely used in the treatment of vitamin D deficiency rickets. It is not necessary to continue treatment until any leg deformity resolves; this may take several years and orthopaedic correction is rarely required. For the occasional adolescent presenting with symptomatic hypocalcaemia, a tablet preparation containing 10,000 units of cholecalciferol is available and is the most appropriate for this age group. Following successful healing of rickets, it is important to continue vitamin D in a prophylactic dose of 400 IU/day. Spontaneous healing of rickets may occur during the summer months as a consequence of increased UV-light exposure. Where there are concerns about compliance, single large oral or intramuscular doses of 200,000–600,000 IU have been used without inducing vitamin D toxicity.[25]

PREVENTION

There are a number of means of preventing vitamin D deficiency in at-risk populations.

INCREASING SUNLIGHT EXPOSURE

A study in Cincinnati, Ohio (40° latitude) in 1983 looked at sunshine exposure in exclusively breast-fed infants and found that either 30 min/week sunshine exposure, solely wearing a nappy, or 2 h/week fully clothed, but without a hat, was sufficient to prevent vitamin D deficiency irrespective of the maternal vitamin D status.[26] Vitamin D levels in the infants correlated with sunlight exposure and maternal vitamin D levels.

In the UK (50–60° latitude), there is insufficient sunlight of the correct wavelength between mid-October and April such that winter vitamin D levels are dependent on stores accrued during the previous summer months. This leads to a seasonal variation in vitamin D levels in unsupplemented populations. It is estimated that to maintain adequate plasma levels of vitamin D above 8 mcg/l in the winter, summer levels of plasma vitamin D should be above 16 mcg/l.[27]

The duration and timing of sunlight exposure has an effect and different skin types influence local synthesis of vitamin D, as the amount of melanin in the skin has an inverse correlation with vitamin D synthesis. Young age, timing and duration of sunlight exposure relate to an increased risk of development of skin cancer, particularly malignant melanoma. Measures taken to increase sunlight exposure, therefore, may promote the increasing incidence of this disease. Measures to reduce the risks associated with sunlight exposure such as the use of high sun-protection factor lotions can adversely affect circulating concentrations of 25-hydroxyvitamin D.[28]

The wearing of the Hijab by Muslim women renders them more susceptible to vitamin D deficiency; however, this is a time-honoured and essential custom with specific benefits pertinent to their culture. The changing of cultural practices and encouragement of sunlight exposure has potentially harmful effects and does not make a suitable universal prevention policy for vitamin D deficiency.

FORTIFICATION OF FOOD PRODUCTS WITH VITAMIN D

Since the 1920s in the UK, margarine has been fortified with vitamin D, and cheap or free cod liver oil was provided and encouraged by child welfare services. In the 1930s, cows' milk was supplemented as required by law, along with a number of weaning foods. During the Second World War, a fortification programme was introduced with analogous benefit, relying on heavily subsidised national dried milk (not less than 280 IU/oz of milk powder). There was a significant reduction in the prevalence of rickets in the post-war period. However, during the 1950s, there was an epidemic of infantile hypercalcaemia with significant mortality and neurological deficit[29] which was attributed to over-consumption of vitamin D. Fortification was subsequently limited to a restricted number of foods only, the calciferol content of dried milk and infant cereals was reduced by half and the use of 400 IU vitamin D supplements was recommended.

Vitamin D dietary intake is currently primarily provided from margarines, cereals (some breakfast cereals are fortified) and oily fish, meats, eggs and milk products. Infant formulas are fortified with vitamin D; however, weaning foods currently are not. Unlike the US and France where cows' milk is routinely supplemented with vitamin D, without the development of hyper-calcaemia in infants who are likely to receive significantly more sunlight exposure than in the UK, there is no plan to introduce similar supplementation here. A previous suggestion of fortification of chapatti flour with vitamin D was rejected by the UK Committee for Medical Aspects of Food because of concern that older Asian men would be at risk of vitamin D intoxication due to the large quantities consumed. Such a strategy would also not prevent vitamin D deficiency in infants who do not consume chapattis.

VITAMIN D SUPPLEMENTATION

Vitamin D supplementation has been demonstrated to be a safe and effective way of preventing vitamin D deficiency in at-risk populations.

In the 1970s with the resurgence of rickets widely identified in the children of South Asian immigrants, the nation-wide public health initiative 'STOP RICKETS CAMPAIGN' with promotion of vitamin D supplements for pregnant and lactating women as well as weaning infants was successful in heralding a decline in the incidence in this population.

The Greater Glasgow Health Board Campaign local initiative initially comprised training of healthcare professionals and targeting the Asian population through community groups, schools, newspapers, leaflets and films produced by the health education unit. Vitamin D supplements were made available to Asian school children at the discretion of school medical officers.

Goel et al. in 1981[30] described pre- and post-campaign surveys reporting a reduced prevalence of rickets between 1974 and 1979 amongst 200 children of Indian or Pakistani parentage in local Glasgow schools and in prevalence of rickets amongst children admitted to hospital. In the post-campaign survey, unsupplemented children had 3 times the incidence of biochemical rickets and 4 times the incidence of radiological rickets than regular vitamin D takers. In 1979, 50% of children were taking regular vitamin D supplements as compared to none in 1974.

Between 1970 and 1980, surveys in Lancashire examining the Asian community for evidence of vitamin D deficient rickets demonstrated a striking improvement in biochemical markers in children, but not adults, as a direct result of supplementation.[31]

The recent increase in the prevalence of vitamin D deficiency forces us to re-examine our current guidelines for vitamin D supplementation. Essentially, the guidelines for vitamin D supplementation developed by the UK Committee for Medical Aspects of Food on behalf of the Department of Health have altered very little in the last 20 years.[32] The UK Committee for Medical Aspects of Food currently recommends:

- Vitamin D supplementation of all pregnant and lactating women (10 mcg (400 IU)/day)

- Supplementation of all infants except those receiving at least 500 ml infant formula (7–8.5 mcg (280–340 IU)/day)

- Breast-fed babies may delay supplements until 6 months of age if the mother was in good vitamin status during pregnancy

- Where there is any doubt about mother's vitamin status, supplementation of breast-fed infants should begin at 1 month

- Asian children should take supplements until 5 years of age.

Vitamin D supplementation in pregnancy and lactation

Maternal vitamin D stores are essential to the development of adequate stores in the fetus; and, as little vitamin D is available in breast milk (25 IU/l or less), the provision of vitamin D supplementation during pregnancy is important to prevent deficiency in the infant. A 400 IU daily dose of vitamin D should theoretically result in normal concentrations of 25-hydroxyvitamin D_3 and 1,25-dihydroxyvitamin D. However, a recent study from Denmark undertaken in veiled Moslem women indicates that, in the absence of sunlight exposure, a dietary intake of 600 IU vitamin D per day is insufficient to maintain adequate 25-hydroxyvitamin D levels and the authors suggested that 1000 IU/day would be more effective.[33] There are, however, problems in compliance with vitamin D supplementation particularly when intended to be taken daily. A recent health programme in Norway,[34] consisting of free samples of 10 mcg (400 IU) vitamin D daily combined with information, failed to reduce vitamin D deficiency to acceptably low levels in Pakistani mothers. An alternative is to give 25 mcg (1000 IU) daily during the third trimester, which has been shown to produce normal 25-hydroxyvitamin D levels in mothers and infants at term.[35] Another proposal is a single high dose of vitamin D of 100,000–200,000 IU given during months 6–7 of pregnancy, which appears sufficient to cover both maternal and fetal needs.[36]

Studies in Finland have indicated that vitamin D supplementation of 25 mcg (1000 IU)/day in breast feeding Caucasian mothers is insufficient to protect the infant from deficiency during winter months.[37] This indicates the importance of ensuring breast-fed infants should be supplemented as well. There is no evidence to suggest that infants would come to harm if supplemented in addition to their mothers. Breast milk contains less vitamin D than formula milk and even supplementing overweight fully formula-fed infants on 150 ml/kg/day with 7 mcg (280 IU)/day of vitamin D is unlikely to lead to intakes greater than 23 mcg (920 IU)/ day.

Vitamin D supplementation of infants

As regards infants, it is clear that national recommendations about vitamin D supplements are not being followed. This is not helped by the fact that the UK Committee for Medical Aspects of Food guidelines only advocate early introduction of vitamin D supplements if there is 'doubt about the mother's vitamin status'. It is also apparent that relying on vitamin D fortification of formula feeds is inadequate to overcome the impact of maternal vitamin D deficiency as even these infants are presenting with hypocalcaemic symptoms in the early months after birth. It is important, therefore, to ensure that fetal stores are optimised by supplementation of at-risk mothers.

It would be an easier policy to implement if all infants were given 400 IU vitamin D daily whether breast or formula fed. Alternatively, if poor daily compliance is a problem, an annual dose (4 mg, 150,000 IU) at the beginning of autumn, appears to provide protection against vitamin D deficiency without vitamin D overload.[38]

Vitamin D supplementation of older children

It is commonly assumed that older children will receive an adequate vitamin D intake as a consequence of diet and sunlight exposure. However, the American Academy of Pediatrics has recently issued new guidelines[39] advocating an intake of 200 IU daily for children of all ages. Recent work from Finland on peripubertal girls indicates that 400 IU daily during the winter months was insufficient to normalise 25-hydroxyvitamin D levels and an intake of 800 IU was required to achieve this.[40] There is currently no UK policy for this age group; in view of the regular presentation of clinical symptoms in South Asian adolescents, particularly girls, this needs to be considered.

IMPLEMENTING VITAMIN D SUPPLEMENTATION

As the UK Committee for Medical Aspects of Food guidelines have been in existence for 20 years, one could question why we are witnessing a resurgence of symptomatic vitamin D deficiency. A recent survey of healthcare professionals caring for women and children at primary and secondary care tiers in the West Midlands demonstrated that, although two-thirds of professionals felt vitamin D deficiency to still be a cause for concern, only a very small minority were routinely supplementing at-risk groups. The majority of professionals were not familiar with the UK Committee for Medical Aspects of Food recommendations (unpublished data). Another key factor has been the change in the delivery of child health surveillance in the past decade which has moved from child health clinics to GP surgeries. Previously, mothers attending child health clinics would be able to obtain vitamin ADC drops for their infants in addition to exchanging milk tokens for infant formula. However, vitamin ADC drops remain only available through health clinics whereas infant formula is now supplied from pharmacies. Lack of supplies of the vitamin drops has also been a problem in some areas.

The most suitable preparation of vitamin D for pregnant mothers remains to be clarified, particularly as there is a perception that the Department of Health ADC vitamin drops are contra-indicated due to a potential teratogenic effect of vitamin A even though the quantity of vitamin A in the drops (200 mcg) is low and equivalent to that provided by two glasses of full cream milk.

It remains unacceptable that a readily preventable condition still contributes to significant morbidity and we look to the Scientific Advisory Committee on Nutrition (SACN), as the recent successors of the UK Committee for Medical Aspects of Food to clarify the recommendations as well as local public health departments and primary care trusts to drive local initiatives forward.

Key points for clinical practice

- Health professionals need to be aware that vitamin D deficiency rickets will always be a risk in the UK unless vitamin D supplementation is provided.

- There is insufficient sunlight for adequate cutaneous vitamin D synthesis for nearly half the year in the UK,

- Asymptomatic vitamin D deficiency is very common in Asian children and adults.

- The mode of presentation with vitamin D deficiency varies with age.

- Adolescents are more likely to present with hypocalcaemia and muscle weakness than rickets.

- Maternal vitamin D deficiency is a key factor in the presentation with hypocalcaemia in infancy.

- Low dietary calcium intake may also aggravate the impact of vitamin D deficiency.

- Abnormal infant diets (*e.g.* prolonged, exclusive breast feeding or vegan diets) are a risk factor.

- A low plasma phosphate is a consequence of secondary hyperparathyroidism and does not indicate the need for phosphate supplements.

- The biochemical picture may resemble pseudohypoparathyroidism.

- The most appropriate treatment is with calciferol rather than alfacalcidol or calcitriol.

- Vitamin D deficiency is preventable if Department of Health guidelines are followed.

- Paediatricians should ensure that all breast-fed infants receive vitamin D supplements.

- New arrangements for the provision of cheap, easily accessible vitamin D supplements are required.

References

1. Garland CF, Comstock GW, Garland FC, Helsing KJ, Shaw EK, Gorham, ED. Serum 25-hydroxyvitamin D and colon cancer: eight year prospective study. *Lancet* 1989; **18**: 1176–1178.
2. Boucher BJ. Inadequate vitamin D status: does it contribute to the disorders comprising syndrome 'X'? *Br J Nutr* 1998; **79**: 315–327.
3. Wilkinson RJ, Llewelyn M, Toossi Z *et al*. Influence of vitamin D deficiency and vitamin D receptor polymorphisms on tuberculosis among Gujarti Asians in West London: a case control study. *Lancet* 2000; **355**: 618–621.
4. Lehtonen-Veromaa MK, Mottonen TT, Nuotio IO, Irjala KM, Leino AE, Viikari JS. Vitamin D and attainment of peak bone mass among peripubertal Finnish girls: a 3–y prospective study. *Am J Clin Nutr* 2002; **76**: 1446–1453.
5. Muhe L, Lulseged S, Mason KE, Simoes EA. Case-control study of the role of nutritional rickets in the risk of developing pneumonia in Ethiopian children. *Lancet* 1997; **349**: 1801–1804.
6. Malabana A, Veronikis IE, Holick MF, Redefining vitamin D insufficiency. *Lancet* 1998; **351**: 805–806.
7. Guillemant J, Taupin P, Le HT *et al*. Vitamin D status during puberty in French healthy male adolescents. *Osteoporos Int* 1999; **351**: 805–806.
8. Holick MF. Vitamin D: the underappreciated D-lightful hormone that is important for skeletal and cellular health. *Curr Opin Endocrinol Diabetes* 2002; **8**: 87–98.
9. Callaghan A, Booth IW, Moy RGD, Shaw NJ, Debelle G. Rickets return. *Arch Dis Child* 2002; **86 (Suppl 1)**: A35.
10. Ashraf S, Mughal MZ. The prevalence of rickets among non-Caucasian children. *Arch Dis Child* 2002; **87**: 263–264.
11. Krieter SR, Schwartz RP, Kirkham Jr HN, Charlton PA, Calikoglu AS, Davenport ML. Nutritional rickets in African American breast-fed infants. *J Pediatr* 2000; **137**: 153–157.
12. Lawson M, Thomas M. Vitamin D concentrations in Asian children aged 2 years living in England: population survey. *BMJ* 1999; **318**: 28.
13. Alfaham M, Woodhead S, Pask G, Davies G. Vitamin D deficiency: a concern in pregnant Asian women. *Br J Nutr* 1995; **73**: 881–887.
14. Iqbal SJ, Featherstone S, Kaddam IM, Mortimer J, Manning D. Family screening is effective in picking up undiagnosed Asian vitamin D deficient subjects. *J Hum Nutr Dietetics* 2001; **14**: 371–376.
15. Guillemant J, Le HT, Maria A, Allemandou A, Peres G, Guillemant S. Wintertime vitamin D deficiency in male adolescents: effect on parathyroid function and response to vitamin D3 supplements. *Osteoporos Int* 2001; **12**: 875–879.
16. Zlotkin S. Limited vitamin D intake and use of sunscreens may lead to rickets. *BMJ* 1999; **318**: 1417.
17. Clemens TL, Adams JS, Henderson SL, Holick MF. Increased skin pigment reduces the capacity of skin to synthesise vitamin D_3. *Lancet* 1982; **I**: 74–76.
18. Agarwal KS, Mugal MZ, Upadhyay P, Berry JL, Mawer Eb, Puliyel JM. The impact of atmospheric pollution on vitamin D status of infants and toddlers in Delhi, India. *Arch Dis Child* 2002; **87**: 111–113.
19. Clements MR, Johnson L, Fraser DR. A new mechanism for induced vitamin D deficiency in calcium deprivation. *Nature* 1987; **324**: 62–65.
20. Awumey EMK, Mitra DA, Hollis BW, Kumar R, Bell NH. Vitamin D metabolism is altered in Asian Indians in the Southern United States: a clinical research centre study. *J Clin Endocrinol Metab* 1998; **83**: 169–173.
21. Thacher TD, Fischer PR, Pettifor JM. The usefulness of clinical features to identify active rickets. *Ann Trop Paediatr* 2002; **22**: 229–237.
22. Narchi H, Jamil ME, Kulaylat N. Symptomatic rickets in adolescence. *Arch Dis Child* 2001; **84**: 501–503.
23. Rao S, Parfitt AM, Kleerekoper M, Pumo BS, Frame B. Disassociation between the effects of endogenous parathyroid hormone on adenosine 3′,5′-monophosphate generation and phosphate reabsorption in hypocalcaemia due to vitamin D depletion: an acquired disorder resembling pseudohypoparathyroidism type II. *J Clin Endocrinol Metab* 1985; **61**: 285–290.

24. Thacher TD, Fischer PR, Pettifor JM *et al.* A comparison of calcium, vitamin D, or both for nutritional rickets in Nigerian children. *N Engl J Med* 1999; **341**: 563–568.
25. Shah BR, Finberg L. Single day therapy for vitamin D deficiency rickets: a preferred method. *J Pediatr* 1994; **125**: 487–490.
26. Specker BL, Valanis B, Hertzberg V, Edwards N, Tsang RC. Sunshine exposure and serum 25-hydroxyvitamin D concentrations in exclusively breast fed infants. *J Pediatr* 1985; **107**: 372–376.
27. Lawson DE, Paul AA, Black AE, Cole TJ, Mandal AR, Davie M. Relative concentrations of diet and sunlight to vitamin D state in the elderly. *BMJ* 1979; **2**: 303–305.
28. Matsuoka LY, Wortsman J, Hanifan N, Holick MF. Chronic sunscreen use decreases circulating concentrations of 25-hydroxyl-vitamin D. A preliminary study. *Arch Dermatol* 1988: **124**: 1802–1804.
29. Wharton BA, Darke SJ. Infantile hypercalcaemia. In: Jelliffe EFP, Jelliffe DB. (eds) *Adverse Effects of Foods*. New York: Plenum, 1982; 397–404.
30. Goel KM, Sweet EM, Campbell S, Attenburrow A, Logan RW, Arneil GC. Reduced prevalence of rickets in Asian children in Glasgow. *Lancet* 1981; **2**: 405–407.
31. Stephens WP. Observations on the natural history of vitamin D deficiency amongst Asian immigrants. *Q J Med* 1982: **51**: 171–188.
32. Department of Health. *Weaning and the Weaning Diet*, Report on Health and Social Subjects 45. London: HMSO, 1994.
33. Glerup H, Mikkelsen K, Poulsen L *et al.* Commonly recommended daily intake of vitamin D is not sufficient if sunlight exposure is limited. *J Intern Med* 2000; **247**: 260–268.
34. Brunvand L, Henriksen C, Haug E. Vitamin D deficiency among pregnant women from Pakistan. How best to prevent it? *Tidsskr Nor Laegeforen* 1996: **116**: 1585–1587.
35. Brooke OG, Brown IR, Bone CD *et al.* Vitamin D supplements in pregnant Asian women: effects on calcium status and fetal growth. *BMJ* 1980; **280**: 751–754.
36. Hellouin de Menibus C, Mallet E, Henocq A, Lemeur H, L'Hostis C. Neonatal hypocalcaemia. Results of vitamin D supplement in the mother. Study on 13,377 newborn infants. *Bull Acad Natl Med* 1990; **174**: 1051–1059.
37. Ala Houhala M. 25-Hydroxyvitamin D levels during breastfeeding with or without maternal or infantile supplementation of vitamin D. *J Pediatr Gastroenterol Nutr* 1985; **4**: 22–26.
38. Oliveri B, Cassinelli H, Mautalen C, Ayala M. Vitamin D prophylaxis in children with a single dose of 150,000 IU of vitamin D. *Eur J Clin Nutr* 1996; **50**: 807–810.
39. Gartner LM, Greer FR. Prevention of rickets and vitamin D deficiency: new guidelines for vitamin D intake. *Pediatrics* 2003; **111**: 908–910.
40. Lehtonen-Veromaa M, Mottonen T, Nuotio I, Irjala K, Viikari J. The effect of conventional vitamin D(2) supplementation on serum 25(OH)D concentration is weak among peripubertal Finnish girls: a 3–y prospective study. *Eur J Clin Nutr* 2002; **56**: 431–437.

Joseph G. Mallon Howard I. Maibach

7

Head lice: diagnosis, treatment, and clinical resistance

Head lice typically affect school-aged children (5–11 years old); however, any age group can be affected. Diagnosis is via identifying a living, moving louse or by finding many eggs within 6.5 mm of the scalp. Diagnostic difficulties include determining viable from non-viable eggs, and the task of identifying active from extinct infestations, and dealing with a degree of parental anxiety when the possibility of head lice is mentioned. Current treatment guidelines suggest permethrin, malathion, carbaryl, and benzyl benzoate as viable treatment options depending on local resistance patterns. The safety and efficacy of several other pediculicides have not been determined. Treatment resistance and treatment failure have been reported with continuing frequency. The need for on-going research and development of new and existing treatments for *Pediculitis capitis* and refining our biological knowledge is apparent.

HEAD LICE

Head lice commonly affect primary school children (5–11 years old) but the incidence varies throughout the year and the parasite can be found in all age groups.[1] The hysteria caused by *P. capitis*, or head lice can lead to a disproportionate response that may cause harm to the patient. It is estimated that US children lost 12–24 million days of school in 1998 because of 'no-nit' policies, which exclude children who have any nits (egg cases) on inspection.[2] It is necessary to establish clear diagnostic criteria, analyze treatment results versus resistance, and to identify those individuals who should be treated.

Joseph G. Mallon MD
Department of Dermatology, University of California, San Francisco, CA 94143-0989, USA
E-mail: jgemallon@yahoo.com

Prof. Howard I. Maibach MD
Department of Dermatology, University of California, San Francisco, CA 94143-0989, USA
Tel: +1 415 476 2468; Fax: +1 415 753 5304; E-mail: himjlm@itsa.ucsf.edu (for correspondence)

Table 1 Diagnostic keys

- Finding many eggs within a quarter inch (6.5 mm) of the scalp[2]
- Finding a living moving louse – time consuming but definitive

DIAGNOSIS

Diagnostic criteria are outlined in Table 1. The presence of eggs alone is not sufficient for diagnosis as eggs may retain a viable appearance for weeks after death. As most infestations have existed for weeks rather than days before they are discovered, contacts over the previous month should be traced. It is possible to contract lice by relatively prolonged head-to-head contact with an infected person, which typically means that the louse is passed between people who know each other well.[3] The difficult areas regarding diagnosis are outlined in Table 2.

TREATMENT RESULTS

Several medications are effective in the treatment of head lice; however, there is no single drug that is universally accepted as the gold standard. Location, drug-resistance patterns, and concurrent drug therapy can all alter the effectiveness of head lice treatment. Several randomized clinical trials have analyzed the effectiveness and safety profile of individual treatment modalities as shown in Table 3. The reader is referred to the Cochrane website for additional details.[5]

Table 2 Difficulty in diagnosis

- Examination under conditions of high anxiety
- Significant time requirement
- Presence of hair casts, which are not lice[4]
- Presence of non-viable eggs (nits)
- Task of identifying active from inactive infestations

Table 3 Head lice treatments

Name	Safety profile	Effectiveness
Malathion	Intermediate	Good
Pyrethroids (permethrin)	Good	Intermediate
Carbaryl	Good	Good
Gamma benzene hexachloride	Poor (with misuse)	Poor
Ivermectin	Little data on this condition	?
Cromamiton	Good	?
Benzyl benzoate	Excellent	Good
Wet combing	Good	Poor – requires extensive care-giver effort

Data summarized from Downs[1] and Roberts.[2]

Table 4 Pediculicidal efficacy

Authors	Drug/Tx	Result (% louse free 7 days after treatment)	Comments
Mathias et al.[6]	Malathion (0.5%) in isopropanal (Prioderm) Lindane (1%)	93% (n = 27/29) 88% (n = 29/33)	Prospective randomized trial of children. Eligibility required children to have the presence of live lice or no fewer than 20 nits or both within 1.3 cm in diameter on the scalp prior to treatment. The limited power of the study could have missed a large difference in efficacy
Taplin et al.[7]	Permethrin (1%) Lindane (1%) Placebo	100% (n = 29/29) 67% (n = 20/30) 9% (n = 3/34)	Placebo-controlled, double-blinded, randomized study. Eligibility required children to have the presence of live adult lice and nymphs, and the presence of at least 20 viable nits prior to treatment. No prior treatments were used in the week prior to or during the therapy. The higher than expected treatment failure with lindane may have been due to lindane resistance
Roberts et al.[8]	Malathion (5%) Bug-Busting	78% (n = 31/40) 38% (n = 12/32)	Randomized controlled trial. Eligibility required children to have the presence of live (moving) lice, no treatment with insecticide lotion in the previous 2 weeks, and no broken skin on the scalp. Malathion was twice as effective as manual removal of lice (P = 0.0006).

Malathion and Pymethrin are both effective in the treatment of head lice, although there are many viable alternatives.[2] If infestation recurs within one month after treatment, a different topical insecticide can be used. Although malathion is effective, its strong smell deters many patients.

Pyrethroids such as permethrin are the mainstay of treatment in many countries.[2] Sufficient treatment should be applied to wet the entire scalp, though it need not be applied to the ends of long hair below the level of the shirt collar. Hair should be washed with regular shampoo to remove the insecticide at the end of the recommended application period. If permethrin or pyrethrins are used, two applications performed one week apart are recommended.[2] Results of pediculicidal efficacy are shown in Table 4.

TREATMENT RESISTANCE

The emergence of resistant strains of *P. capitis* to commonly used insecticides has long been suggested. Proposed criteria for resistance are shown in Table 5.

Table 5 Proposed criteria for clinical resistance

Stronger evidence	
	Live lice on scalp
	Healthcare worker dosing
	Separation of individual from other individuals with lice
Softer evidence	
	In vitro observation

Due to alleged resistance, especially of eggs, two applications performed 7 days apart has been recommended for permethrin but not for malathion. More than three applications of the same product within 2 weeks is not recommended.[1] By thoroughly coating the scalp it is unlikely that the medication will evaporate quickly. A large residual load is left on the scalp to enhance its pediculicidal activity. By the time insecticide resistance is clinically evident, the resistance gene pool may be too large to remove. Resting the insecticide and assuming that the rogue phenotype will naturally die out is at best speculative.[1] Reports of resistance to lindane and DDT have led to the development of malathion, permethrin, and carbaryl. Carbaryl in the UK is a prescription only medication. Its limited use may be a reason why we have not seen much resistance develop to this medication.[9] Resistance needs to be identified early with *in vitro* tests, biochemical assays or molecular biology. The clinical correlation between *in vitro* observation and clinical end-point is far from complete.

An English study concluded that multiresistant lice were found showing *in vitro* resistance to permethrin as high as 87%, with concurrent resistance to malathion of 64%. Resistance to DDT was 100% and only carbaryl was found to allow survival of fewer than 5% of tested lice *in vitro*.[10] A proposed mechanism of resistance suggests that if the binding site of the drug is altered than no pyrethroid or DDT can bind irrespective of the concentration of drug given. This family of chemicals could become obsolete. It is a common pyrethroid resistance mechanism adopted by many other insect species and termed *kdr* gene resistance.[1] An altered acetylcholinesterase molecule that only weakly binds to malathion or carbaryl may explain the super-resistance to malathion that cannot be overcome by higher doses of malathion and the increase in carbaryl tolerance seen within *in vitro* studies carried out in some regions of the UK.[1] Head lice resistant to lindane have not been biochemically assessed. In other insect species, enhanced detoxification by glutathione-S-transferase is commonly seen.[1] Glutathione-S-transferase is thought partially responsible for resistance to organophosphates such as malathion, but does not appear to play a role in pyrethroid resistance; monooxygenase-based resistance and *kdr* appear to be responsible for pyrethroid resistance.[11]

TREATMENT FAILURE

Treatment failure can be attributed to causes other than resistance. Many of these causes are listed in Table 6. Compliance can be readily dealt with by healthcare worker dosing, albeit infrequently performed.

Table 6 Causes of treatment failure

- Poor compliance or improper use of an insecticide
- Lack of nit removal
- New exposure to lice
- Use of an out-of-date preparation
- Using an insufficient amount of the pediculicide
- Shortened treatment period
- Application of antilice product to wet hair
- Re-infestation

Results of well-controlled trials (including healthcare worker dosing) cannot be extrapolated to standard patient usage; however, the data have the potential for clarifying the relationship of *in vitro* and *in vivo* resistance.

WHO TO TREAT?

The issue of who should be treated, for how long, and with what agents remains debatable. For children 2 years of age and younger or if parents prefer not to use an insecticide, wet combing is an alternative; albeit less effective method.[2] In the UK, malathion is a more popular treatment option, while in the US permethrin is likely to be first-line treatment. Most experts agree that effective treatment can be achieved if the pediculicide is applied carefully and in sufficient quantity on two occasions, 1 week apart. A nit comb should be used during that interval, and the patient should be checked for surviving lice and nymphs between treatments and for the following week.[10] Because no pediculicide is 100% ovicidal, grooming and nit removal in the period between treatments are essential.[10] Applying a conditioner, a crème rinse, a detangler, or a light oil can facilitate combing the hair.[10] All family members and close contacts over the preceding months should be examined for evidence of infestation. Screening with a nit comb is more effective than when done by hand. It is often difficult to detect an early infestation because these patients are usually asymptomatic, and lice and nits are hard to find with a standard comb. The majority of infestations go undetected for several weeks. When in doubt, it is better to treat all close contacts that may be carriers than to treat the same child repeatedly.[10] However, careful, albeit time-consuming, examinations will decrease the number of individuals requiring treatment.

Other methods to treat head lice infestation include petroleum jelly, olive oil, or mayonnaise to the scalp and covering the scalp overnight with a shower cap. This method reportedly kills lice through asphyxiation, immobilization, and/or inability to feed. Head shaving is also used; however, this treatment is effective for male children but is not socially acceptable for the female population in which the majority of head lice infestation occurs.[12]

Malathion appears to be a safe alternative to pyrethrins and permethrins for topical application. Lindane is no longer package-labelled as a first-line therapy by the US Food and Drug Administration (FDA) because of the inability to control misuse – with resulting toxicity.

The safety and efficacy of ivermectin is not well established; it is not package-labelled by the FDA for treating head lice; however, a single oral dose of ivermectin 200 mmmg/kg has been reported to be effective for treatment of head lice. Current recommendations suggest that ivermectin should not be used in children weighing less than 15 kg.[11]

Opinion is sharply divided on the need for disinfecting personal and household items.[13]. The US Centers for Disease Control (CDC) recommends that anything touched by the patient in the previous 2 days should be hot-washed, dry-cleaned, sealed in plastic for 2 weeks, or vacuumed, whereas authorities in the UK advise against environmental cleaning. Use of insecticide sprays to disinfect furnishings is not recommended.[2]

Head lice infestation in schools is a common occurrence and an area of heightened anxiety among school administrators, teachers, and parents.[14] Current recommendations suggest that a child can return to school immediately after completion of the first application of a normally effective insecticide or the first wet combing session, regardless of the presence of nits.[2] Exclusion of children from school because of head lice results in anxiety, fear, social stigma, overtreatment, loss of education, and economic loss if parents miss work.[2] Non-infested children may be excluded from school because of presumed pediculosis more frequently than are infested children.[15] Clear treatment guidelines drawn up by healthcare professionals with an interest in head lice and taking into account regional/national resistance patterns should be implemented.[1] Society will benefit significantly when this common clinical entity is scrutinized with care of the Mellenby studies in World War II on scabies biology.[16]

Key points for clinical practice

- Confront the social stigma and hysteria regarding head lice.
- Establish clear protocol for head lice treatment.
- Management should not harm the patient.
- Products with more than one insecticide will take longer to produce resistance.
- The best insecticide will depend on local resistance patterns (see text for details on criteria for documenting clinical resistance).
- Apply physical treatments such as wet combing and nit removal, after dosing with insecticidal agents.
- Do not resort to potentially dangerous remedies such as kerosene or pet shampoos.
- If you continue to be infested with live lice after treatment, discontinue the pesticide and try another agent or different class of medication.
- Avoid spending too much time 'cleansing' the environment; head lice need human blood to survive.
- In cases of treatment failure, consult with a physician experienced in head lice treatment.
- Consider healthcare worker dosing when compliance is an issue (see text for details).

References

1. Downs AMR. Managing head lice in an era of increasing resistance to insecticides. *Am J Clin Dermatol* 2004; In press.
2. Roberts RJ. Head lice. *N Engl J Med* 2002; **346**: 1645–1650.
3. Dodd C. Treatment of head lice (Editorial). *BMJ* 2001; **323**: 1084.
4. Webster GF, Kligman AM. A method for the assay of inflammatory mediators in follicular casts. *J Invest Dermatol* 1979; **73**: 266–268.
5. Dodd CS. Interventions for treating head lice (Cochrane review). In: *The Cochrane Library*, 3. Oxford, England: Update Software, 2001.
6. Mathias RG, Huggins DR, Leroux SJ, Proctor EM. Comparative trial of treatment with Prioderm lotion and Kwellada shampoo in children with head lice. *Can Med Assoc J* 1984; **130**: 407–409.
7. Taplin D, Meinking BA, Castillero PM, Sanches R. Permethrin 1% crème rinse for the treatment of *Pediculus humanus* var *capitis* infestation. *Pediatr Dermatol* 1986; **3**: 344–348.
8. Roberts RJ, Casey D, Morgan DA, Petrovic M. Comparison of wet combing with malathion for treatment of head lice in the UK: a pragmatic randomized controlled trial. *Lancet* 2000; **356**: 540–544.
9. Downs AMR, Stafford KA, Harvey I, Coles GC. Evidence for double resistance to permethrin and malathion in head lice. *Br J Dermatol* 1999; **141**: 508–511.
10. Witkowski JA, Parish LC. Pediculosis and resistance: the perennial problem. *Clin Dermatol* 2002; **20**: 87–92.
11. Bartels CL, Peterson KE, Taylor KL. Head lice resistance: itching that just won't stop. *Ann Pharmacother* 2001; **35**: 109–112.
12. Hipolito RB, Mallorca FG, Zoraya O, Zuniga-Macaraig, Apolinario PC, Sherman JW. Head lice infestation: single drug versus combination therapy with one percent permethrin and trimethoprim/sulfamethoxazole. *Pediatrics* 2001; **107**: e30.
13. Orkin M, Maibach HI. Current concepts in parasitology. This scabies pandemic. *N Engl J Med* 1978; **298**: 496–498.
14. Orkin M, Maibach HI. *Cutaneous Infestation and Insect Bites*. New York: Marcel Dekker, 1985.
15. Pollack RJ, Kiszewski AE, Spielman A. Overdiagnosis and consequent mismanagement of head louse infestations in North America. *Pediatr Infect Dis J* 2000; **19**: 689–693.
16. Mellanby K. *Scabies*, 2nd edn. Hampton, UK: E.W. Classey, 1972.

Jennifer E. Weiss Norman T. Ilowite

8

Juvenile idiopathic arthritis

Juvenile idiopathic arthritis (JIA) is an umbrella term referring to a group of disorders characterised by chronic arthritis. JIA is the most common chronic rheumatic illness in children and is a significant cause of short- and long-term disability. It is a clinical diagnosis made in a child less than 16 years of age with arthritis (defined as swelling or limitation of motion of the joint accompanied by heat, pain or tenderness) for at least 6 weeks duration with other identifiable causes of arthritis excluded. The incidence of JIA is fairly similar world-wide and ranges form 5–18 per 100,000 with a prevalence of 30–150 per 100,000.

Three separate systems are currently used to classify patients under 16 years of age with chronic arthritis. They are the American College of Rheumatology (ACR), the European League Against Rheumatism and the International League Against Rheumatism (ILAR) classification systems. The ILAR classification system includes 7 sub-types: systemic onset, oligoarticular, polyarticular RF positive and RF negative, enthesitis-related arthritis, psoriatic arthritis and other (Table 1). This classification system was developed to identify clinically homogenous JIA subtypes in order to facilitate communication regarding epidemiology, therapeutics, and outcomes among physicians globally.[1]

AETIOLOGY AND PATHOPHYSIOLOGY

Although the aetiology of JIA remains unclear, it appears that JIA is a complex genetic trait involving the effects of multiple genes related to immunity and

Jennifer E. Weiss MD
Fellow, Pediatric Rheumatology, Schneider Children's Hospital, 269-01 76th Ave, New Hyde Park, NY 11040, USA. E-mail: jluftig@nshs.edu

Norman T. Ilowite MD
Professor of Pediatrics, Albert Einstein College of Medicine and Chief, Pediatric Rheumatology, Schneider Children's Hospltal, 269-01 76th Ave, New Hyde Park, NY 11040, USA
Tel: +1 718 470 3530; Fax: +1 718 831 0182 (for correspondence)

Table 1 The International League Against Rheumatism (ILAR) criteria for juvenile idiopathic arthritis

Systemic arthritis: arthritis with or preceded by daily fever of at least 2 weeks' duration, documented to be quotidian for at least 3 days and accompanied by one or more of the following:
- A. Evanescent, non-fixed, erythematous rash
- B. Generalised lymph node enlargement
- C. Hepatomegaly or splenomegaly
- D. Serositis

Oligoarthritis: arthritis affecting 1–4 joints during the first 6 months of disease
- A. **Persistent oligoarthritis**: arthritis affecting not more than 4 joints at any time during the course of the disease
- B. **Extended oligoarthritis**: arthritis affecting a cumulative total of 5 joints or more after the first 6 months of disease
- C. Exclusions
  1. Psoriasis in a first or second degree relative diagnosed by a dermatologist
  2. Family history of HLA-B27-associated disease
  3. Positive RF test
  4. HLA-B27 positivity with onset of arthritis over 8 years of age
  5. Presence of systemic arthritis as defined above

Polyarthritis-rheumatoid factor (RF) negative: arthritis affecting 5 or more joints during the first 6 months of disease
- A. Exclusions:
  1. Presence of a RF
  2. Presence of systemic arthritis as defined above

Polyarthritis-rheumatoid factor (RF) positive: arthritis affecting 5 or more joints during the first 6 months of disease, associated with a positive rheumatoid factor on at least 2 occasions, at least 3 months apart
- A. Exclusions
  1. Absence of a positive RF on 2 occasions at least 3 months apart
  2. Presence of systemic arthritis as defined above

Enthesitis-related arthritis: arthritis and enthesitis, or arthritis and at least 2 of the following:
- A. Sacroiliac joint tenderness and/or inflammatory spinal pain
- B. Presence of HLA-B27
- C. Family history in first or second degree relative consistent with HLA-B27 associated disease medically confirmed
- D. Anterior uveitis that is usually associated with pain, redness or photophobia
- E. Male older than 8 years at onset of enthesitis or arthritis
- F. Exclusions
  1. Psoriasis in at least first or second degree relative diagnosed by a dermatologist
  2. Presence of systemic arthritis as defined above

Psoriatic arthritis: arthritis and psoriasis or, arthritis and:
- A. A family history of medically confirmed psoriasis in parents or siblings
- B. Dactylitis
- C. Nail abnormalities (pitting or onycholysis)
- D. Exclusions
  1. Positive RF test
  2. Presence of systemic arthritis as defined above

'Other': children with arthritis persisting for at least 6 months but who either:
- A. Do not fit into any category, or
- B. Fit into more than 1 of the categories
- C. Exclusion: patients who meet criteria for other categories

Adapted from Petty et al.[1]

inflammation. Arthritis may be triggered in a genetically predisposed individual by psychological stress, abnormal hormone levels, trauma to a joint, or infection, either bacterial or viral. Several studies have implicated both rubella and parvovirus B19 as possible aetiologies of JIA as rubella virus persists in lymphocytes and establishes a focus of persistent infection in the synovium resulting in chronic inflammation.[2] Highly conserved bacterial heat-shock proteins may be potential disease triggers.[3] Results of studies are inconclusive as to whether or not breast-feeding decreases the risk of developing JIA.

Certain human leukocyte antigens (HLA) class I and class II alleles are associated with an increased risk of JIA. The class II antigens HLA-DRB1*08, HLA-DRB1*11, DQA1*04, DQA1*05, and DQB1*04 are associated with persistent oligoarticular and extended oligoarticular JIA. HLA-DRB1*08 confers an increased risk of rheumatoid factor (RF) negative polyarthritis and HLA-DRB1*11 confers an increased risk of SOJIA. HLAB1*04, which is associated with adult rheumatoid arthritis (RA), is associated with an increased risk of RF-positive polyarticular arthritis. The class I antigen, HLA-B27, and class II antigens HLA-DRB1*01 and DQA1*0101 are associated with enthesitis-related arthritis and juvenile psoriatic arthritis.[4] Other genes conferring risk include cytokine production regulating genes.

There is evidence of immunodysregulation in JIA. Complement activation and consumption promote inflammation, and increasing serum levels of circulating immune complexes (IC) are found with active disease. Anti-nuclear-antibodies (ANA) are found in about 70% of patients with JIA, especially young females with pauciarticular disease. Rheumatoid factor (RF) is positive in up to 20% of patients with JIA.

The T-lymphocyte-mediated immune response is involved in chronic inflammation and T cells are the predominant mononuclear cells in synovial fluid.[5] Patients with JIA have elevated serum levels of IL-1, IL-2, IL-6 and IL-2 receptor (R) and elevated synovial fluid levels of IL-1β, IL-6, and IL-2R, suggesting a Th1 profile.[6] Elevated serum levels of IL-6, IL-2R, and soluble tumour necrosis factor (TNF)-receptor (R), correlate with inflammatory parameters, such as C-reactive protein, in JIA patients with active disease. Serum levels of IL-6 are increased in systemic onset JIA and rise prior to each fever spike, correlating with active disease and elevation of acute phase reactants.[7]

CLASSIFICATION

The disease subtypes, in order of frequency, include oligoarticular JIA (50–60%), polyarticular JIA (30–35%), systemic onset JIA (10–20%), juvenile psoriatic arthritis (2–15%), and enthesitis-related arthritis (1–7%), and are recognised based on their clinical features during the first 6 months of disease. Patients in the 'other' category (11–23%) have arthritis that persists for at least 6 weeks, but either does not fulfil criteria for any other sub-type or fulfils criteria for more than 1 sub-type.[8] Important clinical features necessary for accurate classification are the presence of enthesitis (inflammation at the sites of attachment of ligament, tendon or fascia to bone), fever, rash and serositis.

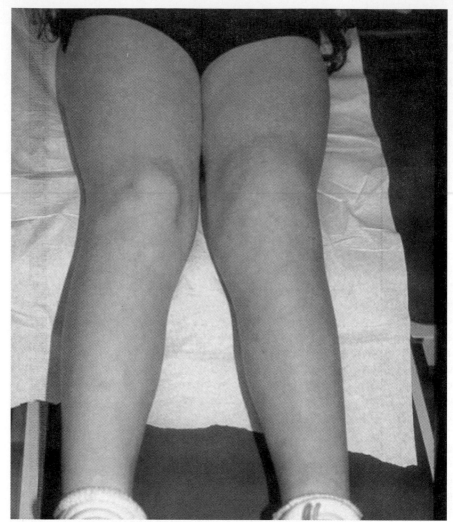

Fig. 1 Swollen left knee in a patient with oligoarticular JIA. Note quadriceps atrophy.

OLIGOARTICULAR JUVENILE IDIOPATHIC ARTHRITIS

Oligoarticular JIA is diagnosed in patients with arthritis in fewer than 5 joints during the first 6 months of disease. These patients tend to have involvement of the large joints of the lower extremities such as knees and ankles. Monoarticular onset affecting just the knee (Fig. 1) is common in half of all children.[8] These patients tend to function remarkably well and often do not complain of pain. They are at high risk for developing uveitis, usually their most serious clinical problem.

A child who develops active arthritis of 5 or more joints after the first 6 months of disease is considered to have extended oligoarticular JIA. Up to 50% of oligoarticular patients may develop extended disease; 30% will do so in the first 2 years after diagnosis. Risk factors for extended disease include ankle and/or wrist arthritis, hand disease, symmetric arthritis, arthritis of 2–4 joints, and an elevated ESR and ANA titre.[9] Extended disease confers a worse prognosis. One retrospective study evaluated JIA patients into adulthood with a median of 16.5 years of follow-up and found an overall remission rate of 12% in extended oligoarticular JIA patients compared to 75% in persistent oligoarticular JIA patients.[10]

POLYARTICULAR JUVENILE IDIOPATHIC ARTHRITIS

Patients with arthritis in 5 or more joints at presentation are diagnosed with polyarticular JIA. This sub-type includes children with RF-negative disease (20–30% of JIA patients) and RF-positive disease (5–10% of JIA patients).[2] Both types affect girls more frequently than boys.

Seronegative (RF⁻) patients often develop polyarthritis in early childhood in contrast to seropositive (RF⁺) patients who develop arthritis during mid-childhood and adolescence. The RF⁻ patients have a variable prognosis. This is a subtype with no strong HLA association, and may represent a group of disorders that can be further dissected.

The RF⁺ patients are primarily adolescent females with symmetric small joint involvement, and severe erosive disease. They may develop sub-cutaneous nodules (non-tender, firm lesions over pressure points and tendon sheaths). These patients share the same HLA associations as adult RF⁺ patients, and probably represent the early expression of adult RA. The arthritis usually involves the large and small joints of the hands (Fig. 2) and feet although the axial skeleton, including cervical spine and temporomandibular joints, may be affected. The second and third metacarpophalangeal joints and the interphalangeal joint of the thumb are frequently involved.[11] Boutonnière (proximal interphalangeal joint flexion and distal interphalangeal joint hyperextension) and swan-neck deformities (proximal interphalangeal joint

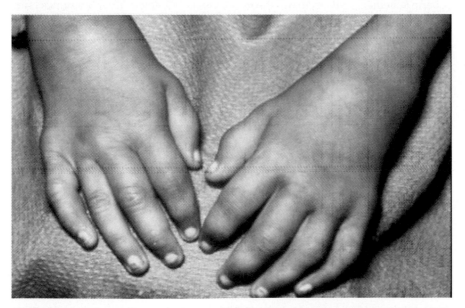

Fig. 2 Polyarthritis of the proximal interphalangeal and distal pharyngeal joints in a polyarticular JIA patient.

hyperextension and distal interphalangeal joint flexion) are common. Chronic uveitis develops less frequently than in oligoarticular disease.

SYSTEMIC ONSET JUVENILE IDIOPATHIC ARTHRITIS

Systemic onset JIA is the only subtype of JIA without a strong age, gender or HLA association. At onset, extra-articular manifestations including rash, fever, lymphadenopathy, hepatosplenomegaly and serositis predominate. Of patients, 10% may present with extra-articular manifestations only and may not develop arthritis for many months. In the right clinical setting, with characteristic fever and classic rash, the diagnosis of probable systemic onset disease may be made, with confirmation of the diagnosis when persistent arthritis develops.[11]

Children with systemic onset JIA typically have 2 weeks of high spiking fever, classically with two peaks daily (double quotidian). When febrile, chills are common and the child is ill-appearing; however, when the fever breaks, the child appears well.[12]

The classic rash is evanescent and consists of discrete, circumscribed, salmon-pink macules 2–10 mm in size that may be surrounded by a ring of pallor or may develop central clearing (Fig. 3). Lesions are more common on the trunk and proximal extremities, including the axilla and inguinal areas. Stress or a warm bath may exacerbate the rash. A linear streak on the skin, known as the Koebner phenomenon, may be elicited by scratching the skin. The rash is rarely pruritic and is never purpuric.[12]

The arthritis associated with systemic onset JIA is polyarticular in distribution and usually manifests within 6 months of systemic features. Both large and small joints are affected.[11]

Laboratory findings in a patient with active systemic onset JIA include severe anaemia, leukocytosis, thrombocytosis, elevated liver enzymes and elevated acute phase reactants. The ANA is rarely positive.[11]

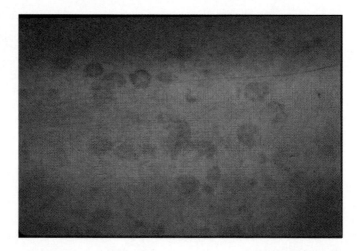

Fig. 3 Salmon-coloured, macular rash of SOJIA. Note perilesional pallor and central pallor of larger lesions.

Systemic onset JIA patients have a variable course with 60–85% of patients going into remission or quiescence and up to 37% developing a chronic, destructive polyarthritis. Systemic features usually resolve within 6 months and the mean period of disease activity is about 6 years.[13] Predictors of a poor prognosis include age less than 6 years at diagnosis, disease duration of greater than 5 years, cardiac disease, elevated immunoglobulin (Ig) A levels and the need for treatment with corticosteroids 6 months into the disease course.[14] Radiographic changes consistent with disease progression are associated with a poor prognosis but not necessarily poor functional status.[13] Patients with severe systemic onset JIA have an increased incidence of amyloidosis (1.4–9%).[10,13] The mortality rate of patients with JIA is less than 0.3% in North America with most deaths in systemic onset JIA patients secondary to macrophage activation syndrome (discussed below), infection due to immuno-suppression, or cardiac complications.[8]

Macrophage activation syndrome is a rare but life-threatening complication of systemic onset JIA characterised by increased activation and demonstration of histiophagocytosis in bone marrow. Triggers include a preceding viral illness and the addition of, or change in, medications, especially non-steroidal anti-inflam-matory medications (NSAIDs), sulfasalazine, and, more recently, etanercept.[15] Patients are acutely ill with hepatosplenomegaly, lymphadenopathy, purpura and mucosal bleeding and may develop multi-organ failure. Pancytopenia, prolongation of the prothrombin time and partial thromboplastin time, elevated fibrin split products and hypertriglyceridaemia are common. The sedimentation rate is often low (a clue to the diagnosis of macrophage-activation syndrome and not exacerbation of systemic onset JIA) due to hypofibrinogenaemia secondary to consumptive coagulopathy and hepatic dysfunction.[16,17] Treatment includes pulse methylprednisolone (30 mg/kg with a maximum of 1 g), which some patients fail to respond to, and cyclosporine A (2–5 mg/kg/day).[16]

ENTHESITIS-RELATED ARTHRITIS

Enthesitis-related arthritis has a prevalence of 12–33 per 100,000,[18] and is most common in males greater than 8 years of age. It has a strong genetic predisposition as evidenced by a positive family history and the presence of HLA-B27 in affected patients. The hallmarks of the disease are pain, stiffness and loss of mobility of the back. Enthesitis is characterised by inflammation at the insertion point of tendon, ligament or fascia to bone. Enthesitis-related arthritis should be suspected in any child with chronic arthritis of the axial and peripheral skeletons, enthesitis and RF or ANA seronegativity. Peripheral arthritis, usually a few joints of the lower extremity, precedes axial involvement and arthritis of the sacroiliac joints may take years to develop. Radiographic changes of the sacroiliac joint include joint space narrowing, erosions, sclerosis, osteoporosis of the pelvis and fusion (late finding).[19]

Extra-articular manifestations include anterior uveitis, aortic insufficiency, aortitis, muscle weakness and low-grade fever. Uveitis may develop in up to 27% of patients and is often unilateral and recurrent. It presents as a red, painful, photophobic eye, often without sequelae.[18] Laboratory data may show mild anaemia, a normal to moderately elevated white blood cell count and a thrombocytosis and elevated sedimentation rate.[18,19]

PSORIATIC ARTHRITIS

Juvenile psoriatic arthritis is chronic inflammatory arthritis with a peak age of onset in mid-childhood. Juvenile psoriatic arthritis is a difficult diagnosis to make as the arthritis may develop many years prior to the rash. Juvenile psoriatic arthritis is an asymmetric arthritis that often affects the knees and ankles and the small joints of the hands and feet. Proximal and distal inter-phalangeal joints along with the tendon sheath are often inflamed resulting in diffuse swelling of the digit, the so-called 'sausage digit'.[20]

Extra-articular manifestations include rash, nail changes uveitis and amyloidosis. One-third of psoriasis patients will develop the rash by 15 years of age.[21] All children with juvenile psoriatic arthritis should have a slit-lamp examination every 6 months, as asymptomatic anterior uveitis is common.

Laboratory data show elevated acute phase reactants, anaemia of chronic disease, and thrombocytosis. A positive ANA may be found, but RFs are usually absent.

EXTRA-ARTICULAR MANIFESTATIONS

UVEITIS

Chronic, anterior, non-granulomatous uveitis (iridocyclitis) develops in up to 21% of patients with oligoarticular JIA and 10% of patients with polyarticular JIA.[8] Uveitis is most common in young girls with oligoarticular disease and a positive ANA. The uveitis is usually asymptomatic although patients may present with conjunctivitis, unequal pupils, eye pain and headache. The uveitis may be present at diagnosis, develop during the course of, or be an initial manifestation of, the JIA. Patients with JIA should be screened routinely (Table 2) in order to prevent delay in diagnosis of uveitis. Patients diagnosed prior to the age of 7 years are considered at low risk 7 years after the onset of JIA, and patients diagnosed at or after 7 years of age are considered low risk 4 years after the onset of JIA and should have yearly ophthalmologic examinations. All high risk patients are at medium risk 4 years after the onset of JIA. Complications of uveitis include posterior synechiae, cataracts, band keratopathy, glaucoma and visual impairment (up to 30%; Fig. 4).[8,22]

Table 2 Frequency of ophthalmological examinations in patients with JIA

	Sub-type at onset	Age at onset	
		< 7 years	≥ 7 years
Oligoarticular	+ANA	H	M
	–ANA	M	M
Polyarticular	+ANA	H	M
	–ANA	M	M
Systemic		L	L

From Yancey et al.[22]
H = High risk. Indicates ophthalmologic examination every 3-4 months.
M = Medium risk. Indicates ophthalmologic examination every 6 months.
L = Low risk. Indicates ophthalmologic examination every 12 months.

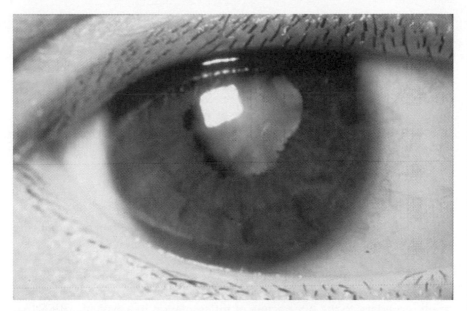

Fig. 4 Posterior synechiae and cataract formation in a JIA patient with iritis.

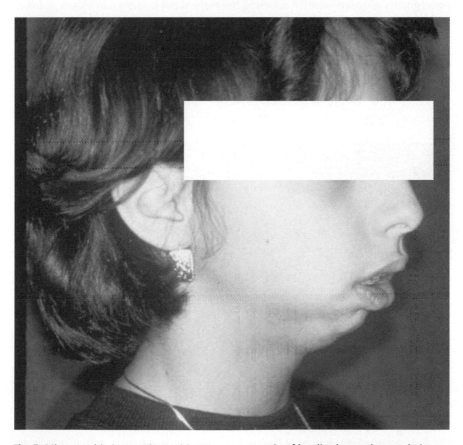

Fig. 5 Micrognathia in a patient with JIA as an example of localised growth retardation.

Treatment of uveitis includes topical steroids and mydriatics to decrease inflammation and prevent posterior synechiae. Glucocorticoid ophthalmic drops may need to be given as often as hourly while the child is awake. Oral corticosteroids at a dose of 2–4 mg/kg/day may be needed in patients failing topical therapy and, in some instances, pulse intravenous methylprednisolone (30 mg/kg) has been used with benefit. Methotrexate, cyclosporine A or a steroid injection under the capsule of the globe may benefit patients unresponsive to glucocorticoid ophthalmic drops. Preliminary case reports have shown infliximab and etanercept to be beneficial in treating refractory uveitis in children and adults.[23,24]

GROWTH DISTURBANCE

Generalised growth retardation and delayed puberty are common in patients with JIA secondary to active disease and treatments such as oral corticosteroids. Localised growth disturbance can result from destruction of a growth centre, as in micrognathia (Fig. 5) or premature closure of the physis, as in brachydactyly of the digits. Overgrowth of an affected extremity may result secondary to the hyperaemia of inflammation in a patient with active arthritis.[25] An example of accelerated maturation of the right carpal bones in a patient with oligoarticular JIA affecting the right wrist is shown in Figure 6. Intra-articular steroid injections are helpful as they control local inflammation thereby reducing the incidence of limb overgrowth and leg length discrepancy.[26]

OSTEOPENIA/OSTEOPOROSIS

Children with JIA are at increased risk for osteopenia and osteoporosis as a consequence of the disease and its treatment (namely corticosteroids) putting

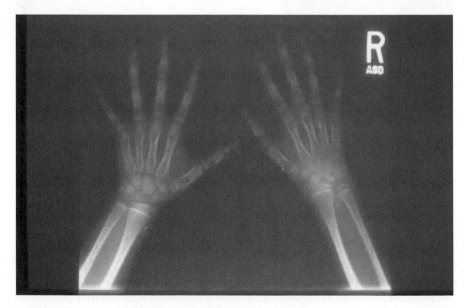

Fig. 6 Accelerated maturation of the right carpal bones in a patient with oligoarticular JIA secondary to active right wrist arthritis.

them at increased risk of fracture. Osteoporosis is defined as the parallel loss of bone mineral and matrix resulting in a bone mineral density more than 2.5 standard deviations (SD) below the mean for age and sex. Osteopenia is a low bone mass for age with a bone mineral density between 1–2.5 SD below the mean for age and sex. Low bone mineral density in children with JIA has been associated with severe disease, younger age, lower body mass index, lower lean body mass, and decreased physical activity. There is also an increased risk in patients with active JIA during their pubertal growth spurt as they may fail to achieve the normal increase in bone mass.[27,28]

The best way to prevent these complications is to control disease activity, encourage appropriate caloric and calcium intake and promote physical activity. Any patient started on oral corticosteroids should be started on 12–1500 mg of calcium and 400 units of vitamin D supplementation.[27,28] In patients that develop osteoporosis on this regimen, the use of bisphosphonates should be considered although there are concerns regarding the safety of these agents in children.

DIFFERENTIAL DIAGNOSIS

The diagnosis of JIA is a clinical one made after exclusion of other identifiable causes of arthritis by a careful history and examination in conjunction with appropriate radiographs and laboratory tests. Important clinical signs such as systemic illness, preceding infection, duration of fever, rash and character of the arthritis will help differentiate JIA from other causes of arthritis. The differential diagnosis of acute arthritis includes entities in the broad categories of reactive arthritis, inflammatory disease, infection, systemic disease, malignancy and trauma (Table 3).

It may be difficult to differentiate systemic onset JIA and polyarticular JIA from other causes of systemic disease with polyarthritis such as acute rheumatic fever, the arthropathy of inflammatory bowel disease (IBD), and other vasculitic and systemic rheumatic diseases. Acute rheumatic fever classically causes migratory arthritis unlike the additive arthritis in JIA. The fever of systemic onset JIA is more spiking in character and longer in duration. JIA patients never have overlying erythema, while this is quite common in acute rheumatic fever. Endocardial disease strongly suggests acute rheumatic fever, but pericarditis can occur in both.

The arthropathy of IBD may present a diagnostic dilemma, as the arthritis may be the first manifestation of the disease. Clues to the diagnosis include gastrointestinal symptoms, weight loss or growth failure, and mucocutaneous abnormalities such as erythema nodosum, aphthous stomatitis, and pyoderma gangrenosum.[21] As a rule, the arthritis should improve when the gastro-intestinal disease is quiescent.

Sarcoidosis is a chronic non-caseating granulomatous disease, uncommon in children, manifesting as fever, arthritis, uveitis, rash and pulmonary disease. The arthritis is characterised by substantial synovial hypertrophy and associated synovial cysts, especially in the ankles and wrists and the uveitis, either anterior or posterior, is granulomatous and nodular with coarse keratic precipitate formation. The fixed macular eruption is unlike the evanescent rash of systemic onset JIA.[29]

119

Table 3 Differential diagnosis of arthritis

Reactive	Post-enteric Reiter's syndrome Rheumatic fever Post-streptococcal
Inflammatory	Juvenile idiopathic arthritis Inflammatory bowel disease Sarcoidosis
Infection	Septic Osteomyelitis Lyme disease Viral Bacterial sacroileitis Discitis
Systemic	Kawasaki disease Behçet's disease Henoch-Schönlein purpura Serum sickness Systemic lupus erythematosus Dermatomyositis Progressive systemic sclerosis

Malignancy	Leukaemia
	Neuroblastoma
	Malignant bone tumours
	  Osteosarcoma
	  Ewing's sarcoma
	  Rhabdosarcoma
	Benign bone tumours
	  Osteoid osteoma

Trauma	Accidental Non-accidental
Miscellaneous	Cystic fibrosis Haemophilia Mucopolysaccharidoses Sphingolipidoses

Patients with other multisystem rheumatic diseases can be distinguished from JIA based on their diagnostic clinical features and supporting laboratory data. Systemic lupus erythematosus (SLE) commonly presents in adolescence with fever and a painful, non-erosive polyarthritis affecting large and small joints.[30] Although the ANA can be positive in SLE, polyarticular and oligoarticular JIA, and both SLE and systemic onset JIA can manifest as polyserositis; malar erythema, nephritis, autoimmune pancytopenia, hypocomplementaemia, presence of anti-double-stranded DNA and other autoantibodies, are unique to SLE. Patients with progressive systemic sclerosis and dermatomyositis may have a mild, symmetric polyarthritis early on, but the diagnosis is easier as symptoms progress. Patients with progressive systemic sclerosis may have limited range of motion secondary to sclerotic changes of the skin that should be distinguished from inflammatory arthritis.

There are numerous causes of oligoarthritis that need to be excluded prior to the diagnosis of oligoarticular JIA. The distinction in most cases can be made based on the history of an antecedent infection and arthritis less than 6 weeks in duration. Septic arthritis needs to be excluded in any patient with acute onset of fever, severe joint pain and an erythematous, hot swollen joint with elevated acute phase reactants. Synovial fluid should be examined and cultured and antibiotics started immediately as septic arthritis can rapidly lead to joint destruction. Bacterial sacroiliitis and discitis are more indolent in nature.

Reactive arthritis is an acute, sterile, inflammatory arthritis that develops when antibodies made against an infectious agent cross-react with the synovial tissue. Postenteric reactive arthritis should be considered in any child with gastroenteritis and arthritis of the large joints of the lower extremity. Reiter's syndrome is a presentation of reactive arthritis that presents with the triad of arthritis, conjunctivitis and urethritis. There is a strong association of HLA-B27 with reactive arthritis and Reiter's syndrome.[21] Patients with sustained fever, arthritis and a preceding streptococcal infection that do not fulfil the Jones' criteria of acute rheumatic fever may be diagnosed with post-streptococcal reactive arthritis.

Lyme disease, caused by *Borrelia burgdorferi*, is a major health problem in endemic areas. Arthritis is a late manifestation of the disease but may be the presenting complaint as the tick bite and initial rash may go unnoticed. The arthritis is episodic with each episode being relatively short-lived. The diagnosis should be confirmed with Lyme serology (ELISA and immunoblot). There are numerous viruses that cause arthritis including parvovirus B19, hepatitis B virus, rubella, varicella, herpes virus, smallpox and human immunodeficiency virus. Identifiable infections should be excluded.

Arthritis of Kawasaki disease usually presents during the subacute phase of the illness and is commonly found in the knees and ankles although the small joints of the hands may be involved. The arthritis may be accompanied by desquamation and subcutaneous oedema of the hands and feet, distinguishing it from systemic onset JIA. Behçet's disease (although rare) should be suspected in patients with recurrent oral and genital mucosal ulceration. When the arthritis of Henoch-Schönlein purpura precedes purpura, nephritis or abdominal involvement, the diagnosis may be difficult. Henoch-Schönlein purpura arthritis rarely manifests with synovial effusions and it is more likely that the inflammation is periarticular.

There are numerous conditions characterised by arthralgia and/or myalgia that may be misdiagnosed as JIA. The presence of bone pain should heighten suspicion for an underlying malignancy. A discrepancy between the blood counts and sedimentation rate (e.g. relative thrombocytopaenia) may be a clue to the diagnosis.[31] Young children with generalised hypermobility pre-dominantly complain of joint pain in the evening, often waking them from sleep, without associated swelling or morning stiffness, contrary to JIA. Overuse syndromes such as patellofemoral syndrome and Osgood-Schlatter are common in adolescents complaining of knee pain exacerbated by exercise. Fibromyalgia and reflex sympathetic dystrophy are chronic pain syndromes with onset in late childhood and adolescence. Musculoskeletal pain, without arthritis, is the predominant feature. These disorders are not inflammatory and the diagnosis is suspect if the patient has evidence of synovitis.

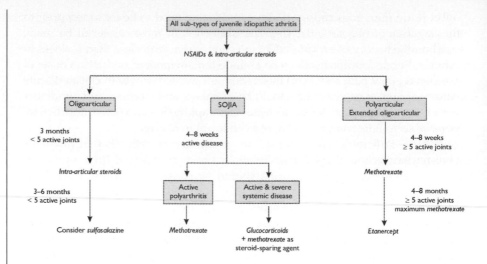

Fig. 7 One suggested treatment algorithm for JIA.

TREATMENT

Objectives of the treatment of JIA include controlling pain and inflammation, preserving function and promoting normal growth, overall development and well-being. Over the past few years, remarkable advances in the treatment of JIA have been made with the advent of new disease modifying anti-rheumatic agents and biopharmaceuticals.

THERAPEUTIC MODALITIES

Physical and occupational therapy are important adjuncts to medication as they help to maintain and improve range of motion, muscle strength and skills for activities of daily living. Splints may be used to support affected joints or work to improve range of motion. Arthroplasty may be needed for patients with severe deforming arthritis of polyarticular JIA.

Non-steroidal anti-inflammatory medications

Initial treatment for most patients with JIA includes intra-articular long-acting corticosteroid injections and NSAIDs (Fig. 7). NSAIDs control pain and inflammation and are usually given for 4–8-weeks before starting a second line agent. Naproxen (15–20 mg/kg div twice a day), tolmentin (20–30 mg/kg div three times a day), diclofenac (2–3 mg/kg div three times a day) and ibuprofen (40 mg/kg/div three times a day) are commonly used and are usually well-tolerated with little gastrointestinal discomfort. The choice of NSAID may be based on medication taste and ease of dosing regimen. Naproxen is prescribed most frequently but should be used with caution in fair-skinned children as they may develop pseudoporphyria cutanea tarda, a scarring photosensitive rash. Indomethacin (1–2 mg/kg/day) is a potent anti-inflammatory medication commonly used to treat enthesitis-related arthritis and systemic onset JIA. When prescribing indomethacin, patients should be warned about the possibility of headaches, trouble concentrating and gastrointestinal upset.[32]

The cyclooxygenase (COX)-2 inhibitors (*i.e.* rofecoxib and celecoxib) selectively inhibit the COX-2 enzyme allowing continued production of COX-1 resulting in a decreased incidence of gastrointestinal side-effects in adults. Although serious gastrointestinal complications are rare in children treated with conventional NSAIDs, COX-2 inhibitors may be useful in selected populations, especially children who have developed significant gastrointestinal symptoms. Studies are underway to assess the efficacy and pharmacokinetics of COX-2 inhibitors in children with JIA.

GLUCOCORTICOIDS

Glucocorticoids are potent anti-inflammatory medications that should be used judiciously in patients with arthritis as the side-effect profile includes cushingoid appearance, hyperglycaemia, immunosuppression, cataracts and glaucoma, adrenal suppression, peptic ulcer, dyslipoproteinaemia, hypertension, avascular necrosis of bone and CNS disturbance. While glucocorticoids are the mainstay of treatment for controlling serious systemic manifestations of systemic onset JIA, use in polyarticular patients should be limited to patients with extreme pain and functional limitation while waiting for a second-line agent to show some effect.[33] In rare instances, pulse methylprednisolone (30 mg/kg) has been used to treat systemic onset JIA patients that have not responded to oral glucocorticoids. Patients should be tapered off steroids as quickly as possible once disease improvement is noted.

Treatment of a few joints with intra-articular long-acting corticosteroid injections is a good way to treat arthritis while minimising systemic side-effects from oral medications. Triamcinolone hexacetomide (20–40 mg/large joint or 1 mg/kg/joint) is commonly used and usually results in improvement after 24–48 h that may last for many months. Side-effects include infection, atrophic skin changes at the injection site and asymptomatic calcifications on radiographs.[33] Injections can be safely given as often as every 3 months.

DISEASE-MODIFYING ANTI-RHEUMATIC AGENTS

The disease-modifying anti-rheumatic agents that have been shown to be effective in JIA include sulfasalazine, methotrexate and etanercept. Other disease-modifying anti-rheumatic agents such as hydroxychloroquine, D-penicillamine and auranofin have failed to show efficacy in double-blind, placebo-controlled trials.[32] Intramuscular or oral gold is rarely used for JIA currently because of poorer response rates and higher incidence of toxicity when compared to methotrexate and other disease-modifying anti-rheumatic agents. Systemic onset JIA patients have been treated with monthly intravenous cyclophosphamide and immunoglobulin with improvement.

Sulfasalazine

Compared with placebo, sulfasalazine was more effective in controlling arthritis and improving laboratory parameters in a double-blind placebo controlled trial.[34] Sulfasalazine is commonly used to treat pauciarticular JIA and HLA-B27 spondyloarthropathies.[35] Its use, however, is limited by side-effects such as headache, rash, gastrointestinal toxicity, myelosuppression, and hypoimmunoglobulinaemia. A complete blood count and liver transaminases need to be monitored prior to the start of the drug, every other week for the first 3 months, monthly for the next 3 months and then every 3 months.[32]

Methotrexate

Methotrexate is the most frequently used second-line agent for patients with JIA,[36] particularly polyarticular and systemic onset JIA. Up to 80% of JIA patients have some clinical response on methotrexate and studies suggest it retards radiographic progression. Extended oligoarticular patients respond best to methotrexate; systemic onset JIA patients may represent a group that does not do as well on this agent.[32] Methotrexate is also helpful in controlling the rash and arthritis of juvenile psoriatic arthritis.

Methotrexate is tolerated quite well in children with doses starting at 0.3 mg/kg/week and increased to a maximum of 1 mg/kg/dose (no more than 25 mg/week orally or 50 mg/m^2 subcutaneously). Gastrointestinal toxicity is the most common adverse event, occurring in 13% of the patients. Additional side-effects include hepatotoxicity, mucocutaneous disorders, teratogenicity, immunosuppression, pulmonary disease, pancytopaenia and an increased risk of lymphoproliferative malignancies.[37] Supplementation with folic acid has been shown to lessen the gastrointestinal and mucocutaneous side-effects without altering the therapeutic effect of methotrexate.[38] Liver enzymes and a complete blood count should be monitored every 1–2 months, although serious, irreversible liver disease is rare in children.[39] The medication should be discontinued if liver enzymes approach 3 times normal. Due to the possible immunosuppressive effects of methotrexate, patients are advised not get live-virus vaccines. Patients in remission for 1 year can have their methotrexate gradually discontinued in order to reduce potential long-term toxicity.[32]

Leflunomide

Leflunomide, an immunosuppressive agent that reversibly inhibits *de novo* pyrimidine synthesis, is used to treat adult RA and is currently being studied for use in JIA. Side-effects include diarrhoea, elevated liver enzymes, mucocutaneous abnormalities and teratogenicity.[32]

BIOPHARMACEUTICALS

Biopharmaceuticals – including etanercept, infliximab, adalimumab, anakinra, and rituximab – have improved the armamentarium for the treatment of patients with rheumatoid arthritis and JIA. All carry a risk of immunosuppression and live-virus vaccines are relatively contra-indicated. Cases of re-activated tuberculosis have been reported in patients using these agents; tuberculin skin test non-reactivity should be demonstrated at the start of therapy. If the tuberculin skin test is positive, patients should complete a course of anti-tuberculosis treatment prior to starting the biopharmaceutical.

Etanercept

Elevated levels of TNF-α and soluble TNF receptor are found in serum of JIA patients. In addition, these patients also have elevated levels of TNF-α in the synovial fluid.[40,41] Etanercept, a soluble TNF receptor, is a fusion protein made up of two recombinant p75 soluble receptors fused with the Fc fragment from human IgG. It binds and inhibits TNF-α and lymphotoxin-α (TNF-β). In a double-blind, placebo-controlled study of polyarticular JIA patients, etanercept was proven effective in controlling pain and swelling and in improving laboratory parameters. There was also evidence that it retards radiographic progression of disease. Etanercept, 0.4 mg/kg (maximum 25 mg) subcutaneously twice weekly results in an excellent response and is highly recommended for patients with extended oligoarticular and polyarticular JIA that have failed first- and second-line agents. Two years post follow-up, patients in the initial clinical trial continued to have an excellent response.[41] Preliminary findings on etanercept in combination with a disease-modifying anti-rheumatic agent have shown it to be well tolerated.[42] In placebo-controlled, clinical trials etanercept was shown to be well-tolerated and no increased incidence of infection was found. As cases of aseptic meningitis secondary to varicella have been reported in patients being treated with etanercept, susceptible children should be immunised 3 months prior to the start of the drug. Any susceptible patient exposed to varicella should be treated with immunoglobulin. Paediatric patients with significant exposure to varicella should temporarily discontinue the etanercept.[32]

Although not currently approved for juvenile psoriatic arthritis, a double-blind, placebo-controlled study of adults with psoriatic arthritis showed remarkable improvement of their arthritis and skin manifestations using etanercept at a dose of 25 mg subcutaneously twice weekly.[40] Etanercept has also shown promise in adults with spondyloarthropathy.

Infliximab

Infliximab is a chimeric monoclonal anti-TNF-α antibody. The variable region of a mouse monoclonal anti-TNF-α antibody is coupled to the constant region of human IgG$_1$. Adult RA patients are treated with infliximab at a dose of 3–10 mg/kg at time 0, 2 and 6 weeks and then every 6–8 weeks. There is little data on dosing, efficacy and pharmacokinetics in paediatric patients. In a recent small, non-randomised, open-label study, etanercept and infliximab (in combination with a disease-modifying anti-rheumatic agent) were found to be equally efficacious in treating patients with juvenile psoriatic arthritis, polyarticular and systemic onset JIA. The incidence of adverse effects was higher and more serious in the infliximab group compared to the etanercept group.[43] Further studies are needed to evaluate the benefits and risks of infliximab in patients with JIA and juvenile psoriatic arthritis.

Investigational therapies

Other biopharmaceuticals, such as anakinra, a recombinant IL-1 receptor antagonist and rituximab, an antibody to B-cell surface antigens, are currently being studied for treatment of chronic arthritis. Autologous stem-cell transplantation has been considered in recalcitrant cases of systemic onset JIA. This treatment option is considered experimental, as it is associated with increased morbidity and mortality, including macrophage activation syndrome. Stem-cell transplantation should only be performed in experienced centres after all other treatment options have failed.[32]

CONCLUSIONS

All patients diagnosed with JIA should be given a trial of NSAIDs and intra-articular corticosteroid injections should be considered. Patients with oligoarticular JIA usually have a good response and need no further intervention. Patients with polyarticular disease will benefit from aggressive therapy with methotrexate in order to improve function and prevent permanent damage. Intra-articular corticosteroids are a good adjunct to treatment. Extended oligoarticular JIA patients and juvenile psoriatic arthritis patients that fail first-line treatment should be treated like polyarticular patients. Systemic onset JIA patients, with active systemic disease, may require oral glucocorticoids for rapid relief of serious systemic manifestations including pericarditis, progressive anaemia, malnutrition and persistent fever. Methotrexate should be considered for articular disease treatment as well as a steroid-sparing agent. Sulfasalazine may be particularly effective in patients with enthesitis related arthritis and extended oligoarticular patients that fail to respond to NSAIDs. Presently, the only biological agent that has been proven to be effective in JIA is etanercept, and should be used in patients with polyarticular disease who fail methotrexate.

Key points for clinical practice

- Juvenile idiopathic arthritis is heterogeneous group of diseases diagnosed in children < 16 years of age with arthritis for at least 6 weeks in duration. Under the International League of Associations for Rheumatology classification system there are 7 sub-types: oligoarticular, polyarticular (rheumatoid factor positive and negative), systemic onset juvenile idiopathic arthritis, enthesitis-related arthritis, juvenile psoriatic arthritis, and 'other'.

- Oligoarticular juvenile idiopathic arthritis has the best prognosis, polyarticular rheumatoid factor positive disease has a poor prognosis if not aggressively treated and systemic onset juvenile idiopathic arthritis and rheumatoid factor negative polyarticular juvenile idiopathic arthritis have a more variable prognosis.

- Complications of juvenile idiopathic arthritis include uveitis, osteopenia and osteoporosis, and growth disturbance.

- It is important that juvenile idiopathic arthritis patients be screened routinely for uveitis, as it may be asymptomatic at onset and, if left untreated, there is a high risk of morbidity, including blindness. The highest risk is among young patients who are anti-nuclear antibody positive with oligoarticular or polyarticular disease.

- Active arthritis and oral glucocorticoids place the patient at an increased risk for osteoporosis.

- Macrophage activation syndrome, a life-threatening complication of systemic onset juvenile idiopathic arthritis, is often triggered by infection or a change in medications, especially non-steroidal anti-inflammatory medications. The sedimentation rate is often low, contrary to flares of systemic onset juvenile idiopathic arthritis.

- The differential diagnosis of acute arthritis includes reactive, infectious, malignancy, trauma, inflammatory and systemic disease.

- Physiotherapy is an integral part of overall treatment for patients with juvenile idiopathic arthritis.

- All juvenile idiopathic arthritis patients should be treated with a trial of non-steroidal anti-inflammatory medications and intra-articular corticosteroid injections should be considered.

- Sulfasalazine may be particularly effective in patients with enthesitis-related arthritis and extended oligoarticular patients that fail to respond to non-steroidal anti-inflammatory disease medications.

- Systemic onset juvenile idiopathic arthritis patients with active systemic disease, despite non-steroidal anti-inflammatory disease medication therapy, may warrant a course of oral glucocorticoids for rapid control of serious systemic manifestations including pericarditis, progressive anaemia, malnutrition and persistent fever while initiating methotrexate as a steroid-sparing agent.

- Polyarticular patients benefit from aggressive treatment with methotrexate in order to improve function and prevent joint damage.

- Etanercept is the only biopharmaceutical that has been proven effective in juvenile idiopathic arthritis, and should be used in patients with polyarticular disease who fail methotrexate.

- Prior to the initiation of a biological agent, especially etanercept, patients should demonstrate tuberculin skin test non-reactivity and be brought up-to-date with all immunisations in agreement with current immunisation guidelines. Patients with a significant exposure to varicella virus should temporarily discontinue etanercept and be considered for prophylactic treatment with varicella zoster immune globulin.

References

1. Petty RE, Southwood TR, Baum J et al. Revision of the proposed classification criteria for juvenile idiopathic arthritis: Durban 1997. *J Rheumatol* 1998; **25**: 1991–1994.
2. Lang BA, Shore A. A review of current concepts on the pathogenesis of juvenile rheumatoid arthritis. *J Rheumatol* 1990; **17 (Suppl 21)**: 1–15.
3. Tucker LB. Juvenile rheumatoid arthritis. *Curr Opin Rheumatol* 1993; 5: 619–628.
4. Thomson W, Barrett JH, Donn R et al. Juvenile idiopathic arthritis classified by the ILAR criteria: HLA associations in UK patients. *Rheumatology* 2002; **41**: 1183–1189.

5. Mangee H, Schauenstein K. Cytokines in juvenile rheumatoid arthritis (JRA). *Cytokine* 1998; **10**: 471–480.
6. Moore TL. Immunopathogenesis of juvenile rheumatoid arthritis. *Curr Opin Rheumatol* 1999; **11**: 377–387.
7. Mangee H, Kenzian H, Gallistl S *et al*. Serum cytokines in juvenile rheumatoid arthritis. *Arthritis Rheum* 1995; **2**: 211–220.
8. Schneider R, Passo MH. Juvenile rheumatoid arthritis. *Rheum Dis Clin North Am* 2002; **28**: 503–530.
9. Al-Matar MJ, Petty RE, Tucker LB, Malleson PN, Schroeder ML, Cabral DA. The early pattern of joint involvement predicts disease progression in children with oligoarticular (pauciarticular) juvenile rheumatoid arthritis. *Arthritis Rheum* 2002; **46**: 2708–2715.
10. Minden K, Niewerth M, Listing J *et al*. Long-term outcome in patients with juvenile idiopathic arthritis. *Arthritis Rheum* 2002; **46**: 2392–2401.
11. Schaller JG. Juvenile rheumatoid arthritis. *Pediatr Rev* 1980; **2**: 163–174.
12. Isdale IC, Bywaters EGL. The rash of rheumatoid arthritis and Still's disease. *Q J Med* 1956; **99**: 377–387.
13. Svantesson H, Akesson A, Eberhardt K, Elbourgh R. Prognosis in juvenile rheumatoid arthritis with systemic onset. A follow-up study. *Scand J Rheumatol* 1983; **12**: 139–144.
14. Spiegel LR, Schneider R, Lang B *et al*. Early predictors of poor functional outcome in systemic-onset juvenile rheumatoid arthritis: a multicenter cohort study. *Arthritis Rheum* 2000; **43**; 2402–2409.
15. Ramanan AV, Schneider R. Macrophage activation syndrome following initiation of etanercept in a child with systemic onset juvenile rheumatoid arthritis. *J Rheumatol* 2003; **30**: 401–403.
16. Sawhney S, Woo P, Murray KJ. Macrophage activation syndrome: a potentially fatal complication of rheumatic disorders. *Arch Dis Child* 2001; **85**: 421–426.
17. Grom AA, Passo MD. Macrophage activation syndrome in systemic juvenile rheumatoid arthritis. *J Pediatr* 1996; **129**: 630–632.
18. Burgos-Vargas R, Petty RE. Juvenile ankylosing spondylitis. *Rheum Dis Clin North Am* 1992; **18**: 123–142.
19. Schaller J, Bitnum S, Wedgwood RJ. Ankylosing spondylitis with childhood onset. *J Pediatr* 1969; **74**: 505–516.
20. Shore A, Ansell BM. Juvenile psoriatic arthritis-an analysis of 60 cases. *J Pediatr* 1982; **100**: 529–535.
21. Petty RE, Malleson P. Spondyloarthropathies of childhood. *Pediatr Clin North Am* 1986; **33**: 1079–1096.
22. Yancey C, White, P, Magilavy D *et al*. Guidelines for ophthalmologic examinations in children with juvenile rheumatoid arthritis. Section on rheumatology and section on ophthalmology. *Pediatrics* 1993; **92**: 295–296.
23. Schwartzman S, Flynn T, Barinstein L, Gartner S, Onel K. Infliximab therapy for resistant uveitis. *Arthritis Rheum* 2002; **46**: S326.
24. Reiff A, Syuji T, Sadeghi S *et al*. Etanercept therapy in children with treatment-resistant uveitis. *Arthritis Rheum* 2001; **44**: 1411–1415.
25. Calabro JJ. Juvenile rheumatoid arthritis. *GP* 1969; **40**: 78–88.
26. Sherry DD, Stein LD, Reed AM, Schanberg LE, Kredich DW. Prevention of leg length discrepancy in young children with pauciarticular juvenile rheumatoid arthritis by treatment with intraarticular steroids. *Arthritis Rheum* 1999; **42**: 2330–2334.
27. Rabinovich CE. Bone metabolism in childhood rheumatic disease. *Rheum Dis Clin North Am* 2002; **28**: 655–667.
28. Cassidy JT. Osteopenia and osteoporosis in children. *Clin Exp Rheumatol* 1999; **17**: 245–250.
29. Cimaz R, Ansell BM. Sarcoidosis in the pediatric age. *Clin Exp Rheumatol* 2002; **20**: 231–237.
30. Klein-Gittelman M, Reiff A, Silverman ED. Systemic lupus erythematosus in childhood. *Rheum Dis Clin North Am* 2002; **28**: 561–577.
31. Cabral DA, Tucker LB. Malignancies in children who initially present with rheumatic complaints. *J Pediatr* 1999; **134**: 53–57.
32. Ilowite NT. Current treatment of juvenile rheumatoid arthritis. *Pediatrics* 2002; **109**: 109–115.
33. Milojevic DS, Ilowite NT. Treatment of rheumatic diseases in children: special considerations. *Rheum Dis Clin North Am* 2002; **28**: 461–482.

34. van Rossum MAJ, Fiselier TJW, Franssen MJAM *et al*. Sulfasalazine in the treatment of juvenile chronic arthritis: a randomized, double-blind, placebo-controlled, multi-center study. Dutch Juvenile Chronic Arthritis Study Group. *Arthritis Rheum* 1998; **41**: 808–816.

35. Ansell BM, Hall MA, Loftus JK *et al*. A multicentre pilot study of sulphasalazine in juvenile chronic arthritis. *Clin Exp Rheumatol* 1991; **9**: 201–203.

36. Cron RQ, Sharma S, Sherry DD. Current treatment by United States and Canadian pediatric rheumatologists. *J Rheumatol* 1999; **26**: 2036–2038.

37. Gianinni EH, Cassidy JT. Methotrexate in juvenile rheumatoid arthritis. Do the benefits outweigh the risks? *Drug Saf* 1993; **9**: 325–339.

38. Hunt PG, Rose CD, McIlvain-Simpson G, Tejani S. The effects of daily intake of folic acid on the efficacy of methotrexate therapy in children with juvenile rheumatoid arthritis. A controlled study. *J Rheumatol* 1997; **24**: 2230–2232.

39. Passo MH, Hashkes PJ. Use of methotrexate in children. *Bull Rheum Dis* 1998; **47**: 1–5.

40. Mease P. Psoriatic arthritis: the role of THF inhibition and the effect of its inhibition with etanercept. *Clin Exp Rheumatol* 2002; **20 (Suppl 28)**: S116–S121.

41. Lovell D, Giannini EH, Reif A *et al*. Long-term efficacy and safety of etanercept in children with polyarticular-course juvenile rheumatoid arthritis. Interim results from an ongoing multicenter, open label extended-treatment trial. *Arthritis Rheum* 2003; **489**: 218–226.

42. Haapasaari J, Kautiainen H, Hannula S, Pohjankoski H, Hakala M. Good results from combining etanercept to prevailing DMARD therapy in refractory juvenile idiopathic arthritis. *Clin Exp Rheumatol* 2002; **20**: 867–870.

43. Lahdenne P, Vähäsalo P, Honkanen V. Infliximab or etanercept in the treatment of children with refractory juvenile idiopathic arthritis: an open label study. *Ann Rheum Dis* 2003; **62**: 245–247.

Richard H. Schwartz Eric A. Voth

The use and toxicity of cannabis in teenagers

Approximately 30% of American high school tenth-graders smoked cannabis (marijuana) in the past 12 months, and 20% of US students of this age have smoked it in the past 30 days.[1] Many tenth-graders who admit to cannabis use report that they began their experimentation before the age of 13 years.[1] A national survey of secondary school children carried out in 2001 by the National Centre for Social Research and the National Foundation for Educational Research that involved more than 9000 pupils in 285 schools in the UK found that 31% of 15-year-olds had smoked cannabis during the previous year.[2] In 1999, 95,000 tenth-grade students from 30 countries answered a co-ordinated set of school surveys conducted by the European School Survey Project on Alcohol and Drugs. Of students from the UK who participated in this multicountry survey, 35% admitted to having smoked cannabis at some time. In 2001, a survey of 15,881 teenagers at 334 primary and secondary schools throughout the UK performed by the Schools Health Education Unit, found that 29% of 14- and 15-year-old males said they had tried cannabis at least once, American and British survey results for 15- and 16-year-old students' use of cannabis, in sum, are now almost identical.

Adolescents who use cannabis frequently during early adolescence may continue to use the drug for a longer period than previously reported. A total of 1228 German adolescents were followed between the age of 14 and 17 years. They were re-evaluated serially for a mean of 20 months. Of these adolescents, 74% used cannabis to some extent over that 3-year period. The higher the baseline use, the higher the probability of heavy use at the time of re-evaluation.[3] Although some or most adolescents who abuse cannabis will reduce or cease smoking the drug by age 30 years, many may have lost valuable and perhaps irreplaceable time in achieving normal developmental

Richard H. Schwartz MD, Inova-Fairfax Hospital for Children, Falls Church, VA, USA. E-mail: rhs738@aol.com (for correspondence)

Eric A. Voth MD. Clinical Assist. Professor of Medicine, University of Kansas, Topeka, Kansas, USA

Table 1 Cannabis terminology

Blunt	A cigar that has been hollowed out and filled with crumbled cannabis
Bong	Air- or water-cooled glass apparatus used for smoking cannabis or tobacco
Bowl	Dainty pipe that holds about a thimbleful of cannabis for purpose of smoking
Buds	Flowering tops of *Cannabis sativa* containing the highest concentration of THC
Cannabis	Medicinal varieties of the hemp plant and its derivatives
Cannabis sativa	Pharmacological hemp plant
Hashish	Heat-pressed cakes of strained cannabis resin and leaf dust. The major form of smoked cannabis in the UK
Hydroponic cultivation	A soil-less system of aqueous cultivation of *C. sativa*
Marijuana	Cured and dried flowering tops and small leaves of *C. sativa*. The major form of smoked cannabis in the US and Canada. Derives from the Central-American word mariguango, which means an intoxicating substance[18]
Spliff	Cannabis cigarette (joint) or fat cigar stuffed with dried cannabis leaf
Sinsemilla	Seedless varieties of highly potent female cannabis plants
THC	Tetrahydrocannabinol, the major psycho-active compound in *C. sativa*

milestone during adolescence and early adulthood. Cannabis plays a powerful regulatory role in mood, motor control, pain perception, appetite, sleep, memory, and cognition.[4]

Since 1995, many general and specialised reviews of cannabis have been published.[4–16] Adverse effects from repeatedly smoking cannabis during adolescence include: (i) an increase risk of motor vehicle and other accidents; (ii) respiratory disease; (iii) developmental delays or difficulties; (iv) school underachievement; and (v) short-term memory defects. Current use of cannabis (within the past month) was associated with a (33%) significantly increased risk in injury for men and with an 86% increase in mortality from poisoning or injury in women.[6]

High-grade cannabis is widely available and is much more potent than a similar quality product several decades ago. Selected strains of hydroponically (soil-free) grown buds now contain more than 10% tetrahydrocannabinol (THC), 4 times the average potency of cannabis products in 1980.[17]

Pro-cannabis groups have created Web sites such as <cannabis.com> or <marijuana.com>. Little information, by contrast, is available on the health and other risks of marijuana use. Of the first 50 entries under 'cannabis' on the browser Web Crawler in 2003, only a single entry was not from a pro-cannabis group or company. Most Internet Web sites serve as advertisements for purchase of cannabis seeds, growing equipment, methods to deceive urine drug tests, and literature or organisations with a decidedly pro-drug philosophy <http://www.ukia.org>. Table 1 lists some of the cannabis terminology used in the UK and US.

CANNABIS – BOTANY

C. sativa, the medicinal variety of the common hemp plant, grows wild in many tropical and temperate climates and is widely cultivated both outdoors and indoors. The primary psycho-active compound produced by *C. sativa* is THC, particularly its delta-9 isomer, which is a unique intoxicating chemical. Cannabis usually has separate male and female plants that are indistinguishable until flowering occurs. Resin-secreting glands that contain the highest amount of sticky THC are most numerous in the smallest leaves and flowering tops of the pistillate (female) plant, but are found in all other parts of the plant of both sexes except the main trunk and roots.

The quantity of THC in a plant varies widely, depending on the pedigree of seed, growing conditions (temperature and sunlight), the composition of the soil or hydroponic solution, and presence or absence of male plants nearby. Indoor horticulture is the primary means of choice for cannabis cultivation in North America. The intensity, angle, and wavelength of artificial light, the number of hours of light and dark per day, the percentage of ambient carbon dioxide, and the control of fungus and insect pathogens all play an important part in the production of choice – highly potent grades of marijuana grown by hydroponic methods indoors.

Ingestion of fresh cannabis leaves or flowers is harmless, because native THC is in the form of THC-carboxylic acid, which must be decarboxylated to psycho-active THC by drying and curing or by heat. After harvesting, the cut plant must be subjected to careful drying and curing.

The Netherlands is currently the source of most of the cannabis smoked in western Europe, and Canada and Mexico are the sources of most of the imported cannabis smoked in the US.

POTENCY OF C. SATIVA

A minimum of 1% THC is necessary for most people to perceive psycho-active effects. Highly potent, sought-after varieties of cannabis known as sinsemilla contain as much as 14% THC and averages more than 8% THC. The intoxicating dose of THC is about 2.5 mg for a 70-kg person. A typical marijuana joint or spliff contains about 1.0 g of cannabis, and good quality marijuana has a potency of at least 7% THC.

Hashish, a cannabis product higher in THC potency than the cannabis leaf, is usually manufactured by sifting the dried small leaves and flowering tops over a silk screen-covered form and under heat and pressure, compressing the collected concentrated resin and leaf dust into slabs or blocks that are then wrapped in muslin and overwrapped in plastic sheets. Because of its fine particulate matter composition, hashish is prone to lose potency over time unless kept airtight. In the UK and the European continent, hashish is the preferred form of smoked cannabis. Although hashish is believed to be much more potent than marijuana, in the US premium grades of marijuana are more potent than hashish, perhaps because THC in hashish decomposes faster.

METABOLISM AND PHARMACOLOGY OF CANNABIS

THC is absorbed into the pulmonary circulation and carried to the systemic circulation where it binds with specific brain receptors (CB1) located primarily in the hippocampus and cerebellum. These brain receptor sites are involved in memory, emotion, cognition, movement and motor co-ordination, and pain perception.[8,19] CB1 and CB2 receptor sites are coupled to G proteins, and their activation decreases production of cAMP and modulation of the ion channel activity. A decade ago, anandamide (arachidonylethanolamide), isolated from porcine brain, was determined to be an endogenous, but considerably weaker, CB1 cannabinoid ligand with affinity for cannabinoid brain binding sites. 2-Arachidonoyl glycerol activates both CB1 and CB2 receptors.

Measurable plasma levels of THC decrease rapidly within a few hours after smoking cannabis products. THC is very lipid-soluble, and concentrates in areas of high lipid content. The significance of this is debatable. There do not seem to be any perceived psycho-active properties of stored THC. In other words, slow release of stored THC does not seem to affect brain function or behaviour. THC is detoxified primarily in hepatocytes by hydroxylation and carboxylation. Only the parent drug and its ultratransient 11-hydroxy metabolite possess any psychotropic effects. Non-toxic metabolites are excreted in faeces (65%) and urine (35%).

9-Carboxy-THC, the terminal metabolite, is measurable in a serum specimen for about 12–24 h and in a urine specimen for 2–3 days in individuals who use cannabis only infrequently. However, using a cut-off point of 20 ng/ml, 9-carboxy-THC can usually be detected in urine specimens for 3–5 days in individuals who use marijuana frequently or daily. It cannot be reliably detected in urine specimens for 1 month, unless the person has smoked or eaten the crude drug on a chronic daily basis. The higher the detection point set for carboxy-THC by the analyser instrument, the fewer consecutive days of its detection in urine. Thus, a cut-off point of 50 ng/ml will generally detect carboxy-THC for 1–2 days after last use in novices, while a detection point of 20 ng/ml will detect it for an additional 1–2 days. For some as yet unexplained reason, about 25% of daily marijuana users continue to excrete measurable amounts of 9-carboxy-THC for a month or more after last verified use of cannabis. No prolonged psychotropic effects have been demonstrated beyond the first 24 h after last use of cannabis except for its impairment of short-term memory.

METHODS OF SMOKING CANNABIS

Cannabis and hashish are usually consumed by smoking in home-rolled cigarettes (joints), dainty pipes (bowls), hollowed-out stones, or air- or water-cooled hookahs, known commonly as bongs. A novel method of smoking marijuana involves hollowing out a tobacco-wrapped cigar and stuffing it with crumbled dried cannabis buds ('blunts'). The preparation and smoking of cannabis often rigidly conform to local social etiquette.

The most effective and rapid method of smoking high-grade cannabis is to use it with a bong or in a spliff. Smoking marijuana in a bong is a more efficient method of extracting THC because THC is more concentrated per inhalation and less is lost in side-stream smoke compared to smoking marijuana cigarettes or pipes. Smoking blunts (hollowed out cigars re-stuffed with crumbled cannabis leaf) is associated with consumption of large amounts of THC. When THC is smoked, it by-passes the liver and is delivered rapidly to the brain. Although dried and cured cannabis can be ingested as an ingredient in many recipes, few adolescents choose oral ingestion as the preferred route of administration of the drug.

More than 70% of 11,996 current marijuana users surveyed in American high schools nation-wide had also smoked tobacco cigarettes in the past 30 days.[20] Although many evidently use both drugs, smoking cannabis differs in many ways from smoking tobacco. An adolescent addicted to nicotine smokes 5–30 tobacco cigarettes daily, while a cannabis-dependent adolescent smokes 2–4 marijuana cigarettes most days of the week. Cannabis smokers do not use a filter to trap particulate matter before inhalation. Tobacco pipe smokers typically do not inhale, while cannabis pipe smokers must deeply inhale to get high. Cannabis smoke is usually deliberately retained for 5 s or more in the lower respiratory tract in order for the bronchioles and alveoli to extract the maximal amount of THC and pass it into the systemic circulation. (An inexperienced marijuana smoker extracts about 10% of the available THC while an experienced smoker extracts 20%.) Although fewer cannabis cigarettes are smoked each day compared to tobacco cigarettes, cannabis smoke contains more particulate matter and tar than cigarette smoke and it is much more irritating to the mucous membranes of the oropharynx and respiratory tree.

ACUTE EFFECTS OF TETRAHYDROCANNABINOL ON THE BODY

Apart from an increase in the heart rate, the only consistent and immediate physical sign of marijuana use in dilation of the conjunctivae (red eyes). During the 2-h period of intoxication, the eyes often have a glassy gaze that can be detected by experienced cannabis smokers but easily overlooked by non-using parents. Xerostomia and xerophthalmia are annoying effects during cannabis use; positional hypotension is unusual in adolescents. The acute toxicity of cannabis is quite low insofar as direct pharmacological harm. Cannabis burns at a higher temperature than does tobacco, leaving a burning or stinging taste in the mouth and throat and often producing a dry, hacking cough. The characteristic smell of burning cannabis lingers on hair and on woollen clothing. Acute and chronic symptoms of irritating smoke on the respiratory conduits include dry stuffy nose, sore throat, hoarse voice, and smoker's cough. Occasionally, these symptoms are bothersome enough to warrant medical attention.

Cannabis is said to be one of the safest of all drugs because there are no reported fatalities directly attributed to its use. However, any intoxicant, including cannabis, can alter behaviours to increase risk taking and diminish vigilance and well-being, particularly during adolescence. There is no conclusive evidence that smoking cannabis products in usual amounts, even frequently, impairs the human immune system. The number and function of T- or B-lymphocytes or immunoglobulins are not impaired, even with chronic daily marijuana use.[21] Although there may be some association of marijuana smoking with leukoplakia and development of squamous cell cancers of the oropharynx, this remains unproven. About 25 years ago, use of cannabis by male adolescents and young adults was reported to cause a reduction in testosterone secretion and sperm production. Such adverse effects have not been validated. There is no proven association between use of cannabis by males and the enlargement of male breast tissue. Cannabis use during pregnancy can cause reductions in birth weight of animals, including humans.[22,23]

THC exerts inconsistent physiological effects to impair vigilance, co-ordination, and reaction time. All three effects, although unproven, may persist for many hours after the self-perceived period of intoxication has ended.[24] Cannabis can alter perception of depth and distance during operation of a motor vehicle. THC-intoxicated drivers may not respond optimally to visual clues such as a sudden change in traffic lights or the unexpected darting out of a child between two parked cars because they are sometimes pre-occupied with drug-induced imagery or loud throbbing music on their car radios. Many experienced cannabis smokers who inhale before or during operation of a motor vehicle believed that they were performing exceptionally well during a time when driving instructors had seen them make careless and dangerous errors during actual driving tests.

One study showed that smoking of cannabis caused reaction time to increase > 36% above that of an unimpaired driver on two tests of driving skills. The Road Tracking Skills test measures a driver's ability to maintain a constant speed of 100 km/h and to drive a steady path. The Car Following Test measures a driver's reaction time and distance between the cannabis smoker's vehicle and a lead vehicle 50 m ahead. (During the test, the lead vehicle executes a series of alternating accelerations and decelerations.) Smoking cannabis without alcohol or other drug use significantly impaired performance on both road tests compared with baseline performance. The cannabis-intoxicated driver needed an additional > 45 m to come to a complete stop when travelling at 96 km/h. There was also a diminished ability to respond to changes in the relative velocities of other vehicles on the test course and to adjust vehicle speed accordingly.[25] Whether cannabis smoking by experienced smokers impairs driving in real-life situations is still unsettled, but evidence is accumulating that real-life driving is impaired in many individuals under the influence of cannabis.

ACUTE TETRAHYDROCANNABINOL EFFECTS ON MIND AND MOOD

THC exerts powerful effects on appetite, causes distortions in the perception of the passage of time (overestimation), and can affect the acquisition of short-term memory. After a few ineffectual attempts to master the technique of smoking cannabis, the user generally finds that the drug induces a 2–3-h state of moderate euphoria, relaxation, enhanced jocularity and camaraderie, and loosening of inhibitions. Silliness and giggles often accompany adolescent peer group use of cannabis, particularly in a secure setting. The effect of smoked cannabis is, however, markedly unpredictable, especially for novices. Consumption of a similar quantity of marijuana of comparable potency on two occasions may produce minimal psycho-active effects on one occasion and a significant effect on another. Soon after the last inhalation of cannabis, there may be an intensified hunger for sweet beverages and snacks known as the 'marijuana munchies'.

After the state of intoxication dissipates, there is often a perceptive moodiness, including physical and mental turpitude, irritability, and emotional lability with easily provoked anger. This is especially evident when a cannabis-smoking teenager is reprimanded about neglected responsibilities such as school homework or house chores. Although novices have reported acute panic reaction and toxic psychosis after the use of cannabis, these are very unusual effects. The link between regular use of cannabis and later mental illness such as schizophrenia, however, has been strengthened by two recent studies.[26,27] Cannabis use among psychologically vulnerable adolescents should be strongly discouraged, because these youths appear to be particularly susceptible to drug abuse and dependence. The theory that individuals with mental illnesses self-medicate with cannabis to control their mental symptoms has been soundly challenged.[26,27]

There is uncontested evidence that intoxication from cannabis adversely effects acquisition of short-term memory but has little effect on retrieval from remote memory.[28] It is more difficult to learn and to retain new material under the influence of cannabis; this is one of the drug's most troublesome adverse effects.[29–33] How long the effect lasts in individuals who smoke cannabis daily remains to be determined.

TETRAHYDROCANNABINOL AFFECTS ON ADOLESCENT BEHAVIOUR

The risk of cannabis use among teenagers is dependent not only on the pharmacological action of the drug but also on the risk-taking behaviours that are magnified during intoxication by any drug, including cannabis. All adolescent cannabis smokers are not equal (Table 2).

Adolescents with multiple risk factors are at higher risk for problematic use of cannabis.[34] On the other hand, adolescents with strong family ties, positive involvement in school and community, high parental and personal expectations, high level of close parental supervision, and a strong sense of religious faith and observance, are less likely to experiment with or abuse cannabis and other drugs.[35,36]

Mixing drugs is the rule when older adolescents 'party' or when they attend rock concerts or 'raves'. Harm is magnified when cannabis is used in large amounts with other intoxicants such as alcohol, stimulants, and hallucinogenic drugs.

Adolescents who smoke cannabis often use a variety of techniques to avoid detection by their parents and siblings. Ophthalmic drops are used to 'get the red out', and mouthwash or breath mints are used to mask the characteristic smell on the breath. Adolescents may store the drug in ingenious hiding places such as carbonated beverage can look-alikes or in secret places in a closet, stereo equipment, or shoe. Those who frequently smoke cannabis are sometimes quite suggestible to impulsive and risky peer group activities

Table 2 Risk factors for progressive drug use in adolescents

Family history of alcoholism or drug abuse
Addiction to nicotine in early adolescence
Alcohol abuse during early adolescence
Conduct disorder, including stealing and repetitive lying
Affiliation with cannabis-smoking peers
Intense enjoyment of impulsive risk-taking and dangerous behaviour
Serious academic underachievement (more than two unsatisfactory final grades)
Dysfunctional family
Divorce during adolescence
Libertarian or liberal parental philosophy toward cannabis
Attention deficit–hyperactivity disorder, especially if untreated
Membership in gang during adolescence
Learning disability
Physical or sexual abuse
Explosive impulse disorder
Low self-esteem
Adoption
Rape

during this THC-induced intoxication. Eleven adolescent cannabis-dependent smokers surveyed in a drug treatment centre admitted to deliberately intoxicating (by blowing marijuana smoke into the animal's nose and mouth), a family dog or cat as a form of group amusement.[37] Some of the ataxic animals were examined by veterinarians and subjected to a diagnostic work-up without learning of the real reason for the acute ataxia. Adolescent cannabis-dependent individuals compared to peers who are non-marijuana smokers, are more likely to be male, underachieve in school subjects, and to use regularly tobacco, alcohol, and other illicit intoxicants such as lysergic acid diethylamide (LSD), methylenedioxymethamphetamine (MDMA or ecstasy), and cocaine.

STAGES OF CANNABIS USE

STAGE 0 – NO USE OR RARE USE

Forces that resist experimentation with cannabis and other intoxicants include strong religious, ethnic, family, personal, and peer-group values that proscribe intoxication from any drug. A fear of getting caught by parents, school authorities, or police may be a deterrent for some. Counterbalancing these resistances are adolescent curiosity, peer pressure, peer modelling, a safe and congenial setting such as a party or rock concert, and use of another intoxicant such as alcohol.

STAGE 1 – REPEATED EXPERIMENTATION WITH CANNABIS AND OTHER DRUGS

During this stage, cannabis is smoked in a secure social setting in the company of friends, some of whom are experienced cannabis users. The novice learns the correct technique of deep inhalation and is prepared for the changes in mood that will soon occur. With further experience, the novice becomes proficient in achieving euphoria ('getting high') and can predictably titrate the desired degree of euphoria by varying potency and quantity of cannabis product. For those that continue towards more frequent and problematic use of cannabis, there is intense enjoyment of the feelings of well-being, serenity, and time distortion that occur with the intoxicated state. In the early part of this stage, adolescents are passive recipients of cannabis at parties and social gatherings.

STAGE 2 – ACHIEVING PROFICIENCY WITH CANNABIS AND PREFERENCE FOR CANNABIS-USING FRIENDS

Having used cannabis with a variety of friends, or even in solitude, the user may become proficient at the terminology of cannabis use, location of cannabis dealers, and purchase of paraphernalia. The adolescent often eagerly shares this expertise with close friends and sometimes with younger siblings. Time and energy that might be expended in normal development and achievement of adolescent goals may be diverted towards cannabis-seeking behaviours.[38] The adolescent who reaches stage 2 of drug use may prefer to associate with like-minded peers and to turn away from friends who do not use drugs. The user may try a mixture of drugs, including alcohol and hallucinogenic drugs, to experience a variety of altered states of consciousness. Counterbalancing the euphoric feelings and entertainment at social gatherings are feelings of guilt and possibly shame because of the need to deceive parents and other authority figures about behaviours that occurred during periods of intoxication. The adolescent must take increasing risks to purchase and conceal the supply of cannabis; this may also increase anxiety levels. Parents may begin to observe subtle undesirable changes in their teenager's mood, goal-direction, participation in family rituals, and reliability and honesty. The adolescence may begin to have academic and school attendance problems, and attire and language may deteriorate.[39] Some teenagers may show none of these signs; others may show a few of them. When drug use is on a fast track, all of these behaviours may occur. Adolescents who smoke cannabis frequently may notice a rebound period or let-down, after the euphoria subsides and usually on the way home. Negative feelings of irritability, apathy, inertia, and depression may be projected onto parents, teachers, friends critical of their frequent use of cannabis, or society in general. In order to modulate these negative feelings, an adolescent may seek to use cannabis or other drugs in solitude.

In the US, studies of adolescent cannabis smokers provided evidence for the 'gateway theory' of drug use.[40] Young adolescents experimented with and became dependent on nicotine in tobacco, then experimented and abused alcohol, and then went on to experiment with and abuse cannabis that served as the gateway for use of cocaine and other 'hard drugs'. This theory has been challenged and modified.[41]

STAGE 3 – DRUG DEPENDENCY

Although most cannabis use is intermittent and time-limited, an estimated 10–20% of American and Australian adolescents who smoke cannabis become dependent on one or more drugs.[42] Cannabis smokers with multiple risk factors for drug abuse appear to have a much higher chance of drug dependency than those with few risk factors, and the former constitute the majority of drug-dependent adolescents. In a large number of cases, these teenagers began to use cannabis because their close friends were using. The combination of group philosophy and group pressure, accompanied by the pleasures of their hedonistic life-style, were the main factors in their decision to begin to use drugs.

A recent report issued by a working party of the Royal College of Psychiatrists and Royal College of Physicians states:[43] 'the evidence that cannabis produces dependence is now beyond dispute. Long term, regular use leads to tolerance and increasing difficulty stopping despite wishing or attempting to do so, and North American population surveys consistently suggest that 5–10% of those who have used cannabis more than once become dependent.' Cannabis abuse in early adolescence and cannabis dependency have been shown to be associated with affiliation with delinquent and substance-using peers, early high school drop-out, unprotected sex, unplanned early parenthood and premature departure from the parental home.[38,44] Pulmonary dysfunction does occur after a few years of heavy use of cannabis. In a study of cannabis-dependent young adult New Zealanders (mean age 21 years), controlled for tobacco use, impaired pulmonary function, wheezing, and exercise intolerance were much more frequent than in the control group.[45]

Table 3 Drug (including cannabis) dependency

305.20 Cannabis abuse

A maladaptive pattern of substance use leading to clinically significant impairment or distress, as manifested by one or more of the following occurring within a 12-month period

1. Failure to fulfil major role obligations at work, school, or home (*e.g.* repeated absences, suspensions, or expulsions from school)

2. Recurrent substance use in situations in which it is physically hazardous (*e.g.* driving an automobile)

3. Recurrent substance-related legal problems (*e.g.* arrests for substance-related disorderly conduct, destruction of property, breaking and entering homes or schools, *etc.*

4. Continued use despite having persistent or recurrent social or interpersonal problems caused or exacerbated by the effects of cannabis (*e.g.* physical fights about the consequences of cannabis intoxication

304.30 Cannabis dependency

The essential feature of cannabis-dependence is a cluster of cognitive and behavioural symptoms indicating that the individual continues use of cannabis despite significant substance-related maladaptive behaviours. There is a pattern of repeated self-administration that can result in tolerance to THC and to compulsive drug-taking behaviour. Whether sudden cessation of daily use of cannabis can produce drug withdrawal syndrome is debatable. Craving for cannabis and/or for the pleasures of the hedonistic life-style is likely to experienced by most individuals with substance dependence

Table 4 Characteristics of adolescent cannabis-abuse/dependency

Apathy and irresponsibility
Academic underachievement (2 or more poor or failing grades)
Preference and defence of cannabis-using friends
School truancy
Deterioration of ethical values (stealing, lying)
Distortion of normal adolescent goals (education, vocational goals)
Alienation and rebelliousness of family and society norms
Promiscuity or multiple sex partners in early adolescence
Running away from home

Table 3 gives the *Diagnostic and Statistical Manual* of the American Psychiatric Association (DSM-IV) criteria for cannabis abuse and dependency.[46] Table 4 lists several of the common characteristics noted in late stage two and stage three of the stages of adolescent drug use.

IMPACT OF ADOLESCENT CANNABIS ABUSE ON THE FAMILY

Frequent drug use by one family member adversely affects every other family member to some degree and the family unit to a large degree. Individual family members adopt their own methods of coping with the turmoil engendered by adolescent drug use. Parents may attempt a variety of techniques to deal with their feelings of hurt, betrayal, anger, confusion, and inadequacy by cajoling, nagging, bribing, pleading, or threatening loss of privileges, overcompensation by spending more time in the office or away from home, or by an increase in their own use of intoxicants. Parents may overprotect their cannabis-abusing teenager by bailing the child out of trouble at school or with law enforcement agencies. The cannabis-abusing adolescent may thus be spared the painful consequences of his or her maladaptive acts. Siblings of the cannabis abuser may become ashamed, frightened, or intimidated by threats of harm should the sibling divulge the drug use to the parents. The adolescent who uses cannabis may apply intense pressure to younger siblings to initiate use of cannabis in order to share the blame and reduce the chance that the parents will find out about the cannabis use. Techniques for successful confrontation of the adolescent cannabis abuser by parents or paediatricians will not be detailed in this article but can be found in several publications.[47,48]

Key points for clinical practice

- 30% of 16-year-old students in the US and UK smoked cannabis during 2002.
- Abusing cannabis during teenage years has high risk of continuation as an adult.
- Cannabis has a powerful effect on emotions and mood, motor control when operating a motor vehicle, appetite, sleep, awareness of the passage of time, and short-term memory.

Key points for clinical practice (continued)

- Adverse effects from smoking cannabis during adolescence include an increase risk of motor vehicle and other accidents, bronchial disease with productive cough, school underachievement, and the possibility of cannabis abuse and dependence.

- High-grade cannabis is much more potent than similar products a few decades ago.

- Cannabis and marijuana Internet web sites are heavily dominated with pro-cannabis messages and sales pitches.

- Hashish is the type of cannabis used primarily in the UK while marijuana cigarettes are the type used primarily in the US.

- Hydroponic (soil-less) cultivation of cannabis is used extensively in the UK, Canada, and the US.

- Sinsemilla cannabis contains about twice the potency of common cannabis and it is about as potent as hashish.

- Cannabis is preferentially smoked by deeply inhaling and retaining the smoke in the respiratory bronchi.

- Intoxication from cannabis lasts about 3 h but motor incoordination may persist for many additional hours.

- Cannabis unquestionably exerts an adverse effect on short-term memory retention: it can interfere with learning during adolescence if it is smoked before school or when studying in the evening.

- Acute organ toxicity of cannabis is quite low, except for the respiratory tract and brain.

- Cannabis exerts frequent but inconsistent, physiological effects to impair vigilance, co-ordination, and reaction time to respond to emergencies during operation of motor vehicles.

- There is growing evidence of a relationship of frequent use of cannabis and the development of schizophrenia in those predisposed to that mental disease.

- All adolescent cannabis smokers are not equal. Those with multiple risk factors have a much greater chance of progressing to cannabis abuse and dependence.

- Experimentation with cannabis is not necessary problematic but who can predict the person who progresses to multiple and frequent drug use.

- Frequent use of cannabis during early adolescence can be associated with delinquent/substance abusing peers, early school underachievement and drop-out, unprotected sex, unplanned early parenthood, and premature departure from the parental home.

- Frequent cannabis use is strongly associated with enormous strains on the family including parents and siblings.

References

1. Johnston LD, O'Malley PM, Bachman JG. *Monitoring the Future: National Survey results on Drug Use, 1975–2001*. Rockville, MD: National Institute on Drug Abuse (NIDA), US Department of Health and Human Services, 2002.
2. Anon. *Drug Use, Smoking, and Drinking among Young People in England in 2001*. London: National Centre for Social Research/National Foundation for Educational Research, 2002.
3. Perkonigg A, Lieb R, Hofler M *et al*. Patterns of cannabis use, abuse, and dependence over time: incidence, progression, and stability in a sample of 1228 adolescents. *Addiction* 1999; **94**: 1663–1678.
4. Iversen LL. (ed) *The Science of Marijuana*. New York, Oxford University Press, 2000; *Understanding Marijuana: a new look at scientific evidence, Mitch Earlywine*. New York: Oxford University Press, 2002.
5. Hall W. Reducing the harms caused by cannabis use: the policy debate in Australia. *Drug Alcohol Depend* 2001; **62**: 163–174.
6. Sidney S, Beck JE, Tekawa IS *et al*. Marijuana and mortality. *Am J Public Health* 1997; **87**: 585–590.
7. <www.drugs.gov.uk/newsandevents/news/cann>.
8. Kumar RN, Chambers WA, Pertwee RG. Pharmacological actions and therapeutic uses of cannabis and cannabinoids. *Anaesthesia* 2001; **56**: 1059–1068.
9. Ashton CH. Pharmacology and effects of cannabis: a brief review. *Br J Psychiatry* 2001; **178**: 101–106.
10. Johns A. Psychiatric effects of cannabis. *Br J Psychiatry* 2001; **178**: 116–122.
11. Hall W, Solowij N. Adverse effects of cannabis. *Lancet* 1998; **32**: 1611–1616.
12. Kalant H, Corrigal W, Hall W, Smart R, EDS. *The Health Effects of Cannabis*. Toronto, Ont: Addiction Research Foundation, 1999.
13. Adams IB, Martin BR. Cannabis: pharmacology and toxicology in animals and humans. *Addiction* 1996; **91**: 1585–1614.
14. Gruber AJ, Pope Jr HG. Marijuana use among adolescents. *Pediatr Clin North Am* 2002; **49**: 1–19.
15. Select Committee on Science and Technology. *Cannabis: The Scientific and Medical Evidence*. 9th Report, HL paper 151; 1997–1998.
16. Schwartz RH. Marijuana, a decade and a half later: still a crude drug with under-appreciated toxicity. *Pediatrics* 2002; **109**: 284–289.
17. El Sohly MA, Ross SA, Mehmedic Z *et al*. Potency of delta-9-THC and other cannabinoids in confiscated marijuana from 1980–1997. *J Forensic Sci* 2000; **45**: 24–30.
18. Siler JF, Sheep WL, Bates LB *et al*. Marijuana smoking in Panama. *Milit Surg* 1933; **73**: 269–280.
19. Ameri A. The effects of cannabinoids on the brain. *Prog Neurobiol* 1999; **58**: 315–348.
20. Chaloupka FJ, Pacula RL, Farrelly MC *et al*. *Do higher cigarette prices encourage youth to use marijuana?* Working Paper 6939. Cambridge, MA: National Bureau of Economic Research, <http://www.nber.org/papers/w6939>.
21. Hollister LE. Marijuana and immunity. *J Psychoactive Drugs* 1992; **24**: 159–164.
22. Zuckerman B, Frank D, Hingson R *et al*. Effects of maternal marijuana and cocaine use on fetal growth. *N Engl J Med* 1989; **320**: 762–768.
23. Hall W, Solowij N, Lemon J. The health and psychological consequences of cannabis use. In: Kalant H, Corrigal W, Hall W, Smart R. (eds) *The Health Effects of Cannabis*. Toronto: Addiction Research Foundation, 1998.
24. Smiley A. *Marijuana: on road and driving simulator studies*. In: Kalant H, Corrigal W, Hall W, Smart R. (eds) *The Health Effects of Cannabis*. Toronto: Addiction Research Foundation, 1998.
25. Institute for Human Psychopharmacology. *Marijuana, Alcohol, and Actual Driving Performance*. NTSA Technology Transfer Series, Monograph Department of Transportation (DOT) 808939. Washington, DC: National Highway Traffic Safety Administration, 1999; 201: 1–4.
26. Zammit S, Allebeck P, Andreasson S *et al*. Self reported cannabis use as a risk factor for schizophrenia in Swedish conscripts of 1969: historical cohort study. *BMJ* 2002; **325**:

1199–1201.

27. Arseneault L, Cannon M, Poulton R *et al*. Cannabis use in adolescence and risk for adult psychosis: longitudinal prospective study. *BMJ* 2002; **325**: 1212–1213.

28. Schwartz RH. Heavy marijuana use and recent memory impairment. *Psychiatry Ann* 1991; **21**: 80–82.

29. Hendin H, Haas AP, Singer P *et al. Living High: Daily Marijuana Use Among Adults*. New York, NY: Human Sciences Press, 1987.

30. Block RL. Does heavy marijuana use impair human cognition and brain function? *JAMA* 1996; **275**: 560–561.

31. Pope HG, Yurgelum Todd D. The residual cognitive effects of heavy marijuana use. *JAMA* 1996; **275**: 521–527.

32. Solowij N, Do cognitive impairments recover following cessation of cannabis use? *Life Sci* 1995; **56**: 2119–2126.

33. Solowij N. *Cannabis and Cognitive Functioning*. Cambridge, UK: Cambridge University Press, 1998.

34. Hammer T, Vaglum P. Initiation, continuation, or discontinuation of cannabis use in the general population. *Br J Addict* 1990; **85**: 899–909.

35. Chilcoat HD, Anthony JC. Impact of parent monitoring on initiation of drug use through late childhood. *J Am Acad Child Adolesc Psychiatry* 1996; **35**: 91–100.

36. Resnick MD, Bearman PS, Blum RW *et al*. Protecting adolescents from harm: findings from the National Longitudinal Study on Adolescent Health. *JAMA* 1997; **278**: 823–832.

37. Schwartz RH. Comments on cannabis intoxication in pets. *Vet Hum Toxicol* 1989; **31**: 262.

38. Lynskey M, Hall W. The effects of adolescent cannabis use on educational attainment: a review. *Addiction* 2000; **95**: 1621–1630.

39. Schwartz RH, Hoffmann NG, Jones R. Behavioral, psychosocial, and academic correlates of marijuana usage in adolescence: a study of a cohort under treatment. *Clin Pediatr* 1987; **29**: 254–270.

40. Kendel DB, Yamaguchi K, Chen K. Stages of progression in drug involvement from adolescence to adulthood: further evidence for the gateway theory. *J Stud Alcohol* 1992; **53**: 447–457.

41. Miller TQ. A test of alternative explanations for the stage-like progression of adolescent substance use in four national samples. *Addict Behaviors* 1994; **19**: 287–293.

42. Hall W, Solowij N. Adverse effects of cannabis. *Lancet* 1998; **352**: 1611–1616.

43. Royal College of Psychiatrists and Royal College of Physicians. *Drugs Dilemmas and Choices*. London: Royal College of Psychiatrists and Royal College of Physicians 2000.

44. Kingree JB, Braithwaite R, Woodring T. Unprotected sex as a function of alcohol and marijuana use among adolescent detainees. *J Adolesc Health* 2000; **27**: 179–185.

45. Taylor RD, Poulton R, Moffitt TE *et al*. The respiratory effects of cannabis dependence in young adults. *Addiction* 2000; **95**: 1669–1677.

46. American Psychiatric Association. *Diagnostic and Statistical Manual of Mental Disorders*, 4th edn. Washington, DC, American Psychiatric Association, 2000.

47. Schwartz RH, Cohen PR, Bair GO. Identifying and coping with a drug-using adolescent: some guidelines for pediatricians and parents. *Pediatr Rev* 1985; **7**: 133–139.

48. Jenny L, Schwartz RH. Adolescent drug dependency and the family. *Virginia Med* 1985; **112**: 711–713.

John P. Kinsella

10

Therapy with inhaled nitric oxide in the newborn

The recent introduction of inhaled nitric oxide therapy to the treatment of newborns with hypoxaemic respiratory failure and pulmonary hypertension has dramatically changed management strategies for this critically ill population. Inhaled nitric oxide (iNO) therapy causes potent, selective, and sustained pulmonary vasodilation and improves oxygenation in term newborns with severe hypoxaemic respiratory failure and persistent pulmonary hypertension.[1–6] Multicentre randomised clinical studies have demonstrated that iNO therapy reduces the need for extracorporeal membrane oxygenation (ECMO) treatment in term neonates with hypoxaemic respiratory failure.[7,8] In this article, I will review an approach to the initial evaluation of the hypoxaemic newborn for treatment with iNO, summarise the clinical experience with iNO in near-term and term newborns, and propose guidelines for the use of iNO in this population. The potential role of iNO in the preterm newborn is currently controversial and its use remains investigational in this population.[9]

RATIONALE FOR INHALED NITRIC OXIDE THERAPY

The physiological rationale for iNO therapy in the treatment of neonatal hypoxaemic respiratory failure is based upon its ability to achieve potent and sustained pulmonary vasodilation without decreasing systemic vascular tone.[10] Persistent pulmonary hypertension of the newborn[11] is a syndrome associated with diverse neonatal cardiac and pulmonary disorders that are characterised by high pulmonary vascular resistance (PVR) causing extrapulmonary right-to-left shunting of blood across the ductus arteriosus and/or foramen ovale.[12] Extrapulmonary shunting due to high pulmonary

John P. Kinsella MD
Division of Neonatology, Box B-070, The Children's Hospital, 1056 E. 19th Ave, Denver, CO 80218-1088, USA. Tel: +1 303 861 6194; Fax: +1 303 764 8117; E-mail: john.kinsella@uchsc.edu

vascular resistance in severe persistent pulmonary hypertension of the newborn can cause critical hypoxaemia which is poorly responsive to inspired oxygen or pharmacological vasodilation. Vasodilator drugs administered intravenously, such as tolazoline and sodium nitroprusside, are often unsuccessful due to systemic hypotension and an inability to achieve or sustain pulmonary vasodilation.[13,14] Thus, the ability of iNO therapy to selectively lower pulmonary vascular resistance and decrease extrapulmonary venoarterial admixture accounts for the acute improvement in oxygenation observed in newborns with persistent pulmonary hypertension of the newborn.[15]

As described in children[16] and adults with severe respiratory failure,[17] oxygenation can also improve during iNO therapy in some newborns who do not have extrapulmonary right-to-left shunting. Hypoxaemia in these cases is primarily due to intrapulmonary shunting caused by continued perfusion of lung units that lack ventilation (*e.g.* atelectasis), with variable contributions from ventilation/perfusion (V/Q) inequality. Distinct from its ability to decrease extrapulmonary right-to-left shunting by reducing pulmonary vascular resistance, low dose iNO therapy can also improve oxygenation by redirecting blood from poorly aerated or diseased lung regions to better aerated distal air spaces ('microselective effect').[18]

In addition to its effects on vascular tone and reactivity, other physiological targets for iNO therapy in hypoxaemic respiratory failure may include direct effects of NO on lung inflammation, vascular permeability, and thrombosis *in situ*. Although some laboratory studies have suggested that NO can potentiate lung injury by promoting oxidative or nitrosative stress,[19] inactivating surfactant and stimulating inflammation,[20] others have demonstrated striking antioxidant and anti-inflammatory effects in models of lung injury.[21–23] Thus, clinical benefits of low-dose iNO therapy may include reduced lung inflammation and oedema, as well as potential protective effects on surfactant function,[24] but these effects remain clinically unproven.

Finally, the diagnostic value of iNO therapy is also important, in that failure to respond to iNO raises important questions about the specific mechanism of hypoxaemia. Poor responses to iNO should lead to further diagnostic evaluation for 'unsuspected' anatomical cardiovascular or pulmonary disease.

EVALUATION OF THE TERM NEWBORN FOR INHALED NITRIC OXIDE THERAPY

HISTORY

Evaluation of the newborn with cyanosis begins with an approach designed to assess the primary cause of hypoxaemia. Marked hypoxaemia in the newborn can be caused by lung parenchymal disease with intrapulmonary shunting, pulmonary vascular disease causing extrapulmonary right-to-left shunting, or anatomic right-to-left shunting associated with congenital heart disease.

This evaluation should begin with the history and assessment of risk factors for hypoxaemic respiratory failure. Relevant history may include the results of prenatal ultrasound studies. Lesions such as diaphragmatic hernia and cystic adenomatoid formation are diagnosed prenatally with increasing frequency. Although many anatomical congenital heart diseases can be diagnosed prenatally, vascular abnormalities (*e.g.* co-arctation, anomalous pulmonary venous return) are more difficult to diagnose using prenatal ultrasound. Thus, a history of a structurally normal heart by fetal ultrasonography should be confirmed with echocardiography in the newborn with cyanosis.

Other historical information which may be important in the evaluation of the cyanotic newborn includes a history of severe and prolonged oligohydramnios causing pulmonary hypoplasia. Prolonged fetal brady- and tachy-arrhythmias and marked anaemia (caused by haemolysis, twin–twin transfusion or chronic haemorrhage) may cause congestive heart failure, pulmonary oedema and respiratory distress. Maternal illness (*e.g.* diabetes mellitus), medications (aspirin causing premature constriction of the ductus arteriosus, association of Ebstein Malformation with maternal lithium use), and drug use may contribute to disordered transition and cardiopulmonary distress in the newborn. Risk factors for infection causing sepsis/pneumonia should also be considered, including premature or prolonged rupture of membranes, fetal tachycardia, maternal leukocytosis, uterine tenderness and other signs of intra-amniotic infection.

Events at delivery may also provide clues to the aetiology of hypoxaemic respiratory failure in the newborn. For example, if positive pressure ventilation is required in the delivery room, the risk of pneumothorax increases. A history of meconium-stained amniotic fluid, particularly if meconium is present below the cords, is the *sine qua non* of meconium aspiration syndrome. Birth trauma (*e.g.* clavicular fracture and phrenic nerve injury) or acute feto–maternal/feto–placental haemorrhage may also cause respiratory distress in the newborn.

PHYSICAL EXAMINATION

The initial physical examination provides important clues to the aetiology of cyanosis. Marked respiratory distress in the newborn (retractions, grunting, nasal flaring) suggest the presence of pulmonary parenchymal disease with decreased lung compliance. However, it is important to recognise that airways disease (*e.g.* tracheo-bronchomalacia) and metabolic acidaemia can also cause severe respiratory distress. In contrast, the newborn with cyanosis alone ('non-distressed tachypnea') typically has cyanotic congenital heart disease (most commonly transposition of the great vessels) or idiopathic persistent pulmonary hypertension of the newborn.

INTERPRETATION OF PULSE OXIMETRY MEASUREMENTS

Right-to-left shunting across the ductus arteriosus causes post-ductal desaturation. Thus, the interpretation of pre-ductal (right hand) and post-ductal (lower extremity) saturation by pulse oximetry provides important clues to the aetiology of hypoxaemia in the newborn. However, it is important to recognise that variability in oximetry readings may be related to differences in available devices and affected by local perfusion.

If the measurements of pre- and post-ductal SaO_2 are equivalent, this suggests either that the ductus arteriosus is patent and pulmonary vascular resistance is sub-systemic (*i.e.* the hypoxaemia is caused by parenchymal lung disease with intrapulmonary shunting or cyanotic heart disease with ductal-dependent pulmonary blood flow), or that the ductus arteriosus is closed (precluding any interpretation of pulmonary artery pressure without echocardiography). It is exceptionally uncommon for the ductus arteriosus to close in the first hours of life in the presence of suprasystemic pulmonary artery pressures.

When the post-ductal SaO_2 is lower than pre-ductal SaO_2 (> 5%), the most common cause is suprasystemic pulmonary vascular resistance in persistent pulmonary hypertension of the newborn. causing right-to-left shunting across the ductus arteriosus (associated with meconium aspiration syndrome, surfactant deficiency/dysfunction, congenital diaphragmatic hernia, pulmonary hypoplasia, or idiopathic). However, the ductal-dependent systemic blood flow lesions (hypoplastic left heart syndrome, critical aortic stenosis, interrupted aortic arch, and co-arctation) may also present with post-ductal desaturation. Moreover, anatomical pulmonary vascular disease (alveolar–capillary dysplasia, pulmonary venous stenosis, and anomalous venous return with obstruction) can cause suprasystemic pulmonary vascular resistance with right-to-left shunting across the ductus arteriosus and post-ductal desaturation.

Finally, the unusual occurrence of markedly lower pre-ductal SaO_2 compared to post-ductal measurements suggest one of two diagnoses – transposition of the great vessels with pulmonary hypertension or co-arctation of the aorta.

LABORATORY AND RADIOLOGICAL EVALUATION

One of the most important tests to perform in the evaluation of the newborn with cyanosis is the chest radiograph (CXR). The CXR can demonstrate the classic findings of respiratory distress syndrome (RDS) (air bronchograms, diffuse granularity, and underinflation), meconium aspiration syndrome, and congenital diaphragmatic hernia. Perhaps the most important question to ask when viewing the CXR is whether the severity of hypoxaemia is out of proportion to the radiographic changes. In other words, marked hypoxaemia despite supplemental oxygen in the absence of severe pulmonary parenchymal disease radiographically suggests the presence of an extrapulmonary right-to-left shunt (idiopathic persistent pulmonary hypertension of the newborn or cyanotic heart disease).

Other essential measurements include an arterial blood gas to determine the blood gas tensions and pH, a complete blood count to evaluate for signs of infection, and blood pressure measurements in the right arm and a lower extremity to determine aortic obstruction (interrupted aortic arch, co-arctation).

RESPONSE TO SUPPLEMENTAL OXYGEN (100% OXYGEN BY HOOD, MASK OR ENDOTRACHEAL TUBE)

Marked improvement in SaO_2 (increase to 100%) with supplemental oxygen suggests an intrapulmonary shunt (lung disease) or reactive persistent pulmonary hypertension of the newborn with vasodilation. The response to mask CPAP is also a useful discriminator between severe lung disease and other causes of hypoxaemia. Most patients with persistent pulmonary hypertension of the newborn have at least a transient improvement in oxygenation in response to interventions such as high inspired oxygen and/or mechanical ventilation. If the pre-ductal SaO_2 never reaches 100%, the likelihood of cyanotic heart disease is high.

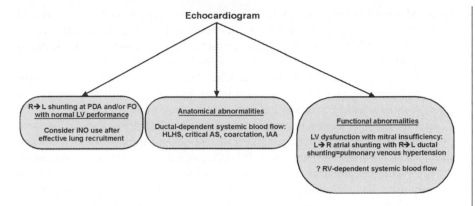

Fig. 1 Echocardiography in the initial evaluation and ongoing management of the hypoxemic newborn.

ECHOCARDIOGRAPHY

The above evaluation should be done regardless of the institutional level of neonatal care. However, the definitive diagnosis in newborns with cyanosis and hypoxaemic respiratory failure often requires echocardiography. Echocardiography has become a vital tool in the clinical management of newborns with cyanosis and hypoxaemic respiratory failure. The initial echocardiographic evaluation is important to rule-out structural heart disease causing hypoxaemia (*e.g.* co-arctation of the aorta and total anomalous pulmonary venous return). Moreover, it is critically important to diagnose congenital heart lesions for which iNO treatment would be contra-indicated. In addition to the lesions mentioned above, congenital heart diseases that can present with hypoxaemia unresponsive to high inspired oxygen concentrations (*i.e.* dependent on right-to-left shunting across the ductus arteriosus) include critical aortic stenosis, interrupted aortic arch, and hypoplastic left heart syndrome. Decreasing pulmonary vascular resistance with iNO in these conditions could lead to systemic hypoperfusion and delay definitive diagnosis.

Echocardiographic evaluation is an essential component in the initial evaluation and ongoing management of the hypoxaemic newborn (Fig. 1). Not all hypoxaemic term newborns have echocardiographic signs of persistent pulmonary hypertension of the newborn. As noted above, hypoxaemia can be caused by intrapulmonary right-to-left shunting or V/Q disturbances associated with severe lung disease and, in unusual circumstances, right-to-left shunting can also occur across pulmonary-to-systemic collaterals. However, extrapulmonary right-to-left shunting at the foramen ovale and/or ductus arteriosus also complicates hypoxaemic respiratory failure, and must be assessed in order to determine initial treatments and to evaluate the response to those therapies.

Persistent pulmonary hypertension of the newborn is defined by the echocardiographic determination of extrapulmonary venoarterial admixture (right-to-left shunting at the foramen ovale and/or ductus arteriosus), not simply evidence of increased pulmonary vascular resistance. Because elevated pulmonary vascular resistance alone does not directly cause hypoxaemia, other echocardiographic signs suggestive of pulmonary hypertension (*e.g.* increased right ventricular systolic time intervals and septal flattening) are less helpful.

Doppler measurements of atrial and ductal level shunts provide essential information when managing a newborn with hypoxaemic respiratory failure. For example, left-to-right shunting at the foramen ovale and ductus with marked hypoxaemia suggests predominant intrapulmonary shunting, and interventions should be directed at optimising lung inflation.

Finally, the measurements made with echocardiography can be used to predict or interpret the response or lack of response to various treatments. For example, in the presence of severe left ventricular dysfunction and pulmonary hypertension, pulmonary vasodilation alone may be ineffective in improving oxygenation. The echocardiographic findings in this setting include right-to-left ductal shunting (caused by suprasystemic pulmonary vascular resistance), and mitral insufficiency with left-to-right atrial shunting.

This constellation of findings suggests that left ventricular dysfunction may be contributing to pulmonary venous hypertension, such as occurs in congestive heart failure. In this setting, pulmonary vasodilation alone (without improving cardiac performance) will not cause sustained improvement in oxygenation. Thus, careful echocardiographic assessment will provide invaluable information about the underlying pathophysiology and will help guide the course of treatment.

Therefore, the initial echocardiographic evaluation determines both structural and functional (*i.e.* extrapulmonary right-to-left shunting in persistent pulmonary hypertension of the newborn, left ventricular performance, etc.) causes of hypoxaemia. Serial echocardiography is important to determine the response to interventions (*e.g.* pulmonary vasodilators) and for re-evaluation in cases where specific interventions have not caused improvement or with progressive clinical deterioration. For example, in a patient with extrapulmonary right-to-left shunting and severe lung disease, pulmonary vasodilation might reverse the right-to-left venous admixture with little improvement in systemic oxygenation. These observations unmask the critically important contribution of intrapulmonary shunting to hypoxaemia.

CANDIDATES FOR INHALED NITRIC OXIDE THERAPY

THE CLINICAL CONDITION

Due to its selective pulmonary vasodilator effects, iNO therapy is an important adjunct to available treatments for term newborns with hypoxaemic respiratory failure. However, hypoxaemic respiratory failure in the term newborn represents a heterogeneous group of disorders, and disease-specific responses have clearly been described.

Several pathophysiological disturbances contribute to hypoxaemia in the newborn infant, including cardiac dysfunction, airway and pulmonary parenchymal abnormalities, and pulmonary vascular disorders. In some newborns with hypoxaemic respiratory failure, a single mechanism predominates (*e.g.* extrapulmonary right-to-left shunting in idiopathic persistent pulmonary hypertension of the newborn, but more commonly, several of these mechanisms contribute to hypoxaemia. For example, in a newborn with meconium aspiration syndrome, meconium may obstruct some airways decreasing V/Q ratios and increasing intrapulmonary shunting. Other lung segments may be over-ventilated relative to perfusion and cause increased physiological dead space. Moreover, the same patient may have severe pulmonary hypertension with extrapulmonary right-to-left shunting at the ductus arteriosus and foramen ovale. Not only does the overlap of these mechanisms complicate the clinical management, but the tendency for time-dependent changes in the relative contribution of each mechanism to hypoxaemia requires continued vigilance as the disease progresses. Therefore, understanding the relative contribution of these different causes of hypoxaemia becomes critically important as the inventory of therapeutic options expands.

Considering the important role of parenchymal lung disease in many cases of persistent pulmonary hypertension of the newborn, pharmacological pulmonary vasodilation alone would not be expected to cause sustained clinical improvement. The effects of inhaled NO may be suboptimal when lung volume is decreased in association with pulmonary parenchymal disease.[25] Atelectasis and air space disease (pneumonia, pulmonary oedema) will decrease effective delivery of iNO to its site of action in terminal lung units. In persistent pulmonary hypertension of the newborn associated with heterogeneous (patchy) parenchymal lung disease, inhaled NO may be effective in optimising ventilation-perfusion matching by preferentially causing vasodilation in lung units which are well ventilated. The effects of inhaled NO on ventilation-perfusion matching appear to be optimal at low doses (< 20 ppm).[17,26] However, in cases complicated by homogeneous (diffuse) parenchymal lung disease and underinflation, pulmonary hypertension may be exacerbated because of the adverse mechanical effects of underinflation on pulmonary vascular resistance. In this setting, effective treatment of the underlying lung disease is essential (and sometimes sufficient) to cause resolution of the accompanying pulmonary hypertension.

CLINICAL CRITERIA

Gestational and postnatal age

Available evidence from clinical trials supports the use of iNO in near-term (> 34 weeks' gestation) and term newborns.[7,8] The use of iNO in infants less than 34 weeks' gestation remains investigational (see below). Clinical trials of iNO in the newborn have incorporated ECMO treatment as an end-point. Therefore, most patients have been enrolled in the first few days of life. Although one of the pivotal studies used to support the new drug application for iNO therapy included as an entry criterion a postnatal age up to 14 days, the average age at enrolment in that study was 1.7 days.[7] Currently, clinical trials support the use of iNO before treatment with ECMO, usually within the first week of life. However, clinical experience suggests that iNO may be of benefit as an adjuvant treatment after ECMO therapy in patients with sustained pulmonary hypertension (*e.g.* congenital diaphragmatic hernia). Thus, postnatal age alone should not define the duration of therapy in cases where prolonged treatment could be beneficial.

Severity of illness

Studies support the use of iNO in infants who have hypoxaemic respiratory failure with evidence of persistent pulmonary hypertension of the newborn, who require mechanical ventilation and high inspired oxygen concentrations. The most common criterion employed has been the oxygenation index. Although clinical trials commonly allowed for enrolment with oxygenation index levels > 25, the mean level at study entry in multicentre trials was about 40.[3,7]

Thus it is unclear whether infants with less severe hypoxaemia would benefit from iNO therapy. However, Davidson et al.[6] reported a controlled clinical trial in which the average oxygenation index at study entry was 24 ± 9. It is important to note that iNO treatment did not reduce ECMO utilisation in this study. Although entry criteria for this trial included echocardiographic evidence of pulmonary hypertension, only 9% of the patients had clinical evidence of right-to-left ductal shunting. Because of the mechanism of action of iNO as a selective pulmonary vasodilator, it is likely that acute improvement in oxygenation caused by decreased pulmonary vascular resistance and reduced extrapulmonary right-to-left shunting would be most predictive of clinical improvement.[7] Therefore, current multicentre studies suggest that indications for treatment with iNO may include an oxygenation index > 25 with echocardiographic evidence of extrapulmonary right-to-left shunting.

TREATMENT STRATEGIES

DOSE

The first studies of iNO treatment in term newborns reported initial doses that ranged from 80 ppm[1] to 6–20 ppm.[2] These laboratory and clinical studies established the boundaries of iNO dosing protocols for subsequent randomised, clinical trials in newborns.[3-5] Increasing the dose to 40 ppm does not generally improve oxygenation in patients who do not respond to the lower dose of 20 ppm.[3] The initial dose in the NINOS trial was 20 ppm, but the dose was increased to 80 ppm if the improvement in PaO_2 was less than 20 torr.[7] In this study, only 3 of 53 infants (6%) who had little response to 20 ppm had an increase in PaO_2 > 20 torr when treated with 80 ppm iNO. Whether a progressive increase in PaO_2 would have occurred with continued exposure to 20 ppm could not be determined with this study design. Roberts et al.[4] initiated treatment with 80 ppm NO and subsequently weaned the iNO concentration if oxygenation improved, thus the effects of lower initial iNO doses could not be evaluated and the effects on ECMO utilisation were not evaluated.

Another trial evaluated the effects of sustained exposure to different doses of iNO in separate treatment groups of newborns. Davidson et al.[6] reported the results of a randomised, controlled, dose-response trial in term newborns with hypoxaemic respiratory failure. In this study, patients were randomised to treatment with either 0 (placebo), 5, 20 or 80 ppm NO. Each iNO dose improved oxygenation compared to placebo, but there was no difference in responses between groups. However, at 80 ppm, methaemoglobinaemia (blood levels > 7%) occurred in 13 of 37 patients (35%) and high inspired NO_2 concentrations (> 3 ppm) were reported in 7 of 37 patients (19%). Thus, iNO at a dose of 80 ppm was not more effective in improving oxygenation than 5 or 20 ppm, and was associated with adverse effects.

The available evidence, therefore, supports the use of doses of iNO beginning at 20 ppm in term newborns with persistent pulmonary hypertension, since this strategy decreased ECMO utilisation without an increased incidence of adverse effects. Although brief exposures to higher doses (40–80 ppm) appear to be safe, sustained treatment with 80 ppm NO increases the risk of methaemo-globinaemia.

DURATION OF TREATMENT

In multicentre, clinical trials of iNO therapy, the typical duration of iNO treatment has been less than 5 days, which parallels the clinical resolution of persistent pulmonary hypertension. However, individual exceptions occur, particularly in cases of pulmonary hypoplasia.[27] If iNO is required for longer than 5 days, investigations into other causes of pulmonary hypertension should be considered (e.g. alveolar capillary dysplasia), particularly if discontinuation of iNO results in suprasystemic elevations of pulmonary artery pressure by echocardiography. In our practice, we discontinue iNO if the FiO_2 is < 0.60 and the PaO_2 is > 60 without evidence of rebound pulmonary hypertension or an increase in FiO_2 > 15% after iNO withdrawal.

In the pre-iNO era, concerns were also raised about delaying ECMO therapy if conventional treatment was prolonged. However, these retro-spective data do not account for recent changes in management strategies, including newer ventilator devices and exogenous surfactant therapy. Moreover, decreased ECMO utilisation with iNO treatment in recent multicentre, controlled trials has not been associated with an increased incidence of chronic lung disease.[7] Indeed, in the most recent trial, iNO treatment was associated with improved pulmonary outcomes.[8] No controlled data are available to determine the maximal safe duration of iNO therapy.

WEANING

After improvement in oxygenation occurs with the onset of iNO therapy, strategies for weaning the iNO dose become important. Numerous approaches have been employed, and little differences have been noted until final discontinuation of iNO treatment. In one study, iNO was reduced from 20 ppm to 6 ppm after 4 h of treatment without acute changes in oxygenation. In another trial, iNO was reduced in a stepwise fashion to as low as 1 ppm without changes in oxygenation.[28]

MONITORING

Early experience suggested that careful monitoring of NO and NO_2 levels should be done with chemiluminescence devices. It has now become clear that NO_2 levels remain low at delivered iNO doses within the recommended ranges, and that electrochemical devices are reliable. The currently available systems use electrochemical cells and appear to be reliable when used appropriately. However, the response time of electrochemical sensors is relatively slow and these devices are not accurate when measurement of acute changes in

NO concentrations are desired.

Methaemoglobinaemia occurs after exposure to high concentrations of iNO (80 ppm).[6] This complication has not been reported at lower doses of iNO (< 20 ppm). However, because methaemoglobin reductase deficiency may occur unpredictably, it is reasonable to measure methaemoglobin levels by co-oximetry within 4 h of starting iNO therapy and subsequently at 24 h intervals.

VENTILATOR MANAGEMENT

Along with iNO treatment, other therapeutic strategies have emerged for the management of the term infant with hypoxaemic respiratory failure. Considering the important role of parenchymal lung disease in specific disorders included in the syndrome of persistent pulmonary hypertension of the newborn (PPHN), pharmacological pulmonary vasodilation alone should not be expected to cause sustained clinical improvement in many cases.[29] Moreover, patients not responding to iNO can show marked improvement in oxygenation with adequate lung inflation alone.[22] High success rates in early studies were achieved by withholding iNO treatment until aggressive attempts were made to optimise ventilation and lung inflation with mechanical ventilation. These early studies demonstrated that the effects of iNO may be suboptimal when lung volume is decreased in association with pulmonary parenchymal disease, for several reasons. First, atelectasis and air space disease (pneumonia, pulmonary oedema) may decrease the effective delivery of iNO to its site of action in terminal lung units. Second, in cases complicated by severe lung disease and underinflation, pulmonary hypertension may be exacerbated because of the adverse mechanical effects of underinflation on pulmonary vascular resistance. Third, attention must be given to minimise overinflation to avoid inadvertent positive end expiratory pressure and gas trapping that may elevate pulmonary vascular resistance from vascular compression. This commonly complicates the management of infants with asymmetric lung disease or airways obstruction as observed in meconium aspiration syndrome (MAS).

In newborns with severe lung disease, high frequency oscillatory ventilation (HFOV) is frequently used to optimise lung inflation and minimise lung injury.[30] In clinical pilot studies using iNO, we found that the combination of HFOV and iNO caused the greatest improvement in oxygenation in some newborns who had severe pulmonary hypertension complicated by diffuse parenchymal lung disease and underinflation (e.g. respiratory distress syndrome, pneumonia).[31,32] A randomised, multicentre trial demonstrated that treatment with HFOV + iNO was often successful in patients who failed to respond to HFOV or iNO alone in severe pulmonary hypertension, and differences in responses were related to the specific disease associated with the various complex disorders (Fig. 2).[3] For patients with pulmonary hypertension complicated by severe lung disease, response rates for HFOV + iNO were better than HFOV alone or iNO with conventional ventilation. In contrast, for patients without significant parenchymal lung disease, both iNO and HFOV + iNO were more effective than HFOV alone. This response to combined treatment with HFOV + iNO likely reflects both improvement in intrapulmonary shunting in patients with severe lung disease and pulmonary hypertension (using a strategy designed to recruit and sustain lung volume, rather than to hyperventilate) and augmented NO delivery to its site of action. Although iNO may be an effective treatment for pulmonary hypertension, it should be

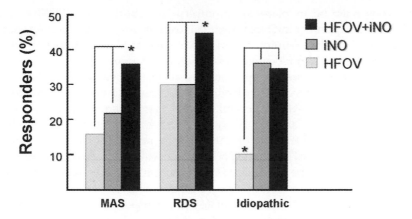

Fig. 2 Lung recruitment with HFOV ventilation augments response to iNO in newborns with PPHN and lung disease. After Kinsella et al.[3] [MAS, meconium aspiration syndrome; HFOV, High frequency oscillatory ventilation; RDS, respiratory distress syndrome; iNO, inhaled nitric oxide]

considered only as part of an overall clinical strategy that cautiously manages parenchymal lung disease, cardiac performance, and systemic haemodynamics.

USE IN NON-ECMO CENTRES AND TRANSPORT WITH INHALED NITRIC OXIDE

Published reports on the use of iNO in ECMO centres have not substantiated early concerns that iNO would adversely affect outcome by delaying ECMO utilisation. In one study, the median time from randomisation to treatment with ECMO was 4.4 and 6.7 h for the control and iNO groups, respectively.[17] Although this difference was statistically significant, there were no apparent adverse consequences caused by the delay. Indeed, iNO treatment may play an important role in stabilising patients before ECMO is initiated, thus improving the chances that ECMO cannulation may proceed without progressive clinical deterioration.[5]

However, the potential dissemination of iNO therapy to non-ECMO centres warrants a cautious approach. Whether the use of iNO for pulmonary hypertension in non-ECMO centres will cause undue delays in initiation of transport to an ECMO centre, increase the risks of transport, or significantly delay ECMO cannot be determined from the currently available evidence from clinical trials. It is likely that promising new therapies for severe hypoxaemic respiratory failure will not be limited to centres which provide all modes of rescue treatment. Although marked improvement in oxygenation occurs in many term newborns with severe pulmonary hypertension, sustained improvement may be compromised in some patients by the nature of the underlying disease leading to progressive changes in lung compliance or cardiovascular dysfunction.[33] When the clinical course is complicated by progression in severity of the cardiopulmonary disease, withdrawal of iNO during transport to an ECMO centre may lead to acute deterioration. In such cases, iNO provides an important therapeutic bridge assuring stability during transport. When progressive deterioration in oxygenation occurs during iNO treatment in institutions which cannot offer more advanced rescue therapy, provisions must be in place to accomplish transport to the ECMO centre without interruption of iNO treatment.[34] Hospitals that are not ECMO centres and cannot guarantee uninterrupted iNO deliver during transport to an ECMO centre should not begin an iNO therapy programme.

Continuing iNO during transport sustains acute improvements in oxygenation and diminishes the oxygenation lability characteristic of persistent pulmonary hypertension of the newborn. Several delivery systems are available to provide iNO during transport, and can be easily incorporated into transport modules. Considering the proliferation of iNO use in non-ECMO centres, prudent integration of functional iNO transport systems within the catchment area of an ECMO centre should be a priority. Finally, the use of HFOV and iNO in non-ECMO centres may pose undue risk for infants who subsequently need to be transported. However, iNO may facilitate these transport missions by decreasing vasolability and stabilising oxygenation en route.

FUTURE APPLICATIONS OF INHALED NITRIC OXIDE THERAPY

CONGENITAL DIAPHRAGMATIC HERNIA

The cause of hypoxaemic respiratory failure in patients with congenital diaphragmatic hernia is complex, and includes pulmonary hypoplasia, surfactant dysfunction, functional and structural abnormalities of the pulmonary vascular bed, and left ventricular dysfunction. Early experience with iNO in this disease showed that some patients had sustained improvement in oxygenation.[17] However, Karamanoukian et al.[35] found little improvement in oxygenation with iNO treatment in patients with diaphragmatic hernia before treatment with ECMO, despite treatment with surfactant. The only randomised, controlled trial of iNO treatment in patients with diaphragmatic hernia found no difference in ECMO utilisation between NO treated and control infants. Although iNO may be an effective therapy in some patients with diaphragmatic hernia and pulmonary hypertension, these patients are poor responders as a group.[36] The lack of apparent efficacy in this disease may be related, in large measure, to the complexity of this disorder.

However, there is a subset of newborns with diaphragmatic hernia who have prolonged pulmonary hypertension despite marked improvements in pulmonary function and gas exchange. A recent study evaluated the role of non-invasive delivery of iNO (using nasal cannula) in newborns with protracted pulmonary hypertension.[37] These investigators found that iNO can be effectively delivered using nasal cannula to newborns with diaphragmatic hernia who have protracted pulmonary hypertension, potentially reducing the duration of mechanical ventilation, while safely treating the pulmonary hypertension.

THE PRETERM NEWBORN

Another area of investigation which is of vital clinical importance involves the role of iNO therapy in preterm newborns with hypoxaemic respiratory failure. Preliminary studies in human preterm neonates with severe hypoxaemic

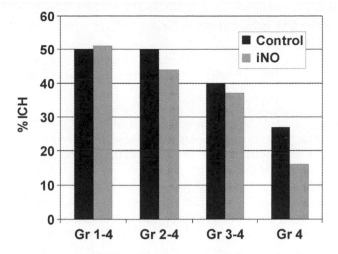

Fig. 3 The incidence of intracranial haemorrhage (ICH) between the control and iNO treated groups.

respiratory failure support the potential role of low-dose iNO as adjuvant therapy. In a small, unmasked, randomised trial of iNO (20 ppm) and dexamethasone treatment, no differences were found in survival, chronic lung disease, or intracranial haemorrhage between iNO treated infants and controls.

To begin to address the potential safety and efficacy of iNO in preterm newborns, we recently conducted a randomised controlled trial of iNO in preterm neonates with severe, hypoxaemic respiratory failure.[38] We randomised 80 preterm newborns of gestational age < 34 weeks with severe hypoxaemic respiratory failure in 12 perinatal centres that provide tertiary care. In all, 48 patients were treated with iNO (5 ppm) and 32 served as controls. Treatment assignment was masked. The primary outcome variable was survival to discharge. Secondary outcome variables included incidence and severity of intracranial haemorrhage, pulmonary haemorrhage, duration of mechanical ventilation, and chronic lung disease at 36 weeks post-conceptional age. In this study, there were no differences between iNO treatment and control groups in baseline characteristics or severity of disease. Inhaled NO acutely improved oxygenation after 60 min of treatment. Survival to discharge was 52% in the iNO group and 47% in controls (P = NS). Total ventilator days for survivors was less for the iNO group (P = 0.046). In contrast to uncontrolled pilot studies, we found no difference in the incidence of intracranial haemorrhage between the control and iNO treated groups (Fig. 3). The incidence of periventricular leukomalacia was also not different between groups (8% of iNO patients and 13% of controls).

Thus, low-dose iNO caused acute improvement in oxygenation in preterm newborns with severe hypoxaemic respiratory failure, without increasing the risk of bleeding complications, including intracranial haemorrhage. Low-dose iNO may be effective as a lung-specific anti-inflammatory therapy to diminish lung neutrophil accumulation and the attendant inflammatory injury which contributes to the evolution of chronic lung disease. Currently, several multicentre clinical trials are underway to test the safety and efficacy of iNO in preterm newborns with respiratory failure.

Key points for clinical practice

- .Inhaled nitric oxide improves oxygenation and decreases extracorporeal life support utilisation in near-term (> 35 weeks' gestation) and term newborns with persistent pulmonary hypertension.

- Available data support the use of inhaled nitric oxide in this population with an oxygenation index > 25. Early, 'prophylactic' use of nitric oxide has not been demonstrated to reduce the need for subsequent 'rescue' nitric oxide treatment or extracorporeal life support.

- Echocardiography is important in determining the contribution of extrapulmonary right-to-left shunting to hypoxaemia in newborns with respiratory failure, and in the evaluation of structural and functional cardiovascular abnormalities.

- Effective lung recruitment is vital to optimise the pulmonary vasodilator effects of inhaled nitric oxide.

- High frequency oscillatory ventilation may be a useful adjuvant therapy to optimise lung recruitment in newborns with severe parenchymal lung disease and pulmonary hypertension; however, it should be used with caution in diseases characterised by gas trapping (e.g. meconium aspiration syndrome).

- From the available information, a reasonable recommendation for starting dose of inhaled nitric oxide in the term infant is 20 ppm, with reductions in dose over time.

- Toxicity is apparent at 80 ppm, causing increases in methaemoglobinaemia and inspired NO_2. High doses (> 20 ppm) of nitric oxide may also prolong bleeding time, but clinically significant increases in bleeding complications have not been reported in term newborns.

- The use of nitric oxide in non-ECMO centres must be done cautiously, with arrangements in place for transport to an ECMO centre without interrupting nitric oxide delivery in patients with sub-optimal acute responses.

- Non-invasive delivery of nitric oxide may be a safe and effective alternative in newborns with congenital diaphragmatic hernia and prolonged pulmonary hypertension.

- There is increasing evidence for the potential role of low-dose nitric oxide (5 ppm) in preterm newborns with hypoxaemic respiratory failure; however, clinical application should currently be limited to controlled trials which target outcomes of both safety and efficacy.

- There is insufficient evidence to support the use of other experimental therapies in persistent pulmonary hypertension such as inhaled ethyl nitrite gas, inhaled prostacyclin, and sildenafil. The proper role of these therapies awaits the results of controlled, clinical trials.

References

1. Roberts JD, Polaner DM, Lang P, Zapol WM. Inhaled nitric oxide in persistent pulmonary hypertension of the newborn. *Lancet* 1992; **340**: 818–819.
2. Kinsella JP, Neish SR, Shaffer E, Abman SH. Low-dose inhalational nitric oxide in persistent pulmonary hypertension of the newborn. *Lancet* 1992; **340**: 819–820.
3. Kinsella JP, Truog WE, Walsh WF *et al*. Randomized, multicenter trial of inhaled nitric oxide and high frequency oscillatory ventilation in severe persistent pulmonary hypertension of the newborn. *J Pediatr* 1997; **131**: 55–62.
4. Roberts JD, Fineman JR, Morin FC *et al*. Inhaled nitric oxide and persistent pulmonary hypertension of the newborn. *N Engl J Med* 1997; **336**: 605–610.
5. Wessel DL, Adatia I, Van Marter LJ *et al*. Improved oxygenation in a randomized trial of inhaled nitric oxide for persistent pulmonary hypertension of the newborn. *Pediatrics* 1997; **100**: e7.
6. Davidson D, Barefield ES, Kattwinkel J *et al*. Inhaled nitric oxide for the early treatment of persistent pulmonary hypertension of the term newborn: a randomized, double-masked, placebo-controlled, dose-response, multicenter study. *Pediatrics* 1998; **101**: 325–334.
7. Neonatal Inhaled Nitric Oxide Study Group. Inhaled nitric oxide in full-term and nearly full-term infants with hypoxic respiratory failure. *N Engl J Med* 1997; **336**: 597–604.
8. Clark RH, Kueser TJ, Walker MW *et al*. Low-dose inhaled nitric oxide treatment of persistent pulmonary hypertension of the newborn. *N Engl J Med* 2000; **342**: 469–474.
9. Kinsella JP, Abman SH. Clinical approach to inhaled nitric oxide therapy in the newborn. *J Pediatr* 2000; **136**: 717–726.
10. Kinsella JP, Abman SH. Recent developments in the pathophysiology and treatment of persistent pulmonary hypertension of the newborn. *J Pediatr* 1995; **126**: 853–864.
11. Levin DL, Heymann MA, Kitterman JA, Gregory GA, Phibbs RH, Rudolph AM. Persistent pulmonary hypertension of the newborn. *J Pediatr* 1976; **89**: 626.
12. Gersony WM. Neonatal pulmonary hypertension: pathophysiology, classification and etiology. *Clin Perinatol* 1984; **11**: 517–524.
13. Stevenson DK, Kasting DS, Darnall RA *et al*. Refractory hypoxemia associated with neonatal pulmonary disease: the use and limitations of tolazoline. *J Pediatr* 1979; **95**: 595–599.
14. Drummond WH, Gregory G, Heymann MA, Phibbs RA. The independent effects of hyperventilation, tolazoline, and dopamine on infants with persistent pulmonary hypertension. *J Pediatr* 1981; **98**: 603–611.
15. Kinsella JP, Neish SR, Ivy DD, Shaffer E, Abman SH. Clinical responses to prolonged treatment of persistent pulmonary hypertension of the newborn with low doses of inhaled nitric oxide. *J Pediatr* 1993; **123**: 103–108.
16. Abman SH, Griebel JL, Parker DK, Schmidt JM, Swanton D, Kinsella JP. Acute effects of inhaled nitric oxide in severe hypoxemic respiratory failure in pediatrics. *J Pediatr* 1994; **124**: 881–888.
17. Gerlach H, Rossaint R, Pappert D, Falke KJ. Time-course and dose-response of nitric oxide inhalation for systemic oxygenation and pulmonary hypertension in patients with adult respiratory distress syndrome. *Eur J Clin Invest* 1993; **23**: 499–502.
18. Rossaint R, Falke KJ, Lopez F, Slama K, Pison U, Zapol WM. Inhaled nitric oxide for the adult respiratory distress syndrome. *N Engl J Med* 1993; **328**: 399–405.
19. Beckman JS, Beckman TW, Chen J, Marshall PA, Freeman BA. Apparent hydroxy radical production by peroxynitrite: implications for endothelial injury from nitric oxide and superoxide. *Proc Natl Acad Sci USA* 1990; **87**; 1620–1624.
20. Robbins CG, Davis JM, Merritt TA *et al*. Combined effects of nitric oxide and hyperoxia on surfactant function and pulmonary inflammation. *Am J Physiol* 1995; **269**: L545–L550.
21. Issa A, Lappalainen U, Kleinman M, Bry K, Hallman M. Inhaled nitric oxide decreases hyperoxia-induced surfactant abnormality in preterm rabbits. *Pediatr Res* 1999: **45**; 247–254.
22. Collet-Martin S, Gatecel C, Kermarrec N, Gougerot-Pocidalo MA, Payen D. Alveolar neutrophil functions and cytokine levels in patients with the adult respiratory distress syndrome during nitric oxide inhalation. *Am J Respir Crit Care Med* 1996; 153: 985–990.

23. O'Donnell VB, Chumley PH, Hogg N, Bloodworth A, Darley-Usmar VM, Freeman BA. Nitric oxide inhibition of lipid peroxidation: kinetics of reaction with lipid peroxyl radicals and comparison with alpha-tocopherol. *Biochemistry* 1997; 36: 15216–15223.

24. Hallman M. Molecular interactions between nitric oxide and lung surfactant. *Biol Neonate* 1997; 71: 44–48.

25. Antunes MJ, Greenspan JS, Holt WJ, Vallieu DS, Spitzer AR. Assessment of lung function pre-nitric oxide therapy: a predictor of response? *Pediatr Res* 1994; 35: 212A.

26. Gerlach H, Rossaint R, Pappert D, Falke KJ. Time-course and dose-response of nitric oxide inhalation for systemic oxygenation and pulmonary hypertension in patients with adult respiratory distress syndrome. *Eur J Clin Invest* 1993; 23: 499–502.

27. Goldman AP, Tasker RC, Haworth SG, Sigston PE, Macrae DJ. Four patterns of response to inhaled nitric oxide for persistent pulmonary hypertension of the newborn. *Pediatrics* 1996; 98: 706–713.

28. Davidson D, Barefield ES, Kattwinkel J *et al.* Safety of withdrawing inhaled nitric oxide therapy in persistent pulmonary hypertension. *Pediatrics* 1999; **104**: 231–236.

29. Kinsella JP, Abman SH. Recent developments in the pathophysiology and treatment of persistent pulmonary hypertension of the newborn. *J Pediatr* 1995; **126**: 853–864.

30. Clark RH. High-frequency ventilation. *J Pediatr* 1994; **124**: 661–670.

31. Kinsella JP, Abman SH. Efficacy of inhalational nitric oxide therapy in the clinical management of persistent pulmonary hypertension of the newborn. *Chest* 1994; **105**: 92S–94S.

32. Kinsella JP, Abman SH. Clinical approach to the use of high frequency oscillatory ventilation in neonatal respiratory failure. *J Perinatol* 1996; *16*: S52–S55.

33. Abman SH, Kinsella JP. Inhaled nitric oxide for persistent pulmonary hypertension of the newborn: the physiology matters! *Pediatrics* 1995; **96**: 1147–1151.

34. Kinsella JP, Schmidt JM, Griebel J, Abman SH. Inhaled nitric oxide treatment for stabilization and emergency medical transport of critically ill newborns and infants. *Pediatrics* 1995; **95**: 773–776.

35. Karamanoukian HL, Glick PL, Zayek M *et al.* Inhaled nitric oxide in congenital hypoplasia of the lungs due to diaphragmatic hernia or oligohydramnios. *Pediatrics* 1994; **94**: 715–718.

36. Neonatal Inhaled Nitric Oxide Study Group. Inhaled nitric oxide and hypoxic respiratory failure in infants with congenital diaphragmatic hernia. *Pediatrics* 1997; **99**: 838–845.

37. Kinsella JP, Parker TA, Ivy DD, Abman SH, Noninvasive delivery of inhaled nitric oxide therapy for late pulmonary hypertension in newborn infants with congenital diaphragmatic hernia. *J Pediatr* 2003; **142**: 397–401.

38. Kinsella JP, Walsh WF, Bose CL *et al.* Inhaled nitric oxide in premature neonates with severe hypoxaemic respiratory failure: a randomised controlled trial. *Lancet* 1999; **354**: 1061–1065.

Sunil K. Sinha Steven M. Donn

11

Weaning and extubation from assisted ventilation

While there is a relative consensus as to when intubation and mechanical ventilation should be started in the presence of respiratory failure, the decisions regarding weaning and extubation during recovery tend to be largely subjective and are predominantly determined by institutional or individual practices or preferences. This inconsistency can lead to babies either being left on the ventilator for too long, or extubated too hastily, thus requiring repeated re-intubation. Both premature extubation as well as prolonged intubation can cause harm; therefore, a process of weaning and extubation that is both expeditious and safe is highly desirable. Although in most situations, especially in those requiring short-term ventilation, there is not as much difficulty in discontinuing mechanical ventilation, this process becomes more difficult when dealing with very premature and extremely low birth-weight babies as well as those recovering from major respiratory failure, who required prolonged ventilatory support. The process of discontinuing mechanical ventilation in such babies has become a major clinical challenge and constitutes a large proportion of the workload in most neonatal intensive care units (NICUs).

PHYSIOLOGICAL CONSIDERATIONS

In the daily vernacular of an NICU, the process of discontinuing mechanical ventilation is usually referred to as weaning. In the strictest sense, however,

Prof. Sunil K. Sinha MD FRCP PhD FRCPCH FIAP
Professor of Paediatrics and Neonatal Medicine, University of Durham, and Directorate of Neonatology, The James Cook University Hospital, Marton Road, Middlesbrough TS4 3BW, UK
Tel: +44 1642 850850; Fax: +44 1642 854830; E-mail: sunil.sinha@stees.nhs.uk (for correspondence)

Prof. Steven M. Donn MD FAAP
Professor of Pediatrics, Director, Section of Neonatal-Perinatal Medicine, C.S. Mott Children's Hospital, University of Michigan Medical Center, Ann Arbor, Michigan 48109–0254, USA

Table 1 Aetiopathogenesis of difficult weaning and failure of extubation

Increased respiratory load	Reduced respiratory capacity
Increased elastic load	*Decreased respiratory drive*
• Unresolved lung disease	• Excessive sedation
• Secondary pneumonia	• CNS infection
• Left-to-right shunt (via PDA)	• Brain lesions such as PVH and PVL
• Abdominal distension	• Hypocapnia/alkalosis
• Hyperinflated lungs	
Increased resistive load	*Muscular dysfunction*
• Thick/copious airway secretions	• Muscular weakness (malnutrition)
• Narrow/occluded endotracheal tube	• Severe electrolyte disturbances
• Upper airway obstruction	• Chronic pulmonary hyperinflation (BPD)
Increased minute ventilation	*Neuromuscular disorders*
• Pain and irritability	• Diaphragmatic dysfunction
• Sepsis/hyperthermia	• Prolonged neuromuscular blockade
• Metabolic acidosis	(in renal failure, concomitant use of aminoglycoside and pheno-barbitone)
	• Myotonic dystrophy
	• Cervical spinal injury

BPD, bronchopulmonary dysplasia; CNS, central nervous system; PDA, patent ductus arteriosus; PVH, periventricular haemorrhage; PVL, periventricular leucomalacia.

weaning is the process of slowly transferring the amount of respiratory support from the ventilator to the patient. This is dependent upon a balance between adequacy of pulmonary gas exchange and performance of the respiratory muscle pump.[1] Failure of the respiratory muscle pump is probably the most common cause of the inability to wean from mechanical ventilation. Intolerance of extubation may, therefore, be the result of either increased load on the respiratory muscles, and/or decreased inspiratory drive and endurance (capacity).[2] The management of such infants requires the identification and correction of all factors that have the potential to impede the tolerance for spontaneous breathing (Table 1). Moreover, it should also be realised that weaning from mechanical ventilation is a dynamic process and is influenced, particularly in newborns, by many factors such as differing stages of lung development, changing status of the underlying lung disease, secondary complications, a unique interaction of the neonatal heart and lungs, and the relationship between central control of respiratory drive and respiratory muscles.

WHEN AND HOW TO WEAN?

Once the infant has clinically 'stabilised' and blood gas values suggest that ventilatory needs are no longer increasing, the general principle should be to decrease the most potentially harmful parameter first. It is also a good practice to limit changes to one parameter at a time and to avoid changes of a large

Table 2 A commonly used protocol for weaning of ventilatory parameters on the basis of blood gas results

	Oxygenation	Ventilation (CO_2)
Determinants	Adequate oxygenation is dependent on FiO_2 and mean airway pressure (PIP, PEEP, Ti)	Adequate ventilation (elimination of CO_2) is dependent on distending pressure (ΔP = PIP – PEEP), rate (frequency), minute ventilation (= V_T x f) and expiratory time (or I:E ratio)
Sequence	Reduce FiO_2 to < 0.4 • If PaO_2 high and $PaCO_2$ normal, decrease PIP (V_T), and PEEP, or T_I • If PaO_2 high and $PaCO_2$ low, decrease PIP (V_T) and rate (if on IMV/SIMV)	• If $PaCO_2$ ↓ and PaO_2 ↑, decrease PIP (V_T) or rate (if on IMV/SIMV) • If $PaCO_2$ ↓ and PaO_2 normal, decrease rate • If $PaCO_2$ and PaO_2 both low, increase PEEP or decrease T_E (longer I:E ratio) or decrease rate (if on IMV)
Practical hints	• If FiO_2 > 0.4, maintain Hgb > 15 g/dl • Avoid 'flip-flop' by making only small changes in FiO_2 at any one time • Avoid too low PIP (V_T) or PEEP to maintain adequate alveolar volume	• Try to maintain normal minute ventilation (240–360 ml/kg/min) • Keep V_T ≥ 4 ml/kg range • Avoid IMV rate lower than 15 breaths/min

FiO_2, fractional inspired oxygen; PIP, peak inspiratory pressure; PEEP, positive end expiratory pressure; Ti, inspiratory time; T_E, expiratory time; ΔP, amplitude (distending pressure); V_T, tidal volume; f, frequency.

magnitude. The commonly used weaning strategies for ventilatory parameters based on arterial blood gas results are described in Table 2.

The classic approach to weaning from conventional ventilation is to extubate from low rate intermittent mandatory ventilation, either directly to supplemental oxygen or continuous positive airway pressure (CPAP). Based on published studies, there is no rationale for trying infants on endotracheal CPAP, because this is only likely to impose considerable work of breathing and contribute to weaning failure.[3] Weaning during synchronised ventilation, however, is conceptually different than it has been for conventional intermittent mandatory ventilation, because many of the parameters previously set by the clinician are now patient-controlled, particularly during patient-triggered (assist-control) ventilation.[4,5] During patient-triggered ventilation, as long as the baby is breathing above the control (back-up) rate, reduction in the rate brings about no change in ventilator cycling or support (Fig. 1). Moreover, because the infant is setting his or her own inspiratory time (in flow cycling), the inspiratory-expiratory ratio cannot be changed. Thus, reduction in peak inspiratory pressure is the primary manoeuvre. Weaning methods in synchronised intermittent mandatory ventilation are similar to intermittent mandatory ventilation (*i.e.* weaning is achieved by decreasing the synchronised intermittent mandatory ventilation rate and peak inspiratory pressure). However, one should avoid using a very low synchronised

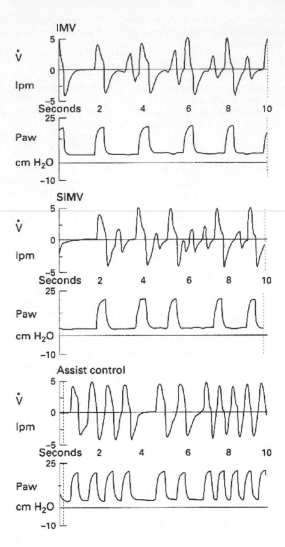

Fig. 1 Flow and pressure waveforms for intermittent mandatory ventilation (IMV), synchronised intermittent mandatory ventilation (SIMV), and assist-control ventilation (A/C). During IMV (top), note mechanical breaths (larger flow waveforms) delivered at fixed intervals, set by the clinician. Spontaneous breaths may occur between mechanical breaths, but may not generate significant positive pressure. During SIMV (middle), spontaneous patient effort above a set threshold can trigger a mechanical breath if it occurs within a 'timing window'. Thus, mechanical breaths occur at a slightly variable interval. Spontaneous breaths between timing windows do not result in triggering and do not generate effective pressure. During assist-control (A/C, bottom) each spontaneous breath which exceeds the trigger threshold is augmented by a machine delivered breath. Thus each breath is identical. The rate will vary according to the patient's own rate, but will not fall below the control back-up rate set by the clinician. Reproduced from Sinha et al.[33] with permission of the publishers.

intermittent mandatory ventilation rate and attempt to maintain a minimum, but adequate, tidal volume delivery (≥4 ml/kg). If babies require continuing minimal support through synchronised intermittent mandatory ventilation, an alternative approach is to use pressure support ventilation in conjunction with

Table 3 Suggested weaning strategies related to commonly used newer modes of ventilation

Modes of ventilation	Weaning strategies
Assist control (A/C) (patient-triggered ventilation)	• Decrease PIP but provide adequate V_T ($\geq$ 4 ml/kg) • Decrease back up rate to 25–30 • May increase trigger sensitivity to condition respiratory muscles • Extubate directly from assist-control or switch to SIMV
Synchronised intermittent ventilation (SIMV)	• Decrease rate • Decrease PIP but provide adequate V_T ($\geq$ 4 ml/kg) • Extubate when stable at low rate (*i.e.* 15 breaths/m) or combine with PSV
Synchronised intermittent ventilation/Pressure support ventilation (SIMV/PSV)	• Add PSV when SIMV rate below 30/min • Adjust level of PSV to give adequate V_T ($\geq$ 4 ml/kg); reduce SIMV slowly • Extubate when stable at low SIMV rate (*i.e.* 15 breaths/m)
High frequency oscillatory ventilation	• Decrease both mean airway pressure and amplitude • As the patient improves, and as amplitude decreases, the patient will do more spontaneous breathing • When achieving most of the CO_2 elimination with spontaneous breathing, and the mean airway pressure has decreased sufficiently, ($<$ 7–8 cmH_2O and FiO_2 0.25–0.3) patient can be extubated

SIMV, synchronised intermittent ventilation; PSV, pressure support ventilation; PIP, peak inspiratory pressure.

synchronised intermittent mandatory ventilation. The major function of pressure support ventilation is to assist respiratory muscle activity and thus reduce the workload. Pressure support ventilation is intended to give the patient an inspiratory pressure 'boost' during spontaneous breathing so as to overcome the imposed work of breathing created by the endotracheal tube, demand valve, and ventilator circuit. However, because it is pressure limited, tidal volume delivery in pressure support ventilation depends on respiratory mechanics and thus may be variable. To overcome this variability, some devices have now combined pressure support with a guaranteed tidal volume delivery, such as volume-assured pressure support.[6] In this mode, the clinician chooses a minimum tidal volume that the patient is to receive during spontaneous breathing. As long as the patient is able to receive this volume, the breath is a simple pressure support breath. However, should the delivered volume not reach the minimal value at the end of inspiration, the breath will transition to a volume cycled breath, and flow will continue, prolonging the inspiratory time until the volume assurance is reached. The mode seems ideally suited to infant weaning, where changes in either pulmonary compliance or respiratory drive occur with relative frequency and often impede the weaning process. Another promising ventilatory strategy is proportional assist ventilation, in which the ventilator generates pressure proportional to the patient's effort.[7] The more the patient 'pulls', the more pressure the machine generates. To do so, the ventilator must be able to sense or estimate patient effort on an on-going basis. This property makes proportional assist ventilation a potentially useful mode for weaning infants from mechanical ventilation. Although the clinical applications of high-frequency ventilation are well described in the literature, there is relatively little research examining it as a weaning process. For example, it has not been shown whether extubation directly from very low high-frequency ventilation settings to either no support or CPAP offers any advantages over switching directly to conventional ventilation. The weaning strategies related to specific modes of ventilation are summarised in Table 3.

DIFFICULT WEANING

Commonly, more than one factor is responsible for weaning failure and these factors might be multifactorial (see Table 1). The management of such infants requires the identification and correction of all factors that have the potential to impede tolerance of spontaneous breathing. Careful adjustment of the ventilator triggering system to its most sensitive level, and appropriate setting of the ventilator inspiratory flow might help to reduce the patient's work of breathing during mechanical ventilation. The maintenance of minute ventilation in a range sufficient to assure adequate removal of carbon dioxide is essential. For the healthy newborn, a tidal volume of 4–6 ml/kg and a respiratory rate of 40–60 breaths/min suggests that the minute ventilation should be approximately 240–360 ml/kg/min in infants with normal lungs.[8] It may be inferred that alveolar hypoventilation will occur if either tidal volume or the respiratory rate is too low. Where available, monitoring of pulmonary function and mechanics might be useful to gain some insight into the reasons for ventilatory dependency in an individual baby.[9] In addition, the nutritional aspects of weaning, particularly in extremely low birth-weight babies, cannot be overlooked, and efforts to provide an adequate energy intake to prevent catabolism might help to prevent weaning failure. Conversely, provision of too much fat or carbohydrate may generate additional carbon dioxide, contributing to ventilatory work.

ADJUNCTS TO WEANING

A number of adjunctive therapies to facilitate extubation and transition to spontaneous breathing have been used for a number of years but remain a subject for further investigation.

Continuous positive airway pressure (CPAP)

CPAP stabilises the upper airway, improves lung function, and reduces apnoea. A number of randomised trials have attempted to investigate the question of whether CPAP, applied 'prophylactically', reduces the need for additional ventilatory support. Although results vary from trial to trial, the cumulative data suggest that infants extubated to nasal CPAP experience a reduction in the frequency of adverse clinical events (apnoea and bradycardia, respiratory acidosis, and increasing oxygen requirement), a decreased need for additional ventilation, and a trend towards a decreased requirement for re-intubation.[10] However, much work still needs to be done to define properly the relationship between CPAP, surfactant replacement therapy, and mechanical ventilation. It is anticipated that several on-going clinical trials may yield information that addresses this issue more fully. CPAP can be applied by nasal prongs or by high flow nasal cannula.

Pharmacological agents

Routine administration of corticosteroids and methylxanthines has been a common practice to help weaning and extubation, particularly in ventilator-dependent babies. The practice of giving corticosteroids, mainly dexamethasone, falls into two main groups:

1. Peri-extubation corticosteroid treatment[11] in infants at increased risk for airway oedema and obstruction, such as those who have received repeated or prolonged intubation.

2. Postnatal corticosteroid treatment as a strategy to prevent chronic lung disease,[12–15] which co-incidentally reduces the duration of intubation and ventilation. However, there are potential hazards of corticosteroid treatment, including possible adverse effects on the developing central nervous system and lungs, and the current recommendation is to restrict their use. Treatment at 7–14 days of age in chronically ventilated infants might give the best outcomes,[16] but there is no consensus regarding its dosing schedule. It seems prudent to use a much lower dose and restrict its use for a maximum of 7–10 days, as being used in the current Australian low-dose BPD trial.[17]

Methylxanthines (theophylline and caffeine) have been used for a long time because of their many theoretical advantages, including increased central respiratory drive and increased diaphragmatic contractility and endurance.[18] A review of the published studies suggests that methylxanthines might increase the chances of successful extubation of some preterm infants, but individual published studies do not allow a firm recommendation to be made for routine use in clinical practice.[19] Moreover, like dexamethasone, there are also concerns about brain injury because of antagonistic properties against adenosine receptors.[20] A large, international, multicentre trial to examine the safety and efficacy of caffeine is underway. Other pharmacological agents often used to facilitate the process of weaning are diuretics and bronchodilators. Like steroids, they have been used as a strategy for treatment of chronic lung disease and have been shown to be beneficial in improving lung function in specific situations, but there are not enough data to recommend their routine use for weaning.

TRIALS OF PREDICTIVE INDICES FOR SUCCESSFUL EXTUBATION

Although an astute clinician might be able to predict the time that an infant is ready to start weaning, extubation failure still occurs in about a third of cases. Attempts have been made to devise some objective parameters which might be used as an adjunct to clinical decision making in identifying the optimal time

Table 4 Clinical trials of predictive indices in weaning

Physiological parameters	Indices	Comments
Pulmonary mechanics[21,22]	• Lung compliance (C_{RS}) (ml/cmH$_2$O/kg) • Lung resistance (R_{RS}) (cm/H$_2$O/L/S) • Resistive work of breathing (g x cm/kg)	• Equivocal results • Poor discriminatory value of individual indices • Uncontrolled studies with fewer numbers
Pulmonary function[23]	• Functional residual capacity (FRC) (ml/kg)	• Measurement made soon after extubation • Threshold value <26 ml/kg for failure sensitivity 71%, specificity 77%
Effect of breathing and respiratory muscle endurance[24–27]	• Spontaneous breath tidal volume (ml/kg) • Minute ventilation (ml/min/kg) [ratio of spontaneous: mechanical breaths] • Mean inspiratory flow (V_T/TI) • Inspiratory pressure/ maximal inspiratory pressure (PI/PI$_{max}$)	• Not discriminatory • Positive predictive value 86% but requires controlled study • Methodological inconsistency • Different 'threshold' values
Composite data[28,29]. (integrated indices)	• Respiratory frequency and tidal volume ratio (f/V_T-breaths/minute/l) • CROP index (compliance, rate, oxygenation and pressure)	• Not assessed in homogenous neonatal population • Not discriminatory as in adults

PI, inspiratory pressure; PI$_{max}$, maximal inspiratory pressure; TI, inspiratory time; V_T, tidal volume.

for extubation. These 'predictive' indices assess different physiological functions of the respiratory system, including the effect of spontaneous breathing and respiratory muscle endurance (Table 4).[21–29] However, despite having potential for clinical applicability, these tools still remain mostly investigative in nature and do not provide a 'threshold' value for either individual or combination of measurements that would consistently discriminate between success and failure of extubation.[30] Recent work with examining spontaneous breathing during mechanical ventilation appears to be one such method. The first study, observational in nature, demonstrated the feasibility of predicting readiness for extubation based on the ratio of spontaneous:mechanical minute ventilation.[24] The second study applied this test to extubation in a randomised, controlled trial comparing it to clinical judgement, and demonstrated that the test was superior in shortening the time to extubation.[25]

EFFICACY OF NEWER VENTILATORY TECHNIQUES ON WEANING

There have been only a few randomised trials which have compared the effect of newer techniques of ventilation primarily on weaning. Most published studies designed to look into the safety and efficacy of these newer modes have included 'duration of ventilation' only as an incidental parameter or surrogate outcome measure of ventilation.[1] Cumulative data from earlier studies indicate that patient-triggered ventilation or synchronised intermittent mandatory ventilation compared to intermittent mandatory ventilation is associated with a shorter duration of ventilation. In comparisons of patient-triggered ventilation (assist-control) to synchronised intermittent mandatory ventilation, again there was a trend towards shorter duration of weaning with the former mode.[31] These findings were not confirmed in a recently published large trial,[32] but this study has been criticised for its methodology and design flaws.[31]

Volume ventilation has only relatively been re-introduced in the NICU, after a less than stellar experience in the early 1980s. One of the first evaluations of volume ventilation was a single-centre, 50 patient, randomised clinical trial which showed that babies receiving volume-limited ventilation had a much shorter duration of mechanical ventilation with fewer complication compared to the group who received pressure-limited ventilation.[34] Although early clinical experience with volume-controlled ventilation seems to be promising, further studies will be required to determine the best applications of each method.[36]

In a similar study, using a pressure-regulated, volume-controlled mode of ventilation, the duration of ventilation was noted to be significantly reduced especially in babies who weighed less than 1 kg.[35]

CONCLUSIONS

Weaning infants from mechanical ventilation involves as much 'art' as 'science' and should be planned according to clearly defined clinical and physiological goals. The measurement of pulmonary mechanics and lung volumes, now available at the bedside, might help in gauging the capacity for weaning, even though its clinical usefulness has not been confirmed in controlled trials. A method that will rapidly and reliably assesses the infant's readiness for extubation would provide clinicians a useful adjunct to their clinical decision making for extubation, and additional clinical investigation in this area is very much needed. Given the availability and variety of newer ventilatory modes that were not available previously, clinicians now have a choice of different weaning techniques which is becoming more extensive every day and clinicians have an obligation to harness all of this new 'power' wisely. The evidence base is as yet not established for most of these techniques, but the time is right to organise randomised clinical trials to answer the myriad of questions that the new technologies have raised.

Key points for clinical practice

- Weaning is a process of transferring the work of breathing from the mechanical ventilator to the patient.

- The process of weaning should be initiated as soon as practical after there are signs of improvement in the underlying condition.

- Successful weaning is dependent on a delicate balance between the respiratory load and respiratory capacity.

- Repeated failure to wean suggests incomplete resolution of the underlying condition, other impediments to weaning, or poor endurance.

- When attempts to wean repeatedly fail, there may be more than one factor requiring meticulous attention.

- The methods of weaning with newer styles of ventilation are specific to different modes and differ from the classical approaches used previously.

- Pharmacological adjuncts such as caffeine and corticosteroids, though effective, should be used cautiously because of potential side-effects and variable therapeutic efficacy.

- Nasal prong continuous positive airway pressure seems to reduce the period of intubation, but there are still many unresolved questions that are under current investigation.

- There is still no single objective 'measure' which will readily predict successful extubation.

- Use of on-line pulmonary mechanics testing and graphics improves the clinical decision-making process regarding weaning and extubation.

References

1. Harris TR, Wood BR. Physiologic principles. In: Goldsmith JP, Karotkin EH. (eds) *Assisted Ventilation of the Neonate*, 3rd edn. Philadelphia, PA: WB Saunders, 1996; 21–68.
2. Lessard MR, Bronchard LJ. Weaning from ventilatory support. *Clin Chest Med* 1996; **17**: 475–489.
3. Davis PG, Henderson-Smart DJ. Extubation from low-rate intermittent positive airways pressure versus extubation after a trial of endotracheal continuous positive airways pressure in intubated preterm infants (Cochrane Review). In: *The Cochrane Library*, Issue 1. Oxford: Update Software, 1999.
4. Donn SM, Sinha SK. Newer modes of mechanical ventilation for the neonate. *Curr Opin Pediatr* 2001; **13**: 99–103.
5. Greenough A. Update on modalities of mechanical ventilation. *Arch Dis Child Fetal Neonat Edn* 2002; **87**: F3–F6.
6. Sinha SK, Donn SM. Volume-controlled ventilation. Variation on a theme. *Clin Perinatol* 2001; **28**: 547–560.
7. Schulze A, Gerhardt T, Musante G *et al*. Proportional assist ventilation in low birth weight infants with acute respiratory disease. A comparison to assist-control and conventional mechanical ventilation. *J Pediatr* 1999; **135**: 339–344.

8. Bhutani VK, Sivieri EM, Abbasi S. Evaluation of pulmonary function in the neonate. In: Polin RA, Fox WW. (eds) *Fetal and Neonatal Physiology*. Philadelphia, PA: WB Saunders, 1998; 1143–1164.

9. Sinha SK, Nicks JJ, Donn SM. Graphic analysis of pulmonary mechanics in neonates receiving assisted ventilation. *Arch Dis Child* 1996; **75**: F213–F218.

10. Ho JJ, Subramaniam P, Henderson-Smart DJ, Davis PG. Continuous distending pressure for respiratory distress syndrome in preterm infants (Cochrane Review). In: *The Cochrane Library*, Issue 2. Oxford: Update Software, 2003.

11. Davis PB, Henderson-Smart DJ. Intravenous dexamethasone for extubation of newborn infants (Cochrane Review). In: *The Cochrane Library*, Issue 1. Oxford: Update Software, 1999.

12. Kovacs L, Davis GM, Faucher D, Papageorgiou A. Efficacy of sequential early systemic and inhaled corticosteroid therapy in the prevention of chronic lung disease of prematurity. *Acta Paediatr* 1998; **87**: 792–798.

13. Papile LA, Tyson JE, Stoll BJ *et al*. A multicenter trial of two dexamethasone regimens in ventilator dependent premature infants. *N Engl J Med* 1998; **338**: 1112–1118.

14. Bhutta T, Ohlsson A. Systematic review and meta-analysis of early postnatal dexamethasone for prevention of chronic lung disease. *Arch Dis Child* 1998; **79**: F26–F33.

15. Halliday HL, Ehrenkranz RA. Early postnatal (< 96 hours) corticosteroids for preventing chronic lung disease in preterm infants (Cochrane Review). In: *The Cochrane Library*, Issue 1. Oxford: Update Software, 1999.

16. Halliday HL, Ehrenkranz RA. Moderately early (7–14 days) postnatal corticosteroids for preventing chronic lung disease in preterm infants (Cochrane Review). In: *The Cochrane Library*, Issue 1. Oxford: Update Software, 1999.

17. Neonatal Formulary. *The Northern Neonatal Network*, 3rd edn. London: BMJ Publishing Group, 2000.

18. Laubscher B, Greenough A, Dimitriou G. Comparison effects of theophylline and caffeine on respiratory function of prematurely born infants. *Early Hum Dev* 1998; **50**: 185–192.

19. Henderson-Smart DJ, Davis PG. Prophylactic methylxanthine for extubation in preterm infants (Cochrane Review). In: *The Cochrane Library*, Issue 1. Oxford: Update Software, 1999.

20. Dux E, Fastbom J, Ungerstedt U, Rudophi K, Fredholm BB. Protective effect of adenosine and a novel xanthine derivative propentofylline on the cell damage after bilateral carotid occlusion in the gerbil hippocampus. *Brain Res* 1990; **516**: 248–256.

21. Balsan MJ, Jones JG, Watchko JF, Guthrie RD. Measurements of pulmonary mechanics prior to the elective extubation of neonates. *Pediatr Pulmonol* 1990; **9**: 238–243.

22. Veness-Meehan KA, Richter S, Davis JM. Pulmonary function testing prior to extubation in infants with respiratory distress syndrome. *Pediatr Pulmonol* 1990; **9**: 2–6.

23. Dimitriou G, Greenough A, Laubscher B. Lung volume measurements immediately after extubation by prediction of 'extubation failure' in premature infants. *Pediatr Pulmonol* 1996; **21**: 250–254.

24. Wilson Jr BJ, Becker MA, Linton ME, Donn SM. Spontaneous minute ventilation predicts readiness for extubation in mechanically ventilated preterm infants. *J Perinatol* 1998; **18**: 436–439.

25. Gillespie LM, White SD, Sinha SK, Donn SM. Usefulness of 'minute ventilation test' in predicting successful extubation in newborn infants: a randomised controlled trial. *J Perinatol* 2003; **23**: 205–207;

25a El-Khatib MF, Baumeister B, Smith PG, Chatburn RL, Blumer JL. Inspiratory pressure/maximal inspiratory pressure: does it predict successful extubation in critically ill infants and children? *Intensive Care Med* 1996; **22**: 264–268.

26. Dimitriou G, Greenough A, Endo A *et al*. Prediction of extubation failure in preterm infants. *Arch Dis Child Fetal Neonat Edn* 2002; **86**: F32–F35.

27. Khan N, Brown A, Venkataraman ST. Predictors of extubation success and failure in mechanically ventilated infants and children. *Crit Care Med* 1996; **24**: 1568–1579.

28. Baumeister BL, el-Khatib M, Smith PG, Blumer JL. Evaluation of predictors of weaning from mechanical ventilation in pediatric patients. *Pediatr Pulmonol* 1997; **24**: 344–352.

30. Farias JA, Alia I, Retta A *et al*. An evaluation of extubation failure predictors in mechanically ventilation infants and children. *Intensive Care Med* 2002; **28**: 752–757.

31. Greenough A, Milner AD, Dimitriou G. Synchronised mechanical ventilation for respiratory support in newborn infants (Cochrane Review). In: *The Cochrane Library*, Issue 1. Oxford: Update Software, 1999.

32. Baumer JH. International randomised controlled trial of patient triggered ventilation in neonatal respiratory distress syndrome. *Arch Dis Child* 2000; **82**: F5–F10.

33. Donn SM, Greenough A, Sinha SK. Patient triggered ventilation. Arch Dis Child Fetal Neonat Edn 2000; **83**: F225–F226.

34. Sinha SK, Donn SM, Gavey J, McCarty M. A randomised trial of volume-controlled versus time-cycled, pressure-limited ventilation in preterm infants with respiratory distress syndrome. Arch Dis Child 1997; **77**: F202–205.

35. Piotrowski A, Sobala W, Kawczynski P. Patient-initiated, pressure-regulated, volume-controlled ventilation compared with intermittent mandatory ventilation in neonates: a prospective randomised study. Intensive Care Med 1997; **9**: 975–981.

36. Donn SM, Sinha SK. Invasive and noninvasive neonatal mechanical ventilation. Respir Care 2003; **48**: 426–441.

Charles J. Coté

12

Effective and safe sedation for infants and toddlers undergoing procedures

This chapter is intended for non-anaesthesiologists. It should be understood that there are many ways of accomplishing the same end-point so this review will stress process and procedures that improve the safety of sedating children. This chapter covers: (i) the history of sedation guidelines and current recommendations; (ii) the demographics and issues related to adverse outcomes in children sedated by non-anaesthesiologists with emphasis on prevention; (iii) the pharmacology of commonly used sedating analgesic medications; and (iv) commonly used sedation regimens that may be effective in the majority of children for specific procedures.

INTRODUCTION

It is often difficult to gain the co-operation of children through reasoning alone. Therefore, to carry out a procedure in paediatric patients safely some degree of pharmacological assistance is usually required. The choice of sedative/analgesic regimen depends upon the painfulness of the procedure as well as whether or not there is a need for complete immobility. For example, some children may be undergoing procedures such as a bone marrow aspiration, which is somewhat painful, and therefore may require opioid plus anxiolytic plus local anaesthetic, but some degree of movement is tolerable, whereas another may be undergoing magnetic resonance imaging (MRI) where any motion at all would alter the quality of, or not allow, the study to be completed successfully. The selection of drug, the route of administration and dosage need to be tailored to the procedure being performed as well as patient

Charles J. Coté MD
Professor of Anesthesiology and Pediatrics, The Feinberg School of Medicine at Northwestern University, Vice Chairman, Director of Research, Department of Pediatric Anesthesiology, Children's Memorial Hospital, Chicago, IL 60614, USA
E-mail ccote@northwestern.edu

Table 1 ASA Physical Status Classification

Class I	A normally healthy patient
Class II	A patient with mild systemic disease
Class III	A patient with severe systemic disease
Class IV	A patient with severe systemic disease that is a constant threat to life
Class V	A moribund patient who is not expected to survive without the operation.

characteristics, *i.e.* each patient's drug selection must be individually based on a careful review of their medical and surgical history and how the sedating medications might affect them.

The guiding principle for providing safe sedation means that there is a protective safety net. This means a 'systems' approach so that all candidates for sedation are evaluated, prepared, and monitored in a similar fashion. This approach has allowed the safety of general anaesthesia to improve from a mortality rate of 1:10,000 in the 1960s to approximately 1:200,000 anaesthetics in 2003.[1] A 'systems' approach means the following:

1. Appropriate presedation evaluation of underlying medical conditions and how those conditions would affect the child's response to the sedating/analgesic medications (*e.g.* congenital heart disease, impaired liver or renal function.

2. Current medications and how these might alter choice or dose of sedating medications (*e.g.*, erythromycin or rifampin [cytochrome 450 3A4 inhibitors or inducers] alteration in midazolam metabolism).[2,3]

3. A careful physical examination including a focused examination of the airway (*e.g.* tonsillar hypertrophy or midfacial hypoplasia increase the likelihood of drug induced airway obstruction).[4]

4. Assessment of potential risk using the American Society of Anesthesiologists (ASA) Physical Status classification (Table 1). Physical status 3 and 4 patients require special consideration.

5. A review of the child's past experiences with sedating medications and how they responded (*e.g.* the child who has had many procedures often requires increasing doses of medications or combinations of medications to achieve the desired state of sedation).

6. Appropriate fasting from solids and liquids to decrease the likelihood of pulmonary aspiration while avoiding hypovolaemia (Table 2).

7. Informed consent so that the parents understand that sedation has risks.

8. Appropriate monitoring equipment including continuous pulse oximetry (provides an early warning of developing desaturation), electrocardiograph (provides a back-up for the pulse oximeter, *i.e.* if both devices show the same heart rate then the data on the pulse oximeter is likely not an artefact but a true measurement of haemoglobin saturation), intermittent blood pressure measurement (useful for following trends and

Table 2 Recommended preprocedural sedation fasting

Age (months)	Recommendation
0–5	No milk or solids for 4 h*
6–36	No milk or solids for 6 h*
> 36	No milk or solids for 8 h*

*Clear liquids (water, apple juice, Jell-O, *etc.*) may continue for up to 2 h before the procedure.
Breast milk is considered 'milk' and should be with-held for 4 h before the procedure.
Data from Committee on Drugs, American Academy of Pediatrics.[15]

Table 3 Age and size appropriate equipment for managing emergencies

SUGGESTED EMERGENCY EQUIPMENT	
Intravenous equipment	Intravenous catheters 24-, 22-, 18-, and 16-gauge
	Tourniquets
	Alcohol wipes
	Adhesive tape
	Assorted syringes, 1 ml, 3 ml, 6 ml, and 12 ml
Intravenous tubing	Paediatric drip (60 drops/ml)
	Paediatric burette type
	Adult drip (10 drops/ml)
	Extension tubing
Intravenous fluid	Lactated Ringer's solution
	Normal saline
Three-way stopcocks	
Paediatric i.v. boards	
Assorted i.v. needles, 22-, 20-, and 18-gauge	
Intra-osseous bone marrow needle	
Sterile gauze pads	

AIRWAY MANAGEMENT EQUIPMENT	
Face masks	Infant, child, small adult, medium adult, large adult
Breathing bag & valve set	
Oral airways	Infant, child, small adult, medium adult, large adult
Nasal airways	Small, medium, large
Laryngoscope handles	
Laryngoscope blades	Straight (Miller) No. 1, 2, 3
	Curved (Macintosh) No. 2, 3
Endotracheal tubes:	2.5, 3.0, 3.5, 4.0, 4.5, 5.0, 5.5, 6.0 uncuffed;
	6.0, 7.0, 8.0 cuffed
Stylettes (appropriate sizes for endotracheal tubes)	
Surgical lubricant	
Suction catheters (appropriate sizes for endotracheal tubes)	
Nasogastric tubes	Yankauer-type suction
Nebuliser with medication kits	
Gloves	

Data from Committee on Drugs, American Academy of Pediatrics.[15]

potential anaphylactoid reactions), end expired carbon dioxide monitoring (particularly useful for assessing patient respirations in difficult environments such as CAT scan or MRI.

9. A standardised sedation record for recording all drugs, doses, routes of administration, patient responses, and vital signs.

10. Calculation of all medications on a mg/kg basis with strict attention to upper limits particularly for local anaesthetics.

11. Both the sedation and recovery facilities must be equipped with age and size appropriate equipment for managing emergencies (Table 3).

12. An immediately available emergency drug cart including drugs to antagonise opioids and benzodiazepines (Table 4).

13. An appropriately staffed and equipped recovery area.

14. Rigorous discharge criteria such that the child is returned to presedation level of consciousness (Table 5).

15. Provision to the family of emergency call-back numbers and appropriate instructions regarding observation after discharge (particularly important for infants who will be in car seats – the child could potentially resedate and develop airway obstruction).

16. Appropriately trained and skilled healthcare providers whose only responsibility is to observe the patient, recognise adverse responses in a

---

Table 4 Suggested emergency drugs

- Oxygen
- Glucose (50%)
- Atropine
- Epinephrine (1:1000; 1:10,000)
- Phenylephrine
- Dopamine
- Diazepam
- Isoproterenol
- Calcium chloride or calcium gluconate
- Sodium bicarbonate
- Lidocaine (cardiac lidocaine, local infiltration)
- Naloxone hydrochloride
- Diphenhydramine hydrochloride
- Hydrocortisone
- Methylprednisolone
- Succinylcholine
- Aminophylline
- Racemic epinephrine
- Albuterol by inhalation
- Ammonia spirits
- Flumazenil

The choice of emergency drugs may vary according to individual need.
Data from Committee on Drugs, American Academy of Pediatrics.[15]

Table 5 Recommended discharge criteria

Cardiovascular function and airway patency are satisfactory and stable

The patient is easily arousable, and protected reflexes are intact

The patient can talk (if age-appropriate)

The patient can sit up unaided (if age-appropriate)

For a very young or handicapped child, incapable of the usually expected responses, the presedation level of responsiveness or a level as close as possible to the normal level for that child should be achieved

The state of hydration is adequate.

Data from Committee on Drugs, American Academy of Pediatrics.[15]

timely manner, and intervene so that the patient is successfully rescued. These individuals must understand the pharmacology of the drugs administered, the expected side-effects, and have the necessary skills to manage hypoventilation, airway obstruction, perform bag/mask ventilation, and advanced cardiopulmonary resuscitation.

The literature suggests that most accidents associated with the administration of procedural sedation are preventable when a systematic approach is undertaken.[5–12]

THE ORIGINS OF SEDATION GUIDELINES

The Section on Anesthesiology of the American Academy of Pediatrics (AAP) along with the American Academy of Pediatric Dentistry (AAPD), the Committee on Hospital Care and the Committee on Drugs (COD) of the AAP published the first sedation guideline in 1985.[13,14] The impetus for developing this document was the result of several paediatric deaths during dental procedures. However, there seemed to be some confusion following this initial guideline as to whom they applied (*i.e.* just dentists or anaesthesiologists). Therefore, the guideline was revised in 1992 and the title changed to reflect the fact that the guidelines applied to all children that were being sedated for procedures.[15] The 1992 guideline was the first to require continuous pulse oximetry and a clear 'systems approach' was outlined (see above). In addition, the administration of prescription sedating medications at home prior to a procedure was prohibited.

In the US, in this interim, the Joint Commission on Healthcare Organizations (JCAHO) took interest in the sedation process and developed its regulations for sedation services in hospital facilities. It should be noted that JCAHO standards only applied to hospitals and not to private offices or free-standing facilities other than surgery centres. The JCAHO initially made the Chief of Anaesthesiology responsible for all sedated patients within an institution! This, obviously, got the attention of the ASA which then formed a task force that developed the ASA's first guideline for sedation by non-anaesthesiologists published in 1996.[16] This only addressed the level of sedation described as 'conscious sedation'. The ASA task force felt that this phrase was confusing and changed 'conscious sedation' to 'sedation/analgesia'. The JCAHO then modified their regulations so that the Chief of Anaesthesiology or his/her designee was responsible for developing 'within institution' sedation guidelines but that the chief of each division within that hospital would be responsible for their own people who provided sedation/analgesia. The JCAHO further modified their regulations using language developed through the ASA,[17] such that in the year 2000 new terminology was developed and instead of the phrase 'anxiolysis' we have the phrase 'minimal sedation'. Instead of the phrases 'conscious sedation' or 'sedation/analgesia' we now have the phrase 'moderate sedation'; 'deep sedation' remained unchanged. The caveat was that with 'moderate sedation' there would be no interference with the patient's ability to exchange air and there would be cardiovascular stability, whereas with 'deep sedation' the patient may or may not maintain a patent airway and may or may not have cardiovascular stability (Table 6).[18]

The JCAHO also introduced the **'concept of rescue'**. By this they meant that if the intended level of sedation was 'minimal', then 'the clinician who is

---

Table 6 Definitions of sedation

Minimal sedation

A drug-induced state during which patients respond normally to verbal commands. Although cognitive function and co-ordination may be impaired, ventilatory and cardiovascular function are unaffected

Moderate sedation/analgesia ('conscious sedation')

A drug-induced depression of consciousness during which patients respond purposefully* to verbal commands, either alone or accompanied by light tactile stimulation. No interventions are required to maintain a patent airway, and spontaneous ventilation is adequate. Cardiovascular function is usually maintained

Deep Sedation/analgesia

A drug-induced depression of consciousness during which patients cannot be easily aroused but respond purposefully* following repeated or painful stimulation. The ability to independently maintain ventilatory function may be impaired. Patients may require assistance in maintaining a patent airway, and spontaneous ventilation may be inadequate. Cardiovascular function is usually maintained

General anaesthesia

A drug-induced loss of consciousness during which patients are not arousable, even by painful stimulation. The ability to independently maintain ventilatory function is often impaired. Patients often require assistance in maintaining a patent airway, and positive pressure ventilation may be required because of depressed spontaneous ventilation or drug-induced depression of neuromuscular function. Cardiovascular function may be impaired

*Reflex withdrawal from a painful stimulus is NOT considered a purposeful response.

Because sedation is a continuum, it is not always possible to predict how an individual patient will respond. Hence, practitioners intending to produce a given level of sedation should be able to rescue patients whose level of sedation becomes deeper than initially intended. Individuals administering moderate sedation/analgesia ('conscious sedation') should be able to manage patients who enter a state of deep sedation/analgesia, while those administering deep sedation/analgesia should be able to manage patients who enter a state of general anaesthesia.

providing the sedation must have the necessary skills to rescue the patient should they become 'moderately sedated'. If the patient's intended level of sedation is 'moderate sedation', then 'the practitioner must have the skills to rescue the patient should they become deeply sedated'. Likewise, if a patient's intended level of sedation is 'deep sedation', then 'the practitioner must have the skills to rescue the patient should they slip into a state of general anaesthesia'.[18] Obviously, for the paediatric patient and many adult patients, the primary effect of sedating medications is to compromise respirations either in terms of decreased respiratory rate and excursion, or airway obstruction and desaturation. Thus, the JCAHO requires that practitioners administering or directing sedation must have the skills to perform bag/mask ventilation to unobstruct an obstructed airway, to treat laryngospasm, and perhaps even the skill of endotracheal intubation if the intended level of sedation is deep sedation.

In the year 2000, the ASA formed a new task force and published a revised sedation guideline for non-anaesthesiologists[19] and then in 2002 the AAP published an addendum[20] to their 1992 guideline which now clarified the definitions so that all the major organisations in the US (ASA, AAP, and JCAHO) now use the same uniform definitions for the various levels of sedation.[20] In addition, the AAP addendum stressed that the guideline applied to all patients that are sedated regardless of the venue, *i.e.* it is meant to apply to hospitalised patients, patients in a surgery centre, and patients sedated in a private office or imaging facility.

Interest in sedation processes has also been the subject of concern in a variety of countries other than the US,[21] and perhaps the best known recent guideline is the Scottish Intercollegiate Guidelines Network which presented the general principles of preparation for sedation, specific sedation techniques, requirements for those individuals who were providing sedation, and then, in particular, addressed specific information related to dentistry, radiology, emergency medicine, information for parents, and how to audit the provision of such services.[22] Obviously, the implementation of such guidelines can be a very cumbersome and expensive process, and that in part explains the reluctance of the medical community to adopt sedation guidelines voluntarily. In the US the JCAHO has provided an important piece of this process, because its regulations have forced hospitals and physicians to comply with these guidelines. This, in turn, has likely reduced the incidence of life-threatening complications associated with the sedation process simply by reducing the number of individuals who are providing such services, *i.e.* by making the chief of the individual divisions responsible for the physicians within their division, it ensured that those individuals have proper credentials and qualifications. Many physicians who previously provided sedation no longer provide it and instead rely upon the expertise of anaesthesiologists or other sub-specialists trained in advanced airway management skills, such as emergency medicine or intensive care medicine physicians. In addition, many hospitals have developed teams of advance practice sedation nurses who generally have had several years' experience in the postanaesthesia care or in the intensive care unit. These nurses are skilled in rapidly recognising and assessing compromises of respiration and then intervening appropriately.

Clearly all guidelines recognise that there are various levels of sedation. A patient who has received minimal or moderate sedation may require less in the way of vigilance than those who are deeply sedated. However, the consistent feature of all of these guidelines is that if a patient is deeply sedated (*i.e.* at risk for airway compromise and/or progressing to a state of general anaesthesia), then there is need for more frequent vital-sign monitoring as well as an independent observer whose only responsibility is to observe the patient. In other words, a clinician should not be sedating the patient and performing the procedure at the same time. For young paediatric patients there is evidence that the child often progresses to a deeper level of sedation than that intended.[23,24] This suggests that for paediatric patients one should assume from the initiation of sedation that there must be an independent observer and, since the child may become deeply sedated, that part of the healthcare team must consist of an individual who is capable of rescuing the child.

THE DEMOGRAPHICS OF SEDATION ACCIDENTS

In 1994, through the Freedom of Information Act, I requested all adverse drug reports submitted to the FDA regarding paediatric patients. We obtained 629 adverse drug reports, conducted a survey of 1555 paediatric intensive care and emergency medicine physicians as well as 310 paediatric anaesthesiologists, queried the *US Pharmacopoeia*, and received anonymous reports. These were independently reviewed by two paediatric anaesthesiologists, an emergency medicine physician and an intensive care physician for 17 possible contributory factors (systems issues) relating to the adverse event. Each case was debated by

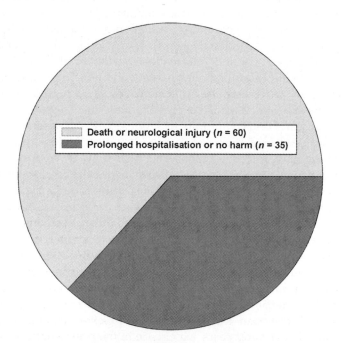

Death or neurological injury (*n* = 60)
Prolonged hospitalisation or no harm (*n* = 35)

Fig. 1 Outcomes of sedation accidents. Pie graph illustrating the outcomes of 95 children following adverse events during sedation by non-anaesthesiologists. Note that 60 out of the 95 patients suffered death or neurological injury indicating the failure to rescue of patients once they developed a respiratory or cardiac complication. Abstracted from data from Coté *et al.*[10]

the four reviewers. A review designed after the ASA Closed Claims Critical Incident Analysis was conducted, *i.e.* 'what went wrong, why did it go wrong, and how could it have been prevented'?[25] Ultimately, 95 cases were selected where all four reviewers agreed upon the contributory factors.[10] The outcomes measures were: death, permanent neurological injury, prolonged hospitalisation, or no harm (Fig. 1). We were astonished by statements within these reports that are included here to illustrate where 'the system' failed.

'An oxygen outlet available but no flow meter...no oxygen for 10 min' (inadequate equipment and planning).

'The child became stridorous and cyanotic on the way home' (premature discharge from medical supervision).

'The child received 6000 mg of chloral hydrate' (drug overdose).

'Drug given at home by a parent' (drug administered without the safety net of medical supervision).

'A 6-week-old infant received Demerol Phenergan and Thorazine for a circumcision – found dead in bed' (inappropriate drug selection for the procedure and age group, prolonged drug half-life, drug overdose, and drug interaction).

'The patient was given 175 µg fentanyl i.v. leading to chest wall rigidity' (they did not understand the pharmacology of the drug so that, in addition to the overdose, they did not use either a muscle relaxant such as succinylcholine or an antagonist such as naloxone).

'The physician administered medication and left the facility leaving the patient with a technician' (abandonment of the patient and inadequately trained person to rescue the patient).

'The patient received tablespoons instead of teaspoons' (a transcription/prescription error).

'The patient was not on any monitors' (inadequate monitoring).

Approximately two-thirds of the children were ≤ 6 years old, the age where pharmacological restraint is most likely to be needed and the majority of the patients were ASA physical status I or II indicating that most had no serious underlying medical conditions. Of the 95 cases, 60 were associated with death or permanent neurological injury (Fig. 1). Two children died before arrival at the healthcare facility emphasising why sedating medications should never be administered without the safety net of medical supervision. Ten others (9 with death or neurological injury) suffered the event in the automobile or at home after discharge. All of these patients had received medications with long half-lives (chloral hydrate, promethazine, chlorpromazine, intramuscular [i.m.] pentobarbital). When examining contributory causes to death or injury, drug overdose (defined as > 125% of the maximum recommended dose), drug interactions (*e.g.* opioid and benzodiazepine), inadequate monitoring, inadequate medical evaluation, and premature discharge were the most common. When examining the drug class, there was equivalent representation of barbiturates, opioids, benzodiazepines and sedatives including 13 children who had received chloral hydrate, suggesting that one class of drugs did not appear to offer advantage over another and that even chloral hydrate could cause an adverse outcome.[26] When examining the route of administration, adverse events were associated with i.v., i.m., oral, rectal, nasal, and inhalational routes of drug administration. Approximately half were associated with a single sedating medication and half received 2–5 sedating medications; there was a significant association with death and neurological injury when 3 or more sedating medications were administered. The majority of events presented with an adverse effect upon respirations or oxygenation; however, a large fraction progressed to cardiac arrest indicating the lack of skills to rescue the patient once a problem was recognised. There was a significantly better outcome when pulse oximetry was used compared to no monitoring. There was a 3-fold increase in morbidity and mortality when procedures were performed in a non-hospital based venue (private office, free-standing radiology facility) compared with a hospital or surgical centre. This suggests a lack of adequate rescue skills in this venue. The specialty with the highest representation was children undergoing dental procedures. In the US, most sedation for dental procedures is provided by dentists since health insurance usually does not cover hospitalisation and anaesthesiology services. This clearly points out a defect in the US healthcare system since dental disease is not given the same recognition as other paediatric healthcare issues. If insurance was provided, the dentists would not be forced to also be the anaesthesiologist.

These data suggest that it is not the drugs and not the route of administration that is important but rather the skills of the individuals involved, continuous monitoring particularly with pulse oximetry, presedation evaluation, and the need for adequate and strict discharge criteria.[10,26] The chloral hydrate deaths following discharge suggest that these children may benefit from an extended period of observation in a step-down unit since re-sedation after discharge is possible (the head falling forward in the car seat possibly resulting in airway obstruction). Clearly, the majority of these adverse outcomes were preventable and these cases illustrate the importance of strict adherence to, and the need for, sedation guidelines.

THE PHARMACOLOGY OF COMMONLY USED SEDATION/ANALGESIC MEDICATIONS

NARCOTICS – LONG ACTING

Morphine

Morphine's duration of action when administered i.v. is 3–4 h and the kinetics are similar to adults in infants older than 3 months of age. It may be administered i.v., i.m., sublingually, or orally. The usual initial dose is 0.05 mg/kg up to 0.3 mg/kg. Since this drug is not very fat soluble, it may take up to 10 min to achieve peak central nervous system (CNS) effect. Therefore, this drug should be titrated to effect with at least 5–8 min between doses. This drug is generally reserved for painful procedures of greater than 30 min duration.

Meperidine (pethidine)

Meperidine is useful for painful procedures of greater than 30 min duration. The usual initial dose is 0.5–2 mg/kg i.v. or i.m. The serum half-life is similar to morphine. This drug is not indicated for the treatment of chronic pain because of the potential for accumulation of toxic metabolites (normeperidine); however, it is a useful opioid for short-term use. Peak values are achieved at 90 min following i.m. injection. Thus, when the i.m. route is used for a procedure, the period of peak narcosis may occur after the procedure has been completed, thus placing the patient at greatest risk for respiratory depression when the physical stimulation to keep them awake is the least.

NARCOTICS – INTERMEDIATE ACTING (AGONISTS/ANTAGONISTS)

Butorphanol and nalbuphine

Opioid agonist-antagonists are useful for a variety of procedures in children. The elimination half-life is approximately 2 h. A reasonable starting i.v. dose is 0.02 mg/kg and then titrate to effect. Since these agents may reverse mu-receptor mediated analgesia from more potent opioids, they should be used as the sole narcotic. The potential for a ceiling on the respiratory depression is an attractive property.

NARCOTICS – SHORT ACTING

Fentanyl

Fentanyl is the most commonly used short-acting opioid and is about 100 times more potent (mg/kg) than morphine. It is highly fat soluble allowing it to penetrate the blood brain barrier rapidly thus resulting in a very rapid onset of action (< 1 min). Its termination of action when administered intermittently is primarily determined by redistribution rather than metabolism. The opioid effects generally last for 30–45 min, but the respiratory depression may last longer. The most important adverse side-effect is that fentanyl can cause chest wall and glottic rigidity, bradycardia, and severe respiratory depression, especially when rapidly administered. Safe administration is achieved by slowly titrating (several minutes between doses) 0.25–0.5 µg/kg per dose (i.v.) with a ceiling of 3–4 µg/kg when administered i.v. The potential for respiratory depression is markedly increased when co-administered with other sedatives and in infants younger than 3 months of age.

Fentanyl is available in a transoral mucosal formulation (the Fentanyl Oralet®/Actique®) offering a painless route of administration (usual dose 10–15 µg/kg). The problem with this formulation is that consumption time is quite variable as are the achieved peak blood levels.[27,28] Generally, uptake from the oral mucosa combined with gastrointestinal absorption results in analgesic concentrations within 15–30 min of completion. One advantage of this route of administration is the prolonged and flat elimination period which extends the analgesic period for several hours. A recent study completed in my institution suggests that similar blood levels may be achieved with equivalent doses of the liquid i.v. formulation administered orally avoiding the problem of variable consumption time.[29] Further studies will be required to examine the usefulness and safety of this route of fentanyl administration for non-operating room venues.

Alfentanil and sufentanil

These synthetic fentanyl analogues have lower lipid solubility and a smaller volume of distribution compared with fentanyl. This results in lower brain concentrations and a more rapid elimination. These medications have dose-independent pharmacokinetics (*i.e.* the larger the dose, the greater the elimination) thus providing a wide margin of safety. Children eliminate alfentanil more rapidly than adults but sufentanil elimination is inversely related to age (teenagers are similar to adults). Clearance of both drugs is markedly delayed in patients with hepatic disease but unaffected by renal disease. As with fentanyl, there is the potential for chest wall and glottic rigidity that is dose-related and a greater likelihood of bradycardia. These drugs are usually used as a supplement to general anaesthesia. There are minimal published data for procedural sedation/analgesia in children. Sufentanil has been administered nasally (2–3 µg/kg) as a non-invasive means for providing short-acting analgesia.

NARCOTICS – ULTRA-SHORT ACTING

Remifentanil

This is the newest approved synthetic opioid which has unique properties because the drug is broken down by non-specific blood and tissue esterases.[30] This implies that drug metabolism would be little affected by either liver or hepatic dysfunction. The most impressive effect is that despite long-term infusions, there is virtually no residual opioid effect 10–12 min after stopping the infusion. The time to 50% reduction in drug effect is approximately 4 min. Although these properties are very attractive, this opioid is so potent and has such a short effective half-life, that it is difficult to manage in patients who are not intubated. This drug must be administered by a continuous i.v. infusion. Chest wall and glottic rigidity as well as bradycardia may be observed. If there is any alteration in the rate of administration (kinked i.v., bolus of another drug, interruption of the carrier i.v. fluid), the patient will rapidly awaken and feel intense pain. At this point in time, it would appear that this drug is best left for the operating room venue.

Tramadol

Tramadol is a new family of drugs that has weak opioid effects and, therefore, minimal effects upon respiration. The major effect seems to be alteration of spinal cord pain receptor activation and alteration of serotonin and norepinephrine re-uptake. The analgesia is similar to that provided by nalbuphine. At present in the US, this drug is not available in an i.v. formulation and there are few data in paediatric patients for procedural analgesia. Once an i.v. formulation becomes generally available, then this medication may be suitable for procedures associated with minimal pain.

SEDATIVES/ANXIOLYTICS

Benzodiazepines

Diazepam

Anxiolysis and amnesia are very important for the sedation process making the benzodiazepines an essential adjunct to procedural sedation. Diazepam is generally used in doses of 0.1–0.3 mg/kg (i.v. or orally) either alone or in combination with other medications; diazepam also may be administered rectally. Its main disadvantage is the long duration of action and the pain it produces with i.v. or i.m. administration. Diazepam should not be administered i.m. because of poor drug absorption. Diazepam should be used with caution in children with severe hepatic dysfunction. Respiratory depression is particularly likely when combined with a narcotic.

Midazolam

Midazolam is a shorter acting water-soluble benzodiazepine which is generally pain free with i.v. or i.m. administration. It is also administered orally and rectally. The beta elimination half-life is significantly shorter than diazepam (106 ± 29 min versus 18 h in children). Midazolam is the most popular sedative in the paediatric age group. Approximately 50% of children will have anterograde amnesia. This drug generally produces a calm, compliant patient who is receptive to most non-threatening interventions but, by itself, it does not usually produce a sleep state even with doses as high as 3.0 mg/kg rectally.[31] This drug seems to have much greater potential for respiratory depression in the elderly than in children.[32] It is my experience that midazolam comes the closest of any sedative to producing a true state of 'moderate sedation – conscious sedation' in children, provided it is not combined with other sedating medications. Unfortunately, the bitter aftertaste of the i.v. preparation is difficult to suppress even with artificial sweeteners. When administered orally, it is best to ask children to swallow as much as possible in the first gulp rather than to ask them to sip it. The nasal route of drug administration is painful and theoretically the drug could traverse along neurovascular tissue directly into the CNS. Since the preservative is neurotoxic, this route of administration would appear less preferable. It should be noted that apnoea may occur when combining midazolam with fentanyl or other medications for sedation. A very important pharmacodynamic effect is that,

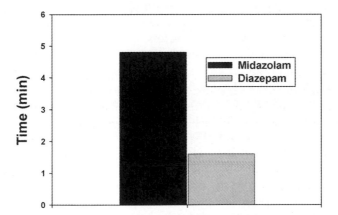

Fig. 2 Time to peak EEG effect. Time to peak electroencephalographic effect (EEG) of diazepam versus midazolam in adult patients. Note that it takes nearly 3 times longer to achieve a peak EEG effect following i.v. midazolam than diazepam. This is likely due to the difference in fat solubility since midazolam is less fat soluble than diazepam; it does not cross biological membranes (*e.g.* into the CNS) as readily. Data abstracted from Buhrer M, Maitre PO, Crevoisier C, Stansky DR. Electroencephalographic effects of benzodiazepines. II Pharmacodynamic modeling of the electroencephalographic effects of midazolam and diazepam. *Clin Pharmacol Ther* 1990; **48**: 555–567.

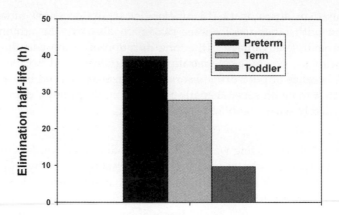

Fig. 3 Beta elimination half-life of the active metabolite of chloral hydrate (trichloroethanol) in preterm infants, term infants, and toddlers. Note the extremely long half-lives in all age groups. Although chloral hydrate is frequently described as a short-acting sedative, these data suggest that chloral hydrate can have profoundly long sedating effects. Data abstracted from Mayers et al.[33]

because midazolam is less fat soluble than diazepam, it takes nearly 3 times longer to achieve a peak EEG effect (adults 4.6 min versus 1.4 min; Fig. 2); thus, it is advisable to wait at least 3 min before administering additional midazolam in order to avoid 'stacking' of doses and overshooting the intended level of sedation.

CHLORAL HYDRATE

Chloral hydrate remains one of the most popular procedural sedatives particularly for infants. The usual dose is 25–75 mg/kg which can be administered orally or rectally. Most practitioners limit the total dose to 100 mg/kg or 2.0 g, whichever comes first. As with most oral sedatives, the peak effect may take 60 min or longer to accomplish. Its bitter taste makes this drug less acceptable to some children. The drug also has a long beta elimination half-life (Fig. 3).[33] The main disadvantage is that chloral hydrate can result in prolonged sedation, particularly in infants. In neonates, the drug half-life is > 24 h (Fig. 3). In addition, late onset or peak sedative effect may occur well after the intended time of desired sedation. A recent case described to me was an infant scheduled for a CAT scan who did not fall asleep nor did the child even appear sleepy after 1 h. The patient was discharged and fell asleep as soon as it was placed in the car seat and the mother started driving home. She returned to the facility and the procedure was carried out successfully! This case had a good outcome but it could easily have been a disaster.

One of this drug's purported attributes is its minimal effect on respiration; however, respiratory depression and deaths have been reported particularly when combined with other sedatives or narcotics. The likely mechanism is inability to unobstruct the airway.[26] One death has occurred following 50 mg/kg administered to an apparently healthy infant at home prior to a scheduled radiological procedure, underscoring the importance of the AAP Guidelines' requirement of only administering sedatives under the safety net of medical supervision.

Irregular absorption may delay the onset of sedation and the practitioner may be tempted to administer a second dose. This second dose may produce satisfactory sedation but result in profound and excessively long sedation following the procedure. One of the deaths reported in our outcomes' study was a child who received two doses of chloral hydrate, was discharged from the hospital, and then found dead at home.[26] Certainly, these cases do not mean that chloral hydrate should not be used; rather, it means that appropriate use in hospital and observation of the child after sedation, particularly for airway patency when asleep, is required.

DEMEROL–PHENERGAN–THORAZINE (DPT)

The 'lytic cocktail' is a commonly used sedation regimen particularly in the cardiac catheterisation laboratory. In North America, this is usually a combination of demerol (meperidine 25 mg/ml), phenergan (promethazine 6.5 mg/ml), and thorazine (chlorpromazine 6.5 mg/ml) administered at a dose of 0.1 ml/kg i.m. A lower dose is recommended for children with cyanotic congenital heart disease. Phenothiazines have α-adrenergic blocking properties which can result in profound hypotension if administered to individuals with a contracted blood volume. Phenothiazines lower the seizure threshold in most individuals; this drug combination should not be used in children with seizure disorders. Dystonic reactions commonly occur with phenothiazine administration.

When one rationally examines this drug combination (two long-acting phenothiazines and a long-acting narcotic) this 'lytic cocktail' makes little sense for patients undergoing non-cardiac catheterisation procedures. In addition, phenothiazines have anti-analgesic properties and potentiate the respiratory depression produced by narcotics. The sedation produced may last for hours longer than the planned procedure (a mean sleep time of 4.7 ± 2.4 h with a reported 19 ± 15 h for 'return to normal').[34] This places the child at risk for late complications particularly if the patient is not carefully monitored. Several children in our sedation accident cohort who died following hospital or office discharge had received this combination of drugs.[26] Some practitioners are administering this drug combination i.v.; if the clinician has i.v. access, there are many other drugs that would make more pharmacodynamic and pharmacokinetic sense. The use of demerol–phenergan–thorazine i.v. should be abandoned and this combination of drugs can no longer be recommended for the vast majority of procedures requiring sedation/analgesia.

ANTIHISTAMINES

Diphenhydramine and hydroxyzine

Antihistamines provide a useful adjunct in the sedation of children. In addition to the antihistaminic properties, the sedation produced is often sufficient to provide a sleeping child for a non-painful procedure. Generally, either diphenhydramine (0.25–1.0 mg/kg i.v., i.m., orally) or hydroxyzine (0.25–1.0 mg/kg i.v., i.m., orally) are combined with another sedating agent such as chloral hydrate (if the chloral hydrate by itself fails).

INTRAVENOUS ANAESTHETIC/INDUCTION AGENTS

Ketamine

Ketamine, a derivative of phencyclidine, is an excellent analgesic and amnestic i.v. anaesthetic agent which binds to opiate receptors. It causes central dissociation of the cerebral cortex and CNS excitation. The degree of sedation may vary from analgesia with moderate sedation to a state of general anaesthesia depending upon the dose and route of administration. Ketamine is administered i.v., i.m., orally, and rectally. Ketamine increases heart rate and systemic blood pressure; cerebral metabolic rate for oxygen also is markedly increased as well as intracranial and intra-ocular pressure by means of cerebral vasodilation. Therefore, ketamine is generally contra-indicated in children with CNS pathology involving intracranial hypertension. Ketamine can result in the production of copious secretions and, therefore, should be administered with an antisialagogue. It may be contra-indicated in children with active upper respiratory infections because the copious secretions may add further to an irritable airway and, therefore, lead to an increased incidence of laryngospasm. Ketamine has been associated with dreaming and hallucinations; concomitant administration of a benzodiazepine or narcotic may reduce these side-effects but also will deepen the level and duration of sedation. Ketamine is associated with purposeless movement and may not be ideal for procedures which require the total lack of movement such as radiation therapy or MRI.

Ketamine has gained wide-spread use in the emergency medicine population where patients with a full stomach are commonly sedated. However, ketamine has been demonstrated to cause an incompetent gag reflex and should be administered with caution to patients with a full stomach or with gastro-oesophageal reflux. Emergency medicine specialists have published a number of papers suggesting that ketamine is different from all other sedating medications and that the dissociative state produced does not fit the standard definitions of sedation.[35] However, ketamine is an intravenous anaesthetic and the effects produced are dose related. Moderate sedation/analgesia ('conscious sedation') may be produced by very low doses titrated i.v. (0.25–0.5 mg/kg). Higher doses (> 1 mg/kg i.v. and > 2 mg/kg i.m.) and in particular when combined with other sedating medications usually produce deep sedation or general anaesthesia. Ketamine has also been administered orally and rectally (6–10 mg/kg).

Ketamine has an excellent safety profile because there is relatively little in the way of respiratory depression. There is no collapse of the hypopharyngeal structures, and cardiovascular stability is maintained. Ketamine's safety profile is such that in non-industrialised countries ketamine is administered by individuals with minimal training in anaesthesiology for major surgical procedures. Nevertheless, despite this strong safety record, individuals who use this medication must recognise that airway obstruction, apnoea, and laryngospasm do occur in 1–2% of patients; therefore, they must have the skills to manage these complications.[36–39] Ketamine is not a drug to be used by the occasional person administering procedural sedation.

Methohexital

Methohexital is a short-acting oxybarbiturate which is an i.v. anaesthetic induction agent often used to sedate children for non-painful procedures such as CAT scans. Doses of 20–30 mg/kg rectally (10% solution, [100 mg/ml], maximum 500 mg) produce a state of light-to-deep sedation in children between 6 months and 6 years of age (20 kg or less). Rectal absorption is rapid but somewhat irregular. About 85% of children loose consciousness within 7–10 min of the first dose. Methohexital can produce seizures in children with temporal lobe epilepsy. The sedation produced will result in airway obstruction if careful attention is not paid to head position (do not allow the head to flex forward); however, with appropriate positioning, the vast majority of patients will maintain normal oxygen saturation even in room air. Children with large tonsils or adenoids may experience airway obstruction. Apnoea may occur when there is rapid rectal drug absorption and is often observed with i.v. administration (0.25–2.0 mg/kg). Methohexital should only be administered by individuals skilled in airway management, and the patients require monitoring for deep sedation or general anaesthesia. Generally, children will remain sedated for 45–60 min if left undisturbed. If it is necessary to insert an i.v. catheter, then local anaesthetic administration or EMLA cream (eutectic mixture of local anaesthetic applied 60 min earlier) will greatly facilitate the insertion of the i.v. catheter without awakening the child. The author has found this drug particularly valuable for CT scans but less useful for MR imaging because of its duration and the noise of the scanner.

Thiopental

Thiopental is a longer acting barbiturate which may be administered safely in patients with temporal lobe epilepsy. For non-painful procedures, a dose of 20–30 mg/kg rectally may be used. The same safety precautions are required as for methohexital, and children will usually sleep slightly longer.

Pentobarbital

This long-acting barbiturate is the most popular barbiturate for sedating children for radiological investigations. Generally, a dose of 5–7 mg/kg i.m. or titrated i.v. doses (2 mg/kg up to 7 mg/kg) produces satisfactory sedation with minimal respiratory compromise. Combination with other sedatives or narcotics will markedly increase the potential for airway obstruction.[40]

Propofol

Propofol is a very versatile sedative-hypnotic anaesthetic agent for the i.v. induction and maintenance of anaesthesia and for procedural sedation. It is very rapidly eliminated through first-pass hepatic degradation. This drug rapidly produces dose-dependent levels of sedation varying from very light sedation to general anaesthesia. Propofol is most safely administered as a constant infusion (by a pump) 'piggy backed' into a constantly running i.v. line which allows careful drug titration. Generally, sedative doses vary between 50–200 µg/kg/min depending on the painfulness of the procedure. Propofol causes a very rapid loss of consciousness, hypotension, and apnoea. Because this drug very rapidly produces a state of general anaesthesia, it should not be used by individuals unskilled in airway management. The role of this drug for procedural sedation should be restricted to individuals with advance airway management skills such as anaesthesiologists, intensive care medicine and emergency medicine specialists. A drawback of propofol is the pain which occurs with i.v. administration, which can be reduced by prior administration of 0.5–1.0 mg/kg lidocaine slowly prior to propofol administration, administering the propofol through a large vein (*e.g.* antecubital), or prior administration of opioid.

LOCAL ANAESTHETICS

The liberal and safe use of local anaesthetic agents is fundamental to the conduct of procedures associated with pain.[41] It is important for the clinician to understand the appropriate use of local anaesthetic agents so as to avoid toxicity. Local anaesthetic overdose causes CNS excitation (seizures) and cardiovascular depression (vasodilatation and decreased cardiac contractility). In children, it is easy to interpret crying as lack of analgesia so that the clinician is tempted to use more local anaesthetic, which may easily lead to local anaesthetic overdose. Toxicity is a function of drug dose, site of injection (vascularity), rate of uptake (use of vasoconstrictor will delay uptake), alteration of toxic threshold (benzodiazepines will raise the CNS toxic threshold but will not alter the cardiotoxic threshold), and technique of administration (direct i.v. administration in a vascular area – always aspirate prior to injecting). All doses should be calculated on a mg/kg basis with upper limits of dose/volume determined prior to the procedure. More local may be used with subcutaneous injection in a relatively non-vascular area than for direct nerve blocks. Table 7 presents the maximum recommended doses of commonly used local anaesthetic agents. Table 8 presents the mg/ml concentration. Table 9 presents the conversion of epinephrine dilution in terms of µg/ml. Long-acting drugs are recommended for providing long-lasting analgesia.

Table 7 Maximum recommended doses and duration of action of commonly used local anaesthetics

Local anaesthetic	Maximum dose (mg/kg)*	Duration of action (min)[†]
Procaine	10	60–90
2-Chloroprocaine	20	30–60
Tetracaine	1.5	180–600
Lidocaine	7	90–200
Mepivacaine	7	120–240
Bupivacaine	3	180–600
Ropivacaine	3	180–600

*These are maximum doses of local anaesthetics. Doses of amides should be decreased by 30% in infants less than 6 months of age. When lidocaine is being administered intravascularly (*e.g.* during intravenous regional anaesthesia), the dose should be decreased to 3–5 mg/kg; there is no need to administer long-acting local anaesthetic agents for intravenous regional anaesthesia, and such a practice is potentially dangerous.
[†]Duration of action is dependent on concentration, total dose, and site of administration, and the patient's age.
Reproduced with permission from Polaner DM, Suresh S, Coté CJ. Pediatric regional anesthesia. Coté CJ, Todres ID, Goudsouzian NG, Ryan JF. (eds) *A Practice of Anesthesia for Infants and Children*, 3rd edn. Philadelphia, PA: WB Saunders, 2001; 636–674.

Table 8 Epinephrine dilution and conversion to µg/ml

Epinephrine dilution	µg/ml
1:100,000	10
1:200,000	5
1:400,000	2.5
1:800,000	1.25

Reproduced with permission from Polaner DM, Suresh S, Coté CJ. Pediatric regional anesthesia. Coté CJ, Todres ID, Goudsouzian NG, Ryan JF. (eds) *A Practice of Anesthesia for Infants and Children*, 3rd edn. Philadelphia, PA: WB Saunders, 2001; 636–674.

Table 9 Local anaesthetic concentration and its conversion to mg/ml

Concentration (%)	mg/ml
3.0	30
2.5	25
2.0	20
1.0	10
0.5	5
0.25	2.5
0.125	1.25

Reproduced with permission from Polaner DM, Suresh S, Coté CJ. Pediatric regional anesthesia. Coté CJ, Todres ID, Goudsouzian NG, Ryan JF. (eds) *A Practice of Anesthesia for Infants and Children*, 3rd edn. Philadelphia, PA: WB Saunders, 2001; 636–674.

TOPICAL ANAESTHETICS

Topically applied, tetracaine, adrenaline, and cocaine is popular for suture of lacerations. Each component of this topical drug combination has the potential for toxicity. Plasma cocaine levels have been found in children to whom topically applied cannabis was applied; however, no cocaine toxicity was demonstrated if applied topically (not on mucosal surfaces). One death from cocaine toxicity has been reported when topically applied cannabis was applied to the oral mucosa.[42] Tetracaine (1.0%, 10 mg/ml), 1:4000 epinephrine (250 µg/ml), and 4.0% cocaine (40 mg/ml) has good efficacy. Limiting the total dose to 1.5 ml/10 kg and absolutely avoid application to any mucus membrane (*i.e.* not to be used in the mouth or nose) reduces the potential for toxicity. Topically applied cannabis should not be applied to areas with limited circulation (*e.g.* digits or the penis). Other topical combinations that have been successfully applied include lidocaine-epinephrine-tetracaine, mepivacaine-epinephrine-tetracaine, and bupivacaine-norepinephrine.

EMLA CREAM

EMLA cream is a eutectic mixture of local anaesthetics (lidocaine and prilocaine) which is applied to the skin with an occlusive dressing for a minimum of 30–60 min prior to the procedure. Prilocaine can cause methaemoglobinaemia if an excessively large amount of drug is applied or if it is applied to mucosal surfaces. A second dressing to cover the EMLA occlusive dressing may prevent the child from accidental ingestion.

COMMON SEDATION REGIMENS

It should be emphasised that no sedation regimen is perfect and that each institution generally develops its own favourite combination of medications that is effective for its population of patients. In addition, the sedation regimens used by anaesthesiologists will markedly differ from those used by non-anaesthesiologists. The following are some regimens that are currently used effectively by non-anaesthesiologists with all the safety measures described above. In most situations inserting an i.v. after topical or infiltration of local anaesthetic provides the ability to titrate drugs to effect and to rescue the patient should that be necessary. Drugs that have an antagonist may provide an additional safety measure.

RADIOLOGY

CAT scan and MRI

For those < 1 year, sleep deprivation with chloral hydrate (50 mg/kg). If sedation is inadequate, then chloral hydrate (25–50 mg/kg up to 100 mg/kg) Note that the half-life in neonates is so prolonged that the lowest effective dose should be chosen (see above). Former preterm neonates < 60 weeks postconceptual age should be admitted for post-procedure apnoea monitoring.

For those > 1 year, sleep deprivation with chloral hydrate (50 mg/kg). If sedation is inadequate, then chloral hydrate (25–50 mg/kg up to 100 mg/kg, maximum 2 g) with diphenhydramine or hydroxyzine (0.25–1.0 mg/kg orally, maximum 10 mg).

For those > 1 year, sleep deprivation, EMLA cream and i.v. pentobarbital (3 mg/kg); wait 3–5 min. If inadequate sedation, additional pentobarbital (2 mg/kg) and wait 3–5 min. If sedation is still inadequate, then pentobarbital (2 mg/kg to maximum of 7 mg/kg or 200 mg) and wait additional 5 min. If sedation is still inadequate, then midazolam (0.05 mg/kg) and wait 5 min. If sedation is still inadequate, then midazolam (0.05 mg/kg). Have midazolam reversal agent (flumazenil, 0.01 mg/kg) immediately available.

An alternate oral regimen for those > 1 year: midazolam (0.5–0.75 mg/kg up to 15 mg) with atropine (0.02–0.03 mg/kg up to 1.5 mg) and ketamine (6–8 mg/kg) orally. Have midazolam reversal agent (flumazenil, 0.01 mg/kg) immediately available.

Invasive radiology procedures

Same as above or the following options:

Intramuscular option

Ketamine (2 mg/kg) and atropine (0.02 mg/kg) i.m. or ketamine (2 mg/kg), atropine (0.02 mg/kg) and midazolam (0.05 mg/kg) i.m. If this fails, then start i.v. and titrate additional ketamine (0.25–0.5 mg/kg) and midazolam

(0.025–0.05 mg/kg) i.v. at 3–5 min intervals as needed. Have midazolam reversal agent (flumazenil, 0.01 mg/kg) immediately available.

Intravenous option
Ketamine (0.5–1.0 mg/kg), atropine (0.02 mg/kg) and midazolam (0.05 mg/kg). Wait 3–5 min. Titrate additional ketamine (0.25–0.5 mg/kg) and midazolam (0.025–0.05 mg/kg) i.v. at 3–5 min intervals as needed. Have midazolam reversal agent (flumazenil, 0.01 mg/kg) immediately available.

Alternate intravenous option
Midazolam (0.05 mg/kg) and fentanyl (1 µg/kg). Wait 3 min. If inadequate sedation, then midazolam (0.025–0.5 mg/kg) and fentanyl (0.5–1 µg/kg). Titrate additional smaller increments at 3–5 min intervals as needed. Have both fentanyl and midazolam reversal agents (naloxone [0.01–0.1 mg/kg] and flumazenil [0.01 mg/kg]) immediately available.

ONCOLOGY

LP/bone marrow aspiration
EMLA cream to venous port at home prior to arrival. Midazolam (0.05 mg/kg), fentanyl (1 µg/kg) i.v. with local infiltration of procedure site. If inadequate sedation after 3 min, titrate additional midazolam (0.025 mg/kg) and fentanyl (0.5 µg/kg) i.v. at 3–5 min intervals as needed. Have both fentanyl and midazolam reversal agents (naloxone [0.01–0.1 mg/kg] and flumazenil [0.01 mg/kg]) immediately available.

Alternatively, EMLA cream to venous port at home prior to arrival. Midazolam (0.05 mg/kg), atropine (0.02 mg/kg) and ketamine (0.5–1.0 mg/kg) i.v. Wait 3–5 min. If inadequate sedation, titrate midazolam (0.025–0.05 mg/kg) and ketamine (0.5 mg/kg) i.v. at 3–5 min intervals as needed. Have fentanyl reversal agent (flumazenil, 0.01 mg/kg) immediately available.

GASTRO-ENTEROLOGY

Upper and lower endoscopy
After EMLA cream or local infiltration, start i.v. Midazolam (0.05 mg/kg), fentanyl (1–2 µg/kg) i.v. with topical local anaesthetic spray or nebulisation of lidocaine to upper airway (important to calculate safe mg/kg local anaesthetic upper limits). After 3–5 min, titrate midazolam (0.05 mg/kg) and fentanyl (1 µg/kg) i.v. If inadequate sedation after 3 min, titrate additional midazolam (0.025 mg/kg) and fentanyl (0.5 µg/kg) i.v. at 3–5 min intervals as needed. Have both fentanyl and midazolam reversal agents (naloxone [0.01–0.1 mg/kg] and flumazenil [0.01 mg/kg]) immediately available.

Alternatively, after EMLA cream or local infiltration start i.v. Midazolam (0.05 mg/kg), fentanyl (1 µg/kg), atropine (0.02 mg/kg), and ketamine (0.5–1.0 mg/kg) i.v. with topical local anaesthetic spray or nebulisation of lidocaine to upper airway. If inadequate sedation after 3 min, titrate additional midazolam (0.025 mg/kg), fentanyl (0.5 µg/kg) and/or ketamine (0.5 mg/kg). If inadequate sedation after 3–5 min, titrate additional midazolam (0.025 mg/kg), fentanyl

(0.5 µg/kg) and/or ketamine (0.5 mg/kg) at 5-min intervals as needed. Have both fentanyl and midazolam reversal agents (naloxone [0.01–0.1 mg/kg] and flumazenil [0.01 mg/kg]) immediately available.

Alternate regimens administered by an anaesthesiologist, or other trained expert (*e.g.* intensive care physician or emergency medicine physician) include combinations of i.v. propofol by continuous infusion, with incremental doses of fentanyl or ketamine and atropine as clinically indicated.

EMERGENCY MEDICINE

Suture of laceration

Option 1
After assessing the risk:benefit ratio of a patient with a full stomach. Midazolam (0.5–0.75 mg/kg, maximum 15 mg) orally. Apply appropriate topical solution (see above) with additional local anaesthetic agent to the laceration as needed (see dose limits above).

Option 2
After assessing the risk:benefit ratio of a patient with a full stomach. Midazolam (0.05 mg/kg), atropine (0.02 mg/kg) and ketamine (2 mg/kg) i.m. Apply appropriate topical solution to wound (see above). Wait 5 min and add additional local anaesthetic agent as needed (see dose limits above). If this is inadequate, start i.v. and titrate additional midazolam (0.025 mg/kg) and ketamine (0.05 mg/kg) i.v. If inadequate sedation/analgesia after 5 min, titrate additional midazolam (0.025 mg/kg) and ketamine (0.05 mg/kg) i.v. at 5-min intervals as needed. Have midazolam reversal agent (flumazenil, 0.01 mg/kg) immediately available.

Option 3
After assessing the risk:benefit ratio of a patient with a full stomach. Midazolam (0.5–0.75 mg/kg, maximum 15 mg) orally and apply appropriate topical solution to wound (see above). After 15 min and after either EMLA cream or local infiltration, start i.v. Inject additional local anaesthetic agent into the wound as needed (see dose limits above). If additional sedation required, fentanyl (0.5–1.0 µg/kg) i.v. If inadequate sedation/analgesia after 2–3 min, titrate additional fentanyl (0.5 µg/kg) i.v. at 3-min intervals as needed. Alternatively, after the first dose of fentanyl one could add ketamine (0.5 mg/kg) and atropine (0.02 mg/kg) i.v. Have both fentanyl and midazolam reversal agents (naloxone [0.01–0.1 mg/kg] and flumazenil [0.01 mg/kg]) immediately available.

Fracture reduction
After assessing the risk:benefit ratio of a patient with a full stomach. Some patients will require general anaesthesia or a regional nerve block for successful reduction. Simple fractures may be reduced with the following regimen. Midazolam (0.5–0.75 mg/kg, maximum 15 mg) orally. After 15 min and after either EMLA cream or local infiltration, start i.v. Fentanyl (1–2 µg/kg) i.v. Wait 3 min. Haematoma block by surgeon (see local anaesthetic limits above). Wait 5 min. Fentanyl (1 µg/kg) i.v. Attempt fracture reduction. If

inadequate sedation/analgesia, titrate fentanyl (0.5–1 µg/kg) i.v. at 3-min intervals as needed. Alternatively, after the second dose of fentanyl one could add ketamine (0.5 mg/kg) and atropine (0.02 mg/kg) i.v. Have both fentanyl and midazolam reversal agents (naloxone [0.01–0.1 mg/kg] and flumazenil [0.01 mg/kg]) immediately available.

BRAIN STEM EVOKED AUDITORY RESPONSE (BEAR)

For those < 1 year, sleep deprivation and chloral hydrate (50 mg/kg). If no sleep, chloral hydrate (25–50 mg/kg up to 100 mg/kg). Note that former preterm infants < 60 weeks postconceptual age generally require post-sedation overnight monitoring for apnoea.

Those > 1 year, sleep deprivation and chloral hydrate (50 mg/kg). If no sleep, chloral hydrate (25–50 mg/kg up to 100 mg/kg, maximum 2 g) and diphenhydramine or hydroxyzine (0.25–1.0 mg/kg orally, maximum 10 mg).

> ## Key points for clinical practice
>
> - The guiding principle for providing safe sedation for children means a protective safety net. This consists of a systematic approach with appropriate presedation evaluation, fasting, physical examination, monitoring during and after the procedure, strict discharge criteria, and skilled personnel capable of rescuing the patient should the patient develop difficulty during sedation.
>
> - The intention of sedation guidelines is not to make life difficult for the practitioner but, rather, to provide a systematic approach as to how best to sedate children safely. A variety of organisations have published guidelines in the US: The American Academy of Pediatrics, The American Society of Anesthesiologists, and the Joint Commission on Accreditation of Healthcare Organization; they have agreed on similar language, thus unifying the concepts of guideline development.
>
> - The choice of sedating agent should be based on patient needs, i.e. opioids generally are used for patients undergoing painful procedures whereas sedatives alone are generally necessary for patients undergoing non-painful procedures. The caveat of the least amount of drug to achieve a successful procedure should always apply.
>
> - For children undergoing procedures where there is risk for pulmonary aspiration, such as emergency medicine patients, the lightest level of sedation that allows the procedure to be accomplished should be chosen.
>
> - Premedications should not be administered at home prior to procedure without the benefit of medical supervision. The reason for this is that the child, particularly the infant, may become sedated in the automobile or during transport, the head fall forward and the child obstruct the airway resulting in an adverse outcome.

Key points for clinical practice (continued)

- Chloral hydrate is generally thought to be a very safe medication with minimal effects on respiration. However, analysis of sedation accidents has revealed a number of children who have suffered adverse outcome and chloral hydrate requires the same degree of vigilance associated with any other medication used for sedating children.

- When faced with the issue of sedating a child, the best approach is to establish intravenous access. This then allows the clinician to titrate drug to effect more precisely than if administering the drug orally or intramuscularly where, once the drug is administered, no further alteration in dosage can be made.

- All children that are sedated require, at a minimum, pulse oximetry, intermittent blood pressure measurement, heart rate and respiratory rate monitoring. If the child is deeply sedated, an independent observer whose only responsibility is to observe the patient must be available.

- Drugs with long half-lives may be associated with prolonged sedation or re-sedation after the patient leaves the facility. Therefore, children who have received chloral hydrate, phenothiazines or intramuscular pentobarbital would best be managed by a prolonged observation period, even after they have met discharge criteria.

- Combinations of medications are frequently used to sedate children. It should be understood that when 3 or more sedating medications are administered, there is a greater potential for adverse outcome.

- A practitioner who administers sedation must have the skills to rescue to patient. This means for the patient who is at risk for airway obstruction, apnoea, or adverse event related to the sedating medications, the physician must have the skills to perform bag/mask ventilation and cardiopulmonary resuscitation.

- Ketamine is a drug that has a wonderful safety profile with minimal effects on respiration, airway patency, and cardiovascular status. However, about 1–2% of children will develop airway obstruction, laryngospasm or apnoea; the practitioner who administers ketamine must have the skills to successfully rescue the patient from these complications.

References

1. Eichhorn JH. Effect of monitoring standards on anesthesia outcome. *Int Anesthesiol Clin* 1993; **31**: 181–196.
2. Olkkola KT, Aranko K, Luurila H *et al*. A potentially hazardous interaction between erythromycin and midazolam. *Clin Pharmacol Ther* 1993; **53**: 298–305.
3. Yuan R, Flockhart DA, Balian JD. Pharmacokinetic and pharmacodynamic consequences of metabolism-based drug interactions with alprazolam, midazolam, and triazolam. *J Clin Pharmacol* 1999; **39**: 1109–1125.

4. Litman RS, Kottra JA, Berkowitz RJ, Ward DS. Upper airway obstruction during midazolam/nitrous oxide sedation in children with enlarged tonsils. *Pediatr Dent* 1998; **20**: 318–320.
5. Innes G, Murphy M, Nijssen-Jordan C, Ducharme J, Drummond A. Procedural sedation and analgesia in the emergency department. Canadian Consensus Guidelines. *J Emerg Med* 1999; **17**: 145–156.
6. Morton NS, Oomen GJ. Development of a selection and monitoring protocol for safe sedation of children. *Paediatr Anaesth* 1998; **8**: 65–68.
7. Poe SS, Nolan MT, Dang D *et al*. Ensuring safety of patients receiving sedation for procedures: evaluation of clinical practice guidelines. *Jt Comm J Qual Improv* 2001; **27**: 28–41.
8. Hoffman GM, Nowakowski R, Troshynski TJ, Berens RJ, Weisman SJ. Risk reduction in pediatric procedural sedation by application of an American Academy of Pediatrics/American Society of Anesthesiologists process model. *Pediatrics* 2002; **109**: 236–243.
9. Coté CJ. Why we need sedation guidelines. *J Pediatr* 2001; **138**: 447–448.
10. Coté CJ, Notterman DA, Karl HW, Weinberg JA, McCloskey C. Adverse sedation events in pediatrics: a critical incident analysis of contributory factors. *Pediatrics* 2000; **105**: 805–814.
11. Malviya S, Voepel-Lewis T, Tait AR. Adverse events and risk factors associated with the sedation of children by nonanesthesiologists. *Anesth Analg* 1997; **85**: 1207–1213.
12. Egelhoff JC, Ball Jr WS, Koch BL, Parks TD. Safety and efficacy of sedation in children using a structured sedation program. *AJR Am J Roentgenol* 1997; **168**: 1259–1262.
13. Committee on Drugs, Section on Anesthesiology, American Academy of Pediatrics. Guidelines for the elective use of conscious sedation, deep sedation, and general anesthesia in pediatric patients. *Pediatrics* 1985; **76**: 317–321.
14. American Academy of Pediatric Dentistry. Guidelines for the elective use of conscious sedation, deep sedation, and general anesthesia in pediatric patients. *ASDC J Dent Child* 1986; **53**: 21–22.
15. Committee on Drugs, American Academy of Pediatrics. Guidelines for monitoring and management of pediatric patients during and after sedation for diagnostic and therapeutic procedures. *Pediatrics* 1992; **89**: 1110–1115.
16. Practice guidelines for sedation and analgesia by non-anesthesiologists. A report by the American Society of Anesthesiologists Task Force on Sedation and Analgesia by Non-Anesthesiologists. *Anesthesiology* 1996; **84**: 459–471.
17. Continuum of depth of sedation. 2000. Internet Communication.
18. Joint Commission on Accreditation of Healthcare Organizations. *Comprehensive Accreditation Manual for Hospitals*. Oakbrook Terrace: 2000.
19. Anon. Practice guidelines for sedation and analgesia by non-anesthesiologists. *Anesthesiology* 2002; **96**: 1004–1017.
20. Anon. Guidelines for monitoring and management of pediatric patients during and after sedation for diagnostic and therapeutic procedures: addendum. *Pediatrics* 2002; **110**: 836–838.
21. Everitt I, Younge P, Barnett P. Paediatric sedation in emergency department: what is our practice? *Emerg Med (Fremantle)* 2002; **14**: 62–66.
22. Scottish Intercollegiate Guidelines Network (SIGN). *Safe Sedation of Children Undergoing Diagnostic and Therapeutic Procedures*. Edinburgh, SIGN, 2003.
23. Dial S, Silver P, Bock K, Sagy M. Pediatric sedation for procedures titrated to a desired degree of immobility results in unpredictable depth of sedation. *Pediatr Emerg Care* 2001; **17**: 414–420.
24. Malviya S, Voepel-Lewis T, Tait AR, Merkel S, Tremper K, Naughton N. Depth of sedation in children undergoing computed tomography: validity and reliability of the University of Michigan Sedation Scale (UMSS). *Br J Anaesth* 2002; **88**: 241–245.
25. Caplan RA, Posner K, Ward RJ, Cheney FW. Peer reviewer agreement for major anesthetic mishaps. *QRB Qual Rev Bull* 1988; **14**: 363–368.
26. Coté CJ, Karl HW, Notterman DA, Weinberg JA, McCloskey C. Adverse sedation events in pediatrics: analysis of medications used for sedation. *Pediatrics* 2000; **106**: 633–644.
27. Dsida RM, Wheeler M, Birmingham PK *et al*. Premedication of pediatric tonsillectomy patients with oral transmucosal fentanyl citrate. *Anesth Analg* 1998; **86**: 66–70.

28. Wheeler M, Birmingham PK, Dsida RM, Wang Z, Coté CJ, Avram MJ. Uptake pharmacokinetics of the Fentanyl Oralet in children scheduled for central venous access removal: implications for the timing of initiating painful procedures. *Paediatr Anaesth* 2002; **12**: 594–599.

29. Wheeler M, Birmingham PK, Lugo RA, Heffner C, Coté CJ. Pharmacokinetics of orally administered intravenous fentanyl in children undergoing general anesthesia. (Submitted).

30. Ross AK, Davis PJ, del Dear G *et al*. Pharmacokinetics of remifentanil in anesthetized pediatric patients undergoing elective surgery or diagnostic procedures. *Anesth Analg* 2001; **93**: 1393–1401.

31. Spear RM, Yaster M, Berkowitz ID *et al*. Preinduction of anesthesia in children with rectally administered midazolam. *Anesthesiology* 1991; **74**: 670–674.

32. Coté CJ, Cohen IT, Suresh S *et al*. A comparison of three doses of a commercially prepared oral midazolam syrup in children. *Anesth Analg* 2002; **94**: 37–43.

33. Mayers DJ, Hindmarsh KW, Sankaran K, Gorecki DK, Kasian GF. Chloral hydrate disposition following single-dose administration to critically ill neonates and children. *Dev Pharmacol Ther* 1991; **16**: 71–77.

34. Terndrup TE, Dire DJ, Madden CM, Davis H, Cantor RM, Gavula DP. A prospective analysis of intramuscular meperidine, promethazine, and chlorpromazine in pediatric emergency department patients. *Ann Emerg Med* 1991; **20**: 31–35.

35. Green SM, Krauss B. The semantics of ketamine [In Process Citation]. *Ann Emerg Med* 2000; **36**: 480–482.

36. Pena BM, Krauss B. Adverse events of procedural sedation and analgesia in a pediatric emergency department. *Ann Emerg Med* 1999; **34**: 483–491.

37. Anon. Nalmefene – a long-acting injectable opioid antagonist. *Med Lett Drugs Ther* 1995; **37**: 97–98.

38. Green SM, Rothrock SG, Lynch EL *et al*. Intramuscular ketamine for pediatric sedation in the emergency department: safety profile in 1022 cases. *Ann Emerg Med* 1998; **31**: 688–697.

39. Green SM, Rothrock SG, Harris T, Hopkins GA, Garrett W, Sherwin T. Intravenous ketamine for pediatric sedation in the emergency department: safety profile with 156 cases. *Acad Emerg Med* 1998; **5**: 971–976.

40. Strain JD, Harvey LA, Foley LC, Cambell JB, Campbell JB. Intravenously administered pentobarbital sodium for sedation on pediatric CT. *Radiology* 1986; **161**: 105–108.

41. Gunter JB. Benefit and risks of local anesthetics in infants and children. *Paediatr Drugs* 2002; **4**: 649–672.

42. Dailey RH. Fatality secondary to misuse of TAC solution. *Ann Emerg Med* 1988; **17**: 159–160.

Peter D. Arkwright   Timothy J. David

13

Eat dirt – the hygiene hypothesis of atopic diseases

Atopic diseases (atopic dermatitis, asthma, allergic rhinitis) are a growing health problem, especially in Western societies. The prevalence of these diseases has more than doubled over the last few generations. Environmental rather than genetic factors are implicated in this recent surge. The hygiene hypothesis, as formulated by Strachan[1] in 1989, attempted to explain this increase in atopic diseases. This chapter critically reviews the hygiene hypothesis as an explanation for the observed changes in prevalence of atopic diseases.

THE HYPOTHESIS

In a brief report published in the *British Medical Journal* in 1989, David Strachan described the prevalence of atopic diseases in a national study of 17,414 British children born during one week in March 1958 and followed up until the age of 23 years.[1] He observed that the prevalence of allergic rhinitis was inversely related to the number of other children in the household, particularly the number of older children. Prevalence of atopic dermatitis in the first year of life was inversely and independently related to the number of older, but not younger, children in the household (Table 1). No data were presented as to the prevalence of asthma in this cohort. Viral infections, particularly those of the

Dr P.D. Arkwright MRCPCH, D Phil
Senior Lecturer in Paediatric Immunology, Academic Unit of Child Health, University of Manchester, Booth Hall Children's Hospital, Charlestown Road, Blackley, Manchester M9 7AA, UK
Tel: +44 161 220 5535; Fax: +44 161 224 1013, E-mail: peter_arkwright@lineone.net (for correspondence)

Prof. T.J. David MD PhD FRCP FRCPCH DCH
Professor of Child Health and Paediatrics, University of Manchester, Honorary Consultant Paediatrician, Booth Hall Children's Hospital, Royal Manchester Children's Hospital, and St Mary's Hospital, Manchester, UK

respiratory tract were said not to be relevant but no data were provided to support this assertion. Strachan concluded that 'unhygienic contact' with siblings might prevent the development of atopy and that 'declining family size, improvements in household amenities and higher standards of personal cleanliness over the last few generations have reduced the opportunity for cross infection in young families' and thus 'may have resulted in the more widespread clinical expression of atopic diseases'.

EXPLANATION OF TERMS AND CONCEPTS

An explanation of certain terms used in this review is important, particularly those which Strachan has used interchangeably to define his hypothesis.

ATOPIC DISEASES

The three atopic diseases are atopic dermatitis, asthma and allergic rhinitis/conjunctivitis. All three diseases are associated with a strong genetic predisposition and raised serum IgE levels.

HYGIENE

Hygeia was the name of the ancient Greek goddess of health and the word hygiene loosely means 'relating to health'. The modern concept of personal hygiene not only includes the prevention of diseases by cross-infection, particularly viral respiratory tract infections, but also the avoidance and removal of dirt.

DIRT

The word dirt is derived from the Old Norse word for excrement. In biological terms, dirt consists of microbes found in faeces and faeces-contaminated soil, especially on farms and in rural environments. Our modern social conditioning of avoiding dirt contrasts with the promotion of dietary supplements that contain a subgroup of normal enteric bacteria thought to be beneficial to health (probiotics; 'pro-life').

PROVING THE HYPOTHESIS

If Strachan's hygiene hypothesis were correct, then one would expect the following to be true:

1. The prevalence of atopic diseases would have indeed increased over the last few generations.

2. Studies should confirm the association between the prevalence of atopic diseases and social factors.

3. Studies should confirm the absence of a protective effect of childhood respiratory illnesses on atopic diseases.

4. If 'good' personal hygiene (avoidance of dirt) is associated with an increased prevalence of atopic diseases, then lack of exposure to certain

Table 1 Prevalence of allergic rhinitis and atopic dermatitis in infancy by position in the household. (summary of data presented in the report by Strachan[1])

	Prevalence of allergic rhinitis in the previous year (aged 23)	Prevalence of atopic dermatitis in the first year of life
# Older children		
0	20.4	6.1
1	15.0	5.2
2	12.5	4.6
3	10.6	3.7
4+	8.6	2.8
# Younger children		
0	17.9	5.3
1	16.9	5.7
2	15.7	5.3
3	13.4	4.6
4+	12.3	5.3

Numbers represent the percentage of children in the subpopulation with atopic disease.

enteric microbes should contribute to the increase in atopic diseases seen in our Western societies.

5. The administration of certain environmental/enteric microbial supplements might prevent or ameliorate atopic diseases.

6. Atopic diseases are essentially immune hypersensitivity reactions (*i.e.* a lack of immune tolerance) to normally innocuous allergens in our environment. If the hygiene hypothesis were correct, it should be possible to show that the environmental microbes in dirt down-regulate this hypersensitivity response and promote immune tolerance to allergens.

The remainder of this review examines the evidence for and against the hygiene hypothesis and the above six predictions.

INCREASING PREVALENCE OF ATOPIC DISEASES

GENERAL TRENDS

Atopic dermatitis
On the basis of several cross-sectional studies from northern Europe, the cumulative incidence of atopic dermatitis in children (up to 7 years of age) was less than 3% if they were born before 1960, 4–8% if born between 1960 and 1970, 8–12% for those born after 1970, and over 15% according to recent studies (Table 2). Although Diepgen emphasised the possible sources of method-ological error in these cross-sectional studies (changes in disease definition, questions, sampling frame and method), the overall consensus is that there has been a true and significant increase in the prevalence of atopic dermatitis over the past three decades in industrialised countries.[2]

Table 2 Epidemiological studies demonstrating an increased prevalence of atopic diseases

Country	Years studied	Atopic disease	Change in prevalence
UK[35]	1946–1970	Atopic dermatitis	5.1% to 12.2%
E. Scotland[36]	1964–1989	Atopic dermatitis	5.3% to 12%
		Asthma	4.1% to 10.2%
		Allergic rhinitis	3.2% to 11.9%
W. Scotland[37]	1972–1996	Asthma	3.0% to 8.2%
		Allergic rhinitis	5.8% to 19.9%
Australia[38]	1982–1997	Asthma	12.9% to 38.6%
		Allergic rhinitis	22.5% to 44%
Norway[39]	1981–1994	Asthma	3.4% to 9.3%
Japan[40]	1985–1997	Atopic dermatitis	15% to 24.1%
Greece[41]	1991–1998	Asthma (current)	1.5% to 6.0%

Asthma

Asthma has only been classified as a single disease entity since 1955 (seventh revision of the *International Classification of Diseases*) and it is not possible to determine changes in the prevalence of this condition prior to this time. However, ever since the 1960s, epidemiologists have noted a progressive increase in morbidity and mortality from asthma in Western societies.[3] Although part of this observed increase is likely to be due to changes in diagnosis and medical care, a number of population surveys suggest that there has been a modest (approximately 50%) increase in the prevalence of all wheezy illnesses among children over the past 30 years (Table 2).

Allergic rhinitis

Allergic rhinitis, which was largely unheard of before the 1940s both by the general public and the medical profession, seems to have increased in prevalence so that it is now one of the most common chronic diseases in Western society. A number of studies document the substantial increase in allergic rhinitis, with an approximate doubling of its prevalence each decade since the 1960s, so that it now affects 15–25% of people in Western communities (Table 2). These studies suggest a more rapid increase in the prevalence of atopic dermatitis and allergic rhinitis than asthma.

GEOGRAPHICAL VARIATION

An international study of the world-wide variation in prevalence of symptoms of atopic eczema, asthma and allergic rhinitis (ISAAC) involving 463,801 children aged 13–14 years from 155 centres in 56 countries provides a most comprehensive set of data.[4] In this study, there was > 60-fold variation in the prevalence of atopic dermatitis between centres (0.3–20.5%). Countries with a prevalence of atopic diseases were highest tended to be Western industrialised countries, while countries with a low prevalence of these diseases were largely non-Westernised countries (Table 3).

Table 3 World-wide variation in the prevalence of atopic diseases[4]

	Least prevalent	Average	Most prevalent
Atopic dermatitis	**0–4%**	**2–10%**	**10–19%**
	China	Thailand	UK
	Georgia	Malaysia	Finland
	Iran	Germany	Sweden
	Uzbekistan	Italy	New Zealand
Asthma	**1–17%**	**8–16%**	**18–36%**
	China	Austria	UK
	India	Iran	New Zealand
	Ethiopia	Argentina	Australia
	Morocco	Estonia	Canada
Allergic rhinitis	**1–11%**	**7–17%**	**12–24%**
	Georgia	France	Argentina
	Estonia	Spain	Canada
	Latvia	Malaysia	Australia
	India	Germany	New Zealand

Only countries where there was data from two or more centres included.

SUMMARY

To summarise this section, there is no doubt that over the last 40 years a significant increase in atopic diseases has occurred, particularly in Western industrialised countries. Because these changes have occurred in one to two generations they cannot be due to a change in genetic susceptibility but must be due to a change within the environment.

PREVALENCE OF ATOPIC DISEASE AND INTERACTION WITH OTHER CHILDREN

FAMILY SIZE

The exposure of a child to other siblings has been shown to inversely affect the prevalence of atopic disease. Studies performed in the decade since Strachan's initial observations have confirmed that his original findings of variation in allergic rhinitis and birth order are real.[5] A negative association between family size and asthma has also been found in independent studies.[6,7] Ponsonby *et al.*,[6] in their Tasmanian study of 6378 children, found no association between family size and atopic dermatitis at 7 years of age, although Lewis and Britton[8] did find a negative association between low birth order and atopic dermatitis at 16 years of age in a British birth cohort of 17,427 children, suggesting that the association between family size and at least atopic dermatitis may depend on the age of the subjects studied.

SOCIO-ECONOMIC CLASS

Socio-economic class is a major factor which has been inversely associated with the frequency of atopic diseases. Williams *et al.*[9] found a significant increase in the prevalence of atopic dermatitis in children in social classes I and II (12–13%) compared with those from social classes IV and V (8–9%). Allergic rhinitis at 16 years (social classes I and II [3–4%]; social classes IV and V [5–8%]), but not asthma at 11 years old (social classes I and II [5–6%]; social classes IV and V [3–6%]) showed similar trends. Williams concluded 'exposures associated with social class are probably at least as important as genetic factors in the expression of childhood eczema'.

LACK OF PROTECTIVE EFFECT OF RESPIRATORY VIRAL INFECTIONS ON THE PREVALENCE OF ATOPIC DISEASES

If children from bigger families consistently have less atopic diseases, then children who attended day-care nurseries may also have less of these illnesses. However, contrary to these expectations, a systematic review of studies shows no relationship between atopy and nursery attendance.[10]

Children from larger families as well as those attending nurseries have significantly more viral respiratory tract infections. Studies specifically addressing the possible link between the frequency of viral upper respiratory tract infections in infancy and early childhood and atopy have shown that these infections do not prevent the development of asthma.[11] In fact, viral lower respiratory tract infections in infancy are associated with an increase, rather than decrease, in childhood asthma prevalence. In a study of 47 infants hospitalised with respiratory syncytial virus bronchiolitis, there was a 12.5-fold increased risk of asthma later in childhood compared with the matched control group of 93 infants.[12] One explanation is that children who are inherently predisposed to asthma develop more severe clinical bronchiolitis in infancy. Sigurs' study also demonstrated that RSV infection does not protect against the subsequent development of chronic asthma.

Thus a decrease in the number of viral respiratory tract infections with smaller sibships in affluent Western societies over the last few generations cannot explain the observed increase in atopic diseases. These data may seem contrary to expectations, and even Strachan in his review of the hygiene hypothesis in 2000 found these data confusing, commenting 'the balance of evidence does not, therefore, suggest a relationship between allergy and early child contacts outside the home, which is difficult to reconcile with the hygiene hypothesis'. However, as defined above, good personal hygiene is not so much the prevention of viral respiratory tract infections by cross-infection, but rather the avoidance of dirt and the microbes it contains. Variations in the prevalence of atopic diseases in relation to the avoidance of dirt is the focus of the next section.

PREVALENCE OF ATOPIC DISEASES AND THE AVOIDANCE OF DIRT

THE MODERN CONCEPT OF GOOD PERSONAL HYGIENE

The concept of 'good personal hygiene' equates with hand washing to remove dirt in order to prevent hand-to-mouth transmission of environmental microbes, particularly enteric bacteria. Could the deliberate avoidance of specific environmental microbes contained in dirt be the reason for the increased propensity to atopic diseases? This section examines the association between childhood exposure to environmental bacteria commonly found in soil and excrement and the prevalence of atopic diseases in our societies.

ATOPIC DISEASES AND EXPOSURE TO FARM ANIMALS

Children living in rural farming communities of Switzerland, Austria and southern Germany have a very low prevalence of atopic diseases (asthma and allergic rhinitis).[13,14] In a cross-sectional survey of 2618 parents with children aged 6–13 years living in these rural areas, Riedler found that the prevalence of asthma and hay fever in infants exposed to stables and unpasteurised farm milk were 1% and 3%, respectively, compared with children exposed at 1–5 years of age (11% and 13%, respectively).[13]

Stables, the lodgings for domestic animals, contain high concentrations of animal excrement (dirt). Unpasteurised milk, by definition, is non-sterile and, therefore, may contain environmental bacteria. What are the data linking the direct exposure to dirt and the prevalence of atopic diseases?

EXPOSURE TO ENDOTOXIN DERIVED FROM ENTERIC BACTERIA AND THE PREVALENCE OF ATOPIC DISEASES

One large group of faecal-derived bacteria contained in dirt is Gram-negative enterobacteria. The outer membrane of these bacteria consists of a family of lipopolysaccharides (endotoxin). In a large study of 812 children aged 6–13 years living in rural areas of Germany, Austria and Switzerland, endotoxin load has been found to be significantly higher in the immediate environment of farming compared with non-farming families. The mattresses of children from farming households had twice the endotoxin load (units/m^2 of mattress surface area) compared with non-farming households.[15] Endotoxin load in this study was shown to be inversely related to allergic rhinitis (odds ratio [OR] 0.53 [range, 0.35–0.81]) and atopic asthma (OR 0.48 [range, 0.28–0.81]).

DIRECT ASSOCIATION BETWEEN EXPOSURE TO CERTAIN ORALLY ACQUIRED INFECTIOUS DISEASES AND ATOPIC DISORDERS

Hepatitis A was endemic in Italy during the 1970s and was usually acquired early in childhood, mostly without inducing symptoms. Its transmission is favoured by faecal contamination of the living environment, poor hygienic food handling, day-care settings, *etc.*, which all facilitate the transmission of many other infections. Serological evidence of previous exposure to hepatitis A virus was associated with a halving of the prevalence of asthma, allergic rhinitis or both in 1659 Italian military students (16.7% [203/1206] in seronegative students to 8.4% [37/443] in seropositive students).[16] A follow-up study by the same group demonstrated an inverse relationship between allergic asthma and the number of oro-faecal microbes (hepatitis A virus, *Helicobacter pylori* and *Toxoplasma gondii*: OR – none 1; one 0.70; two or three 0.37), but not microbes acquired by other routes (measles, mumps, rubella, chickenpox, cytomegalovirus and herpes simplex virus type 1).[17]

Pinworm (*Enterobius vermicularis*) infestation in a cohort of 3107 Taiwanese primary school students has also been associated with a reduced prevalence of childhood asthma (OR 0.25 [range, 0.1–0.63]) and allergic rhinitis (OR 0.61 [range, 0.45–0.84]).[18] These data suggest that the propensity to asthma is inversely related to the number of enteric infections to which the individual has been exposed.

USE OF ORAL ANTIBIOTICS IN INFANCY AND PREVALENCE OF ATOPIC DISEASES

If increased exposure to certain enteric microbes especially in early childhood is associated with a reduction in atopic diseases later, then children who have frequent courses of oral antibiotics which kill gut flora might be expected to have a higher prevalence of atopic diseases. Supporting this hypothesis, a study of 1934 subjects, treatment with oral antibiotics in the first two years of life was associated with a 2.1-fold increase in atopic disease (atopic dermatitis, asthma or allergic rhinitis).[19]

PROBIOTICS AND ATOPIC DISEASES

If exposure to certain enteric microbes prevents atopic diseases, then dietary supplements containing these microbes might ameliorate atopic symptoms. Probiotics (pro-life) have been defined as 'a live microbial food ingredient that is beneficial to health'.[20] The criteria for a micro-organism to be defined as probiotic include that the strain be of human faecal origin, is safe for human use, survives exposure to acid and bile, and adheres to the intestinal mucosa. The genera most frequently used as probiotics are *Lactobacillus* spp. and *Bifidobacterium* spp., normally found in the gut especially of breast-fed infants prior to weaning.[21]

The effect of probiotics has been studied in children with atopic dermatitis. One randomised study involved 27 breast-fed infants with atopic dermatitis who were weaned onto probiotic or non-probiotic formulae.[22] The probiotic group showed a significant reduction in atopic dermatitis compared with the placebo group at 2 months, but by 6 months there was no difference between the two groups. In another prospective trial by the same group, 132 neonates at increased risk of developing atopic dermatitis were studied. Either their mothers prior to delivery or the infants themselves were randomised to receive supplementary Lactobacilli GG or a placebo. At 1 year of age, both the infants whose mothers had been given the probiotics (6/28 [21%], $P = 0.04$) and the infants who had been given the probiotics directly (9/36 [25%]; $P = 0.06$) had a significantly lower prevalence of atopic dermatitis compared with the placebo controls (31/68 [45%]).[23] Further studies are required to clarify the possible role of probiotics in the management of atopic diseases and the fact that infants where atopic dermatitis is most common already have the greatest proportion of these 'probiotic' bacteria in their intestines.[21]

MYCOBACTERIA AND ATOPIC DISEASES

Tuberculosis and BCG

Mycobacteria are ubiquitous in the environment and are present in soil, water and unpasteurised milk. Tuberculosis was until the last few generations one of the most common causes of morbidity and mortality in Europe.[24,25] The increase in atopic diseases over the last few generations has been paralleled by a reduction in mycobacterial infections. A negative association between tuberculin reactivity and the frequency of atopic dermatitis, asthma and allergic rhinitis has been found in 867 Japanese school children.[26] As none of these children had clinical tuberculosis, the size of their skin reaction may relate to either their immune response to BCG or exposure to cross-reacting environmental mycobacteria in earlier childhood. In a retrospective study of 574 Swedish children, those given BCG in the first 6 months of life were no less likely that a control group of having atopic disease (77 [36%] versus 145 [41%], respectively).[27] Thus a single dose of BCG given in the first 6 months of life does not seem to protect against the later development of atopic diseases.

Soil mycobacteria

Mycobacterium vaccae is a non-disease causing soil mycobacterium of the same family as the tuberculosis bacteria. Intradermal administration of a killed suspension of this mycobacterium administered to 41 children with moderately severe atopic dermatitis has been associated with a reduction in the clinical severity score by 48% after 3 months compared with a 3% reduction in the placebo group.[28] In contrast, two small, randomised studies where *M. vaccae* was administered to adults with asthma, one of 43 patients[29] and the other of 24 patients[30] showed no significant differences in the clinical severity of the asthma in the treatment compared with the placebo groups. Further studies are required to determine the nature of the negative association between mycobacteria exposure and the prevalence of atopic diseases.

SUMMARY

In summary, exposure to dirty environments and the environmental microbes they contain are associated with a reduced prevalence of atopic diseases. Some studies have suggested that exposure or administration of microbes contained in dirt (enteric bacteria/endotoxin, probiotics, hepatitis A virus, toxoplasma, pinworm, mycobacteria) protect against or ameliorate atopic diseases.

THE HYPOTHESIS IS CONSISTENT WITH THE CURRENT UNDERSTANDING OF THE IMMUNE MECHANISMS CAUSING ATOPIC DISEASES

Atopic diseases can be thought of as inappropriate and excessive immune responses to antigen challenge. An understanding of the immune mechanisms causing atopic disease requires a working knowledge of the two main immune response pathways, a brief summary of which is given below and in Figure 1.

Th1-TYPE RESPONSES

Cellular responses are critical for the phagocytosis and digestion of small extracellular pathogens (*e.g.* bacteria, fungi and some protozoa such as

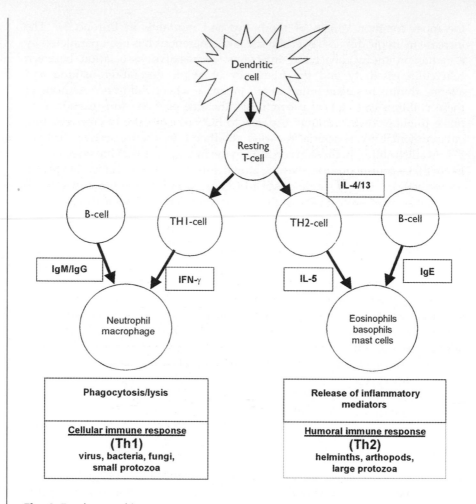

Fig. 1 Fundamental immune responses to environmental microbes.

Pneumocystis carinii and cryptosporidium) as well as immunity to viruses. Antibodies (particularly IgM and IgG) and complement promote phagocytosis of certain extra-cellular pathogens. Interferon-γ (IFN-γ) produced by T helper 1 lymphocytes (Th1 cells) activates neutrophils and macrophages to destroy these pathogens. This cellular Th1-type response is the hallmark of delayed, cell-mediated, hypersensitivity responses, characteristic of a tuberculin reaction, contact dermatitis and chronic atopic diseases.

Th2-TYPE RESPONSES

A humoral/secretory immune pathway induces expulsion of extracellular pathogens too large to be phagocytosed, particularly intestinal helminths and some protozoa, as well as skin infestations with arthropods such as scabies and mites. Inflammatory mediators include histamine, leukotrienes, and kinins released from mast cell, basophil and eosinophil granules. Antibodies (particularly IgE) promote the release of these mediators. T helper 2 (Th2)

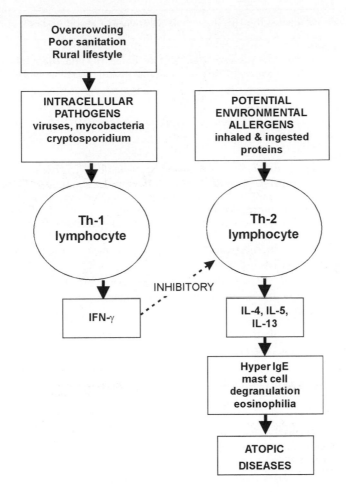

Fig. 2 The Th1/Th2 theory linking the hygiene hypothesis to the observed increase in atopic diseases.

lymphocytes produce cytokines, particularly the interleukins (IL) IL-4, IL-5 and IL-13 that induce this response. Th2-type responses are the hallmark of atopy, acute allergic reactions, allergic rhinitis and acute atopic asthma.

Th1/Th2 IMBALANCE AND ATOPY

During the early 1990s, based largely on experiments done in mice, it was suggested that over-activity of a Th1 or Th2 response was due to lack of feedback inhibition by the other pathway. Atopy was explained as an over-activity of the Th2 pathway associated with a lack of feedback inhibition by the Th1 pathway. As viruses, bacteria, fungi and small protozoa promote a Th1-type response, lack of exposure to these microbes (good personal hygiene) might have led to this Th2/Th1 imbalance and the increased prevalence of atopic diseases (Fig. 2).[31] However, studies performed in humans (Table 4) suggest that this murine-based Th2/Th1 hypothesis of atopic diseases may be too simple and that further refinements are required to comply with our

Table 4 Evidence against the Th1/Th2 imbalance theory of atopic diseases

In vitro evidence
- Chronic atopic dermatitis is associated with increased Th1 and Th2 cytokines[42]
- Transferring IFN-γ producing T cells to an animal model of asthma makes disease worse[43]

Human immunodeficiency diseases
- Patients with IFN-γ pathway defects do not have excessive Th2 activity nor an increase of atopic diseases[44]

Epidemiology
- Recent increase in atopic diseases has been paralleled by an increase in Th1-type diseases (type 1 diabetes,[45] Crohn's disease,[46] and multiple sclerosis[47]
- Recurrent viral infections (Th1 activators) in early childhood do not prevent the development of atopic diseases[5]
- Viral infections (Th1 activators) generally trigger and exacerbate atopic dermatitis and asthma
- World-wide, helminth infections (Th2 activators) are inversely related to the prevalence of allergic diseases[48]

current knowledge of the regulation of the immune system and the pathogenesis of atopic diseases.

ALLERGY = HYPERSENSITIVITY TO USUALLY INNOCUOUS SUBSTANCES = BREAKDOWN IN TOLERANCE

Allergic (hypersensitivity) reactions, by definition imply a lack of tolerance to usually innocuous substances (foods, dander, pollens, *etc.*) and are not usually specific for any one allergen. Patients often have allergic reactions to not one but a number of allergens, and suffer from not just one but often two or three of the atopic disease triad. Lack of immune tolerance is also a feature of autoimmune diseases (*e.g.* insulin-dependent diabetes mellitus and multiple sclerosis). The increase in atopic diseases in Western communities has been paralleled by a similar increase in some these autoimmune diseases (Table 4). Thus clinical, epidemiological and immunological observations suggest a general breakdown in immune tolerance may be at the root cause of atopic as well as autoimmune diseases.

THE EFFECT OF DIRT ON CELLS MEDIATING IMMUNE TOLERANCE

Regulatory T lymphocytes secreting IL-10 and TGF-β1 mediate peripheral tolerance and malfunction of this regulatory pathway is now thought to be important for the balance between allergy and anergy both at the genetic and environmental level (Fig. 3). For example, a genetic predisposition to lower TGF-β1 secretion is associated with an increased frequency of atopic dermatitis in children.[32] In an animal model of asthma, transfer of T lymphocytes which produce TGF-β1 results in amelioration of clinical disease.[33] Furthermore, exposure to environmental microbes (Table 5) associated with an amelioration of symptomatic atopic diseases (*e.g.* endotoxin, *M. vaccae*) can activate this regulatory pathway and increase IL-10 and TGF-β1 production.[15,34]

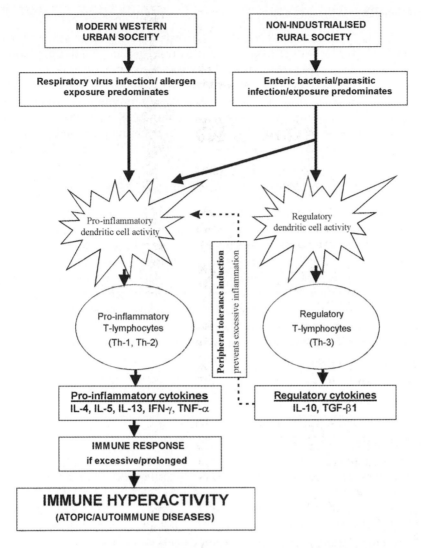

Fig. 3 The refined 'hygiene hypothesis' of atopic and autoimmune diseases.

Table 5 Specific environmental microbes stimulate the activity of T regulatory lymphocytes

Helminths
- Chronic helminth infections are associated with high levels of IL-10[49]

Mycobacteria
- In a mouse model of asthma, *M. vaccae* stimulates T regulatory cell activity and the production of IL-10 and TGF-β1[34]
- In children, larger tuberculin reactions are associated with higher levels of IL-10[26]

Enteric bacteria/probiotics (*Lactobacillus, Bifidobacterium*)
- *In vitro* endotoxin is associated with an increase in IL-10[15]
- Probiotics stimulate the production of IL-10[50]

SUMMARY

In summary, hypersensitivity reactions characteristic of human atopic disease can be mediated by both Th1 and Th2 pathways. They are due to a breakdown in immune tolerance, a process at least partly controlled by specific regulatory T lymphocytes and antigen presenting cells (dendritic cells). Microbes contained in dirt not only stimulate a protective immune response, but also these regulatory pathways. A lack of stimulation of regulatory pathways associated with the avoidance of dirt would explain the increased prevalence of atopic diseases in Western societies and the basis of the hygiene hypothesis.

THE REFINED HYGIENE HYPOTHESIS: EAT DIRT, BE HEALTHY

The evidence detailed in this review provides further support for Strachan's hygiene hypothesis of atopic disease. There is no doubt that the prevalence of atopic diseases has increased significantly, more than doubling over the last few generations. The propensity to atopic diseases does indeed seem to be associated specifically with factors that relate to personal hygiene, especially as applied to Western communities where the prevalence of these diseases is highest. Prevention of cross-infection with viruses, especially respiratory viruses is only one aspect of good personal hygiene. Cross-infection of these viruses does not explain the inverse association between hygiene and atopic diseases. The essence of good personal hygiene is behaviour that reduces exposure to dirt. Dirt by definition contains environmental enteric viruses, bacteria and parasites. Over the last decade, studies have demonstrated that

---

Key points for clinical practice

- There has been a doubling in atopic diseases (atopic dermatitis, asthma and allergic rhinitis) in Western urban societies over the last few generations.

- Over the same period of time, there has been a similar increase in the prevalence of some autoimmune diseases (*e.g.* Crohn's disease, multiple sclerosis and type I insulin-dependent diabetes).

- The hygiene hypothesis proposes that the increase in these inflammatory diseases relates to a lack of exposure to certain environmental microbes.

- Evidence suggests that chronic exposure to certain enteric bacteria and helminths reduces the prevalence of atopic diseases in a community. This explains why atopic diseases are less common in areas where contact with these microbes is more likely (*e.g.* non-industrialised countries, farming and less affluent urban communities).

- Exposure to respiratory infections in childhood does not protect the individual against atopic diseases, indicating that the type of microbe and route of exposure are important factors determining whether or not children will develop these diseases.

Key points for clinical practice (continued)

- The previous hypothesis that a Th1/Th2 imbalance leads to atopic disease is being refined. Th2 hyperactivity is not the sole determinant of chronic atopic diseases. Allergen sensitivity as measured by specific IgE levels (e.g. RAST to house dust mite) is similar (> 30%) in areas with a low and high prevalence of atopic diseases, illustrating the relatively poor positive predictive value of these tests in clinical practice.

- In simple terms, allergy, like autoimmunity is due to a lack of immune tolerance to usually innocuous substances in our environment. Administration of microbes and crude microbial extracts (probiotics, mycobacteria) may prevent and ameliorate clinical atopic diseases by promoting tolerance to potential allergens.

- In the future, it may be possible to prevent and treat atopic and some autoimmune diseases effectively using purified preparations of the active immunoregulatory molecules derived from environmental microbes.

---

reduced exposure to some of these enteric microbes is associated with an increased propensity to atopic diseases; and conversely increased exposure, for example in children living on farms has a protective effect. 'Eat dirt, be healthy' sounds a contradiction in terms, but it may be the key to reversing the modern epidemic of atopic diseases. Dirt has recently been made more palatable by marketing it as 'probiotics'. Time will tell whether select subgroups of enteric microbes are capable of switching off atopic diseases.

References

1. Strachan DP. Hayfever, hygiene and household size. *BMJ* 1989; **299**: 1259–1260.
2. Diepgen TL. Is the prevalence of atopic dermatitis increasing? In: Williams HC. (ed) *Atopic Dermatitis. The Epidemiology, Causes and Prevention of Atopic Eczema.* Cambridge: Cambridge University Press, 2000; 96.
3. Speizer FE, Doll R, Heaf P. Observations on recent increase in mortality from asthma. *BMJ* 1968; **1**: 335–339.
4. ISSAC Steering Committee. Worldwide variation in prevalence of symptoms of asthma, allergic rhinoconjunctivitis, and atopic eczema: ISAAC. *Lancet* 1998; **351**: 1225–1232.
5. Strachan DP. Family size, infection and atopy: the first decade of the 'hygiene hypothesis'. *Thorax* 2000; **55**: S2–S10.
6. Ponsonby AL, Couper D, Dwyer T, Carmichael A. Cross sectional study of the relation between sibling number and asthma, hay fever, and eczema. *Arch Dis Child* 1998; **79**: 328–333.
7. Haby MM, Peat JK, Marks GB, Woolcock AJ, Leeder SR. Asthma in preschool children: prevalence and risk factors. *Thorax* 2001; **56**: 589–595.
8. Lewis SA, Britton JR. Consistent effects of high socio-economic status and low birth order, and the modifying effect of maternal smoking on the risk of allergic disease in childhood. *Respir Med* 1998; **92**: 1237–1244.
9. Williams HC, Strachan DP, Hay RJ. Childhood eczema: disease of the advantaged? *BMJ* 1994; **308**: 1132–1135.
10. Nystad W. Daycare attendance, asthma and atopy. *Ann Med* 2000; **32**: 390–396.
11. Ponsonby AL, Couper D, Dwyer T, Carmichael A, Kemp A. Relationship between early

life respiratory illness, family size over time, and the development of asthma and hay fever: a seven year follow up study. *Thorax* 1999; **54**: 664–669.

12. Sigurs N, Bjarnason R, Sigurbergsson F, Kjellman B. Respiratory syncytial virus bronchiolitis in infancy is an important risk factor for asthma and allergy at age 7. *Am J Respir Crit Care Med* 2000; **161**: 1501–1507.

13. Riedler J, Braun-Fahrländer C, Eder W *et al*. Exposure to farming in early life and development of asthma and allergy: a cross-sectional survey. *Lancet* 2001; **358**: 1129–1133.

14. Leynaert B, Neukirch C, Jarvis D, Chinn S, Burney P, Neukirch F. Does living on a farm during childhood protect against asthma, allergic rhinitis, and atopy in adulthood. *Am J Respir Crit Care Med* 2001; **164**: 1829–1834.

15. Braun-Fahrländer C, Riedler J, Herz U *et al*. Environmental exposure to endotoxin and its relation to asthma in school-age children. *N Engl J Med* 2002; **347**: 869–877.

16. Matricardi PM, Rosmini F, Ferrigno L *et al*. Cross sectional retrospective study of prevalence of atopy among Italian military students with antibodies against hepatitis A virus. *BMJ* 1997; **314**: 999–1003.

17. Matricardi PM, Rosmini F, Riondino S *et al*. Exposure to foodborne and orofecal microbes versus airborne viruses in relation to atopy and allergic asthma: epidemiological study. *BMJ* 2000; **320**: 412–417.

18. Huang SL, Tsai PF, Yeh YF. Negative association of *Enterobius* infestation with asthma and rhinitis in primary school children in Taipei. *Clin Exp Allergy* 2002; **32**: 1029–1032.

19. Farooqi IS, Hopkin JM. Early childhood infection and atopic disorder. *Thorax* 1998; **53**: 927–932.

20. Fuller R. Probiotics in human medicine. *Gut* 1991; **32**: 439–442.

21. Edwards CA, Parrett AM. Intestinal flora during the first months of life: new perspectives. *Br J Nutr* 2002; **88**: S11–S18.

22. Isolauri E, Arvola T, Sutas Y, Moilanen E, Salminen S. Probiotics in the management of atopic dermatitis. *Clin Exp Allergy* 2000; **30**: 1604–1610.

23. Kalliomäki M, Salminen S, Arvilommi H, Kero P, Koskinen P, Isolauri E. Probiotics in primary prevention of atopic disease: a randomised placebo-controlled trial. *Lancet* 2001; **357**: 1076–1079.

24. Galbraith NS, Forbes P, Mayon-White RT. Changing patterns of communicable disease in England and Wales. Part II Disappearing and declining diseases. *BMJ* 1980; **280**: 489–492.

25. Tocque K, Bellis MA, Cheuk MT *et al*. Long-term trends in tuberculosis. Comparison of age-cohort data between Hong Kong and England and Wales. *Am J Respir Crit Care Med* 1998; **158**: 484–488.

26. Shirakawa T, Enomoto T, Shimazu S, Hopkin JM. The inverse association between tuberculin responses and atopic disorders. *Science* 1997; **275**: 77–79.

27. Alm JS, Lilja G, Pershagen G, Scheynius A. Early BCG vaccination and development of atopy. *Lancet* 1997; **350**: 400–403.

28. Arkwright PD, David TJ. Intradermal administration of a killed *Mycobacterium vaccae* suspension (SRL172) is associated with improvement in atopic dermatitis in children with moderate-to-severe disease. *J Allergy Clin Immunol* 2001; **107**: 531–534.

29. Shirtcliffe PM, Easthope SE, Cheng S *et al*. The effect of delipidated deglycolipidated (DDMV) and heat-killed *Mycobacterium vaccae* in asthma. *Am J Respir Crit Care Med* 2001; **163**: 1410–1414.

30. Camporota L, Corkhill A, Long H *et al*. The effects of *Mycobacterium vaccae* on allergen-induced airway responses in atopic asthma. *Eur Respir J* 2003; **21**: 287–293.

31. Cookson WO, Moffatt MF. Asthma: an epidemic in the absence of infection? *Science* 1997; **275**: 41–42.

32. Arkwright PD, Chase J, Babbage S, Pravica V, David TJ, Hutchinson IV. Atopic dermatitis is associated with a low producer TGF-β1 cytokine polymorphism genotype. *J Allergy Clin Immunol* 2001; **108**: 281–284.

33. Hansen G, McIntire JJ, Yeung VP *et al*. CD4(+) T helper cells engineered to produce latent TGF-beta1 reverse allergen-induced airway hyperactivity and inflammation. *J Clin Invest* 2000; **105**: 61–70.

34. Zuany-Amorim C, Sawicka E, Manlius C *et al*. Suppression of airway eosinophilia by killed *Mycobacterium vaccae*-induced allergen-specific regulatory T-cells. *Nat Med* 2002; **8**: 625–629.

35. Taylor B, Wadsworth J, Wadsworth M, Peckham C. Changes in the reported prevalence of childhood eczema since the 1939–45 war. *Lancet* 1984; **2**: 1255–1257.
36. Ninan TK, Russell G. Respiratory symptoms and atopy in Aberdeen schoolchildren: evidence from two surveys 25 years apart. *BMJ* 1992; **304**: 873–875.
37. Upton MN, McConnachie A, McSharry C *et al*. Intergenerational 20 year trends in the prevalence of asthma and hayfever in adults: the Midspan family study surveys of parents and offspring. *BMJ* 2000; **321**: 88–92.
38. Downs SH, Marks GB, Sporik R, Belosouva EG, Car NG, Peak JK. Continued increase in the prevalence of asthma and atopy. *Arch Dis Child* 2001; **84**: 20–23.
39. Nystad W, Magnus P, Gulsvik A, Skarpaas IJ, Carlsen KH. Changing prevalence of asthma in school children: evidence for diagnosis changes in asthma in two surveys 13 years apart. *Eur Respir J* 1997; **10**: 1046–1051.
40. Yura A, Shimiza T. Trends in the prevalence of atopic dermatitis in school children: longitudinal study in Osaka Prefecture, Japan, from 1985 to 1997. *Br J Dermatol* 2001; **145**: 966–973.
41. Anthracopoulos M, Karatza A, Liolios E, Triga M, Triantou K, Priftis K. Prevalence of asthma among schoolchildren in Patras, Greece: three surveys over 20 years. *Thorax* 2001; **56**: 569–571.
42. Hamid Q, Boguniewicz M, Leung DYM. Differential *in situ* cytokine gene expression in acute versus chronic atopic dermatitis. *J Clin Invest* 1994; **94**: 870–876.
43. Hansen G, Berry G, DeKruvti RH, Umetsu DT. Allergen specific Th1 cells fail to counterbalance Th2 cell-induced airway hyperactivity but causes severe airway inflammation. *J Clin Invest* 1999; **103**: 175–183.
44. Lammas DA, Casanova JL, Kumararatne DS. Clinical consequences of defects in the IL-12-dependent interferon-gamma (IFN-γ) pathway. *Clin Exp Immunol* 2000; **121**: 417–425.
45. Stene LC, Nafstad P. Relation between occurrence of type 1 diabetes and asthma. *Lancet* 2001; **357**: 607–608.
46. Barton JR, Gillon S, Ferguson A. Incidence of inflammatory bowel disease in Scottish children between 1968 and 1983: marginal fall in ulcerative colitis, three-fold rise in Crohn's disease. *Gut* 1989; **30**: 618–622.
47. Bach JF. The effect of infections on susceptibility to autoimmune and allergic diseases. *N Engl J Med* 2002; **347**: 911–920.
48. Yazdanbakhsh M, Kremsner PG, van Ree R. Allergy, parasites and the hygiene hypothesis. *Science* 2002; **296**: 490–494.
49. Mahanty S, Nutman TB. Immunoregulation in human lymphocyte filariasis: the role of interleukin-10. *Parasite Immunol* 1995; **17**: 385–392.
50. Pessi T, Sutas Y, Hurme M, Isolauri E. Interleukin-10 generation in atopic children following oral *Lactobacillus rhamnosus* GG. *Clin Exp Allergy* 2000; **30**: 1804–1808.

Philip Hazell

14

Depression

There is evidence that depression is becoming more common with successive generations, and is also presenting at a younger age.[1] It is likely that most people who will ever suffer depression will have experienced their first episode before the age of 20 years. Projections from the World Health Organization and the World Bank suggest that by the year 2020 depression will be the second most common cause of disability after ischaemic heart disease. A significant number of children and adolescents suffer depression, while an even greater number live with an adult who suffers from the disorder. Depression is too common to be considered the exclusive domain of specialist mental health services. Just as general practitioners treat many adults with mild-to-moderate depressive illness, paediatricians may increasingly provide a similar service to children and adolescents. Paediatricians may have a 'head start' over specialist mental health services through their knowledge of the child's development and family circumstances, and by having an existing treatment alliance. Observation of the patient made over several short visits, as occurs in paediatric practice, may also give a more reliable indication of the enduring nature of symptoms than can be gained from cross-sectional assessment. This article provides, in overview, a clinical description of depression in young people, and in particular considers how the condition may present in the paediatric context. Recent research on aetiology will be reviewed, as will current knowledge about treatment effectiveness and prevention.

CLINICAL DESCRIPTION

Children with depressive disorders rarely take on the appearance of classic melancholia (psychomotor slowing, weight loss, early morning wakening, diurnal mood variation) seen in adults. In fact, if they do we should be on the

Prof. Philip Hazell BMedSc, MBChB, PhD, FRANZCP, Cert Accred Child and Adolescent Psychiatry (RANZCP), Child and Youth Mental Health Service, University of Newcastle, Locked Bag 1014, Wallsend, NSW 2287, Australia. Tel: +61 2 492 46386; Fax: +61 2 492 46056;
E-mail: hazell@mail.newcastle.edu.au

Table 1 Symptom criteria used to establish a diagnosis of depression, with comments specific to children and adolescents

Symptom	Commentary
Depressed mood most of the day, nearly every day, as indicated by subjective report or observation made by others	May be irritable rather than depressed mood. Children may not be able to articulate the feeling state very well, and indeed it may be somewhat undifferentiated. Adults may overlook the symptom, especially in the presence of co-morbid problems
Markedly diminished interest or pleasure in all, or almost all, activities most of the day, nearly every day	A discriminating symptom, but may be confused with oppositionality. In addition, some teenagers drop out of previous structured activities because their interest has shifted to socialising, or to solitary activities such as computer games
Fatigue or loss of energy nearly every day	The clinician must exercise judgement over whether the symptom may be better explained by intercurrent medical illness. Symptoms that seem to be in excess of the level of physical morbidity may still raise the possibility of depression
Loss of confidence or self-esteem	As children are easily disheartened by failure and disappointment the symptom is of clinical significance only if it occurs in conjunction with clear depression or irritability
Feelings of worthlessness or excessive or inappropriate guilt (which may be delusional) nearly every day	A discriminating symptom, as guilt is not encountered that often in young people
Recurrent thoughts of death (not just fear of dying), recurrent suicidal ideation, a suicide attempt, or a specific plan for committing suicide	Differentiate from hurtful or manipulative statements made in anger but independent of depressed mood
Diminished ability to think or concentrate, or indecisiveness nearly every day	The problem may come to light because of a decline in academic performance. In the presence of premorbid attentional problems, there needs to be a clear increase in the symptom within the context of the depressive episode
Psychomotor agitation or retardation observable by others and present nearly every day	In the presence of premorbid hyperactivity, there needs to be a clear increase in the symptom within the context of the depressive episode

Table 1 Symptom criteria used to establish a diagnosis of depression, with comments specific to children and adolescents (continued)

Symptom	Commentary
Insomnia or hypersomnia nearly every day	Many teenagers show a normal need for more sleep, plus a tendency to stay up late and to sleep late
Significant weight loss when not dieting or weight gain, or decrease or increase in appetite nearly every day	Consider failure to make expected weight gains. Teenagers sometimes appear to have lost weight when in fact they have had a growth spurt. Change in appetite may be confused with food fads
ASSOCIATED SYMPTOMS OR SIGNS	
Somatic complaints such as headaches and abdominal pains	The clinician must exercise judgement over whether the symptom may be better explained by intercurrent medical illness. Symptoms that seem to be in excess of the level of physical morbidity may still raise the possibility of depression
Anxiety, phobias, school refusal	If present premorbidly, have become more severe in the context of the depressive illness
Hopelessness and helplessness	In excess of the child's circumstances
Lack of reactivity	Affect lifts only temporarily in response to pleasant experiences. In repose the young person still looks depressed

lookout for a physical illness. Symptoms may go unnoticed by adults because of a tendency for depression to have an insidious onset in children, and because the symptoms may fluctuate in intensity. A discriminating indicator of depression in children is the loss of enjoyment derived from previously pleasurable activities. For example, depressed children may no longer accept invitations to play with their friends. They may feel irritable rather than sad. They may criticise themselves and may be pessimistic or hopeless about the future. Problems at school may arise from indecision and difficulties with concentration. Some depressed children may try to avoid school, often on the pretext of ill health. Depressed children tend to lack energy and to have problems sleeping. Morbid thoughts occasionally progress to suicidal thinking and even suicide attempts.[2] Depressed children may be bothered by nuisance stomach-aches or head-aches, and it is these symptoms that may lead to a presentation to the doctor. Anxiety symptoms, including phobias and separation anxiety, are common. If psychotic features are present, they are more likely to involve hallucinations than delusions. The symptom criteria used to diagnose depression are summarised in Table 1. These criteria were developed with adults in mind, and are not entirely satisfactory for use in young people. Comments are made against each symptom to assist the clinician in applying the criteria in the context of children.

COURSE OF ILLNESS

As with adults, depression in children follows a relapsing course. An episode of depression will last, on average, about 7–9 months. There is a 40% probability of relapse within 2 years, increasing to 70% after 5 years. The likelihood of further episodes in adulthood is about 60–70%.[1] The rate of switching to hypomania in young people with depression also seems higher than in adults, with some researchers claiming rates of 20–40%. Depression in young people is not a benign self-limiting disorder. An episode of depression can be quite devastating to a young person's academic and social development, and can also have an adverse effect on family relations, especially if the young person's problems are misunderstood. A third of young people who experience a depressive episode will make a suicide attempt at some stage, and 3–4% will die from suicide.[1]

COMMUNITY PREVALENCE AND CO-MORBIDITY

A recent survey of a nationally representative sample of Australian children found 3.7% of boys and 2.1% of girls aged 6–12 years had experienced a depressive episode in the previous 12 months.[3] The rate among teenagers aged 13–17 years was 4.8% for boys and 4.9% for girls. These prevalence estimates are similar to those found in other Western countries[4] and in non-industrialised countries.[5] Longitudinal data from New Zealand show that depression becomes more common in girls than boys at around 13 years.[6] Depression occurs more frequently in young people living in single-income or blended families, and in families with a low income.[7] In rural areas, depression remains more common among boys than girls in the teenage years. Clinical impressions suggest rates of depression may be high in indigenous youth, but epidemiological studies have not involved enough indigenous youth to enable reliable prevalence estimates. Common co-occurring conditions established by community studies include anxiety disorders, obsessive compulsive disorder, conduct problems, attention-deficit/hyperactivity disorder, and learning difficulties. The rate of co-morbidity is often higher again in clinical settings owing to referral bias, and to the Berkson effect.

PREVALENCE AND DETECTION IN PAEDIATRIC SETTINGS

An American survey found that the prevalence of depression among attendees of a paediatric primary care service was no greater than that found in the general population.[8] However, the prevalence of depression is substantially higher among patients who suffer from chronic medical conditions, particularly epilepsy.[9] Although paediatricians are becoming increasingly involved in the assessment and management of psychosocial disorders,[10] they detect only a small proportion of psychiatric morbidity among clinic attendees.[11] Their specific ability to detect affective disorders has not been systematically studied, but extrapolation from research with adult patients who attend primary care settings would suggest that detection is likely to be low. Detection is somewhat better during routine check-up visits than during acute presentations. An audit found that questioning about depression was documented in less than 5% of charts of adolescents attending an emergency department with pain, weakness, dizziness or hyperventilation,[12] symptoms which should suggest the possibility of an emotional disorder. Detection could be enhanced by the use of simple self-report measures completed by older children and adolescents just prior to their clinic appointment. The Beck Depressive Inventory for Primary Care, for example, consists of seven items that reflect the diagnostic criteria for major depression. These items are: sadness; loss of pleasure (anhedonia); pessimism; past failure; self dislike; self criticalness; and suicidal thoughts or wishes. To avoid false positive diagnoses of depression through contamination by symptoms of physical illness, no somatic symptom items are included in the scale. Each item is rated on a four-point scale from 0 to 3, yielding a total possible score of 21. Scores of 4 and above were found to have 90% specificity and sensitivity for detecting major depression in adolescents attending a community paediatric practice.[13] The use of such instruments is only of value, however, if the clinician is then willing to act on the information by offering intervention or referral. Horwitz *et al.*[14] found that paediatricians only offered intervention to about half the patients in whom they had identified mental health problems. Barriers to intervention may include lack of time, lack of knowledge and skills, or the limited capacity of some specialist child and adolescent mental health services to accept new referrals.

AETIOLOGY

Depression in children usually arises from a combination of genetic vulnerability, suboptimal early developmental experiences, and exposure to stresses. However, depressive syndromes sometimes occur as sequelae to physical illness such as viral infection, and may overlap with fatigue syndromes.[15,16] The heritability of depression may increase with age,[17] but the findings from genetic studies are somewhat inconsistent. What is clear is that, unlike chronic medical conditions such as diabetes, very early onset depression is not associated with a greater genetic risk than later onset depression.[18] Recurrent depression seems to have a stronger familial association than single episode depression. What exactly is being inherited remains uncertain. At the molecular level, one possible candidate is polymorphism of the serotonin transporter gene, although to date research has been confined to adult samples.[19] Hormonal dysregulation may also mediate the symptoms of depression. Dihydroepiandrosterone hypersecretion precedes the onset of depressive disorder in adolescents, and appears to be independent of recent life events and ongoing difficulties.[20] Non-suppression of cortisol release by the administration of dexamethasone is found in populations of children and adolescents with depression at comparable rates to adult samples.[21] Non-suppression occurs despite the fact that depressed children and adolescents do not have the excessive basal levels of cortisol secretion seen in adult patients. Growth hormone may also be dysregulated in juvenile depression, while studies of prolactin secretion in children and adults have produced contradictory results.[21] One magnetic resonance imaging study found lower frontal lobe to total cerebral volume ratios in children and adolescents hospitalised with depression than in normal controls,[22] but only limited conclusions can be drawn from anatomical studies at this stage.

At the intrapsychic level, depression-prone individuals may inherit a cognitive style characterised by an overly pessimistic outlook on events.[23] This cognitive style precedes the onset of depression and appears to be independent of recent life events and ongoing stresses.[20] Stressful life events may trigger the first occurrence of depression, but are rarely sufficient on their own to cause depression. Lower levels of stress are needed to provoke subsequent episodes of illness.[1] This observation has led to the notion of psychological scarring, which suggests that the experience of a depressive episode reduces the individual's resilience to adversity. Enduring problems in the relationship with the primary care-givers is an important risk factor for depression, but such difficulties also predispose to other psychiatric disorders. Relationship difficulties that occur early in development may be more important to the development of depression in boys, while for girls, recent difficulties, especially in the relationship with mother, may be more pathogenic.[24]

ASSESSMENT AND DIAGNOSIS

The core element of assessment is the clinical and developmental history. Factors within the history that make the diagnosis of depression more compelling are previous confirmed episodes of depression, a strong family history of mood disorder, and clear evidence of a decline in function. The duration of symptoms may be hard to determine owing to the insidious onset of the disorder in young people. In addition, regardless of the time-frame specified, young people tend to report their feeling state over the past few days; therefore, it can be difficult to obtain an accurate history of antecedent symptoms. Corroborative history needs to be obtained from the patient and from parents or care-givers, and may be augmented with information provided by the class teacher or student welfare teacher. Discrepancy between the reports of adults and young people is common. Adults tend to under-recognise internalising symptoms and to misattribute externalising symptoms. For example, irritability may be misattributed to 'hormones' or conduct problems. Observations of the mental state are most helpful if combined over several visits or assessments. Even profoundly depressed young people may appear to 'brighten up' when with friends or when engaged in pleasant activities; therefore, such observations do not preclude a diagnosis of mood disorder. The assessment may be supplemented with self-report questionnaires such as the Beck Depression Inventory for Primary Care or the Children's Depression Inventory, or observer-rated measures such as the Children's Depression Rating Scale. Laboratory investigations are only useful for the exclusion of medical illness. The severity and nature of the child's symptoms will determine the need for such investigation.

TREATMENT

Having established a diagnosis of depression, the first important intervention is psycho-education for the child and family. The nature of the condition needs to be outlined, including the risks of relapse. Practical advice should be given on how to counter common symptoms such as sleep problems. Attention needs to be given to pathogenic factors such as family conflict and disruption, and, in the adolescent patient, substance abuse. Young people and parents may want to know whether the problem will go away without treatment. The answer is 'eventually yes', but the young person may have by then experienced secondary complications such as peer problems and academic decline. It is useful to point out that depression is a noxious psychological state from which people of all ages deserve relief.

The type of treatment that is recommended will be determined by the severity of illness, the pattern of co-morbid disorders, the level of suicidality or dangerousness to others, and access to treatment facilities. Most depressive illness in children and adolescents can be treated on an out-patient basis. Reasons for hospitalisation include a high level of suicidality, the need for complex investigation, a lack of response to out-patient treatment, and a need to provide the young person temporary protection from an adverse social environment. The first objective of treatment is remission of symptoms, followed by protection against relapse of the current illness episode, followed by protection against the occurrence of further illness episodes.

The evidence-base for the treatment of depression in young people is expanding, but there are still many gaps in our knowledge. While the responsiveness of adolescents to treatment is closer to that of adults than that of younger children, it is still unwise to assume that results obtained from studies conducted in adult samples will generalise to young people. To obtain information on current evidence, the reader is directed to the chapter on child and adolescent depression in the publication *Clinical Evidence* that may be accessed via the Internet.[25] Table 2 provides a summary statement of the evidence for treatment current at the time of writing. Controlled trials are needed in the following areas: (i) comparative trials of cognitive behaviour therapy versus selective serotonin re-uptake inhibitors; (ii) combined psychotherapy and pharmacotherapy versus psychotherapy or pharmacotherapy alone; (iii) in-

Table 2 Summary of evidence for treatments for depression in adolescents, as of March 2003*

Beneficial
      Cognitive therapy (in mild-to-moderate depression)

Likely to be beneficial
      Interpersonal therapy in mild-to-moderate depression

Trade off
      Selective serotonin re-uptake inhibitors

Unknown effectiveness
      Intravenous clomipramine
      Monoamine oxidase inhibitors
      Lithium
      St John's Wort
      Venlafaxine
      Electroconvulsive therapy
      Family therapy
      Group treatments other than cognitive behavioural therapy
      Long-term effects of psychotherapy

Unlikely to be beneficial
      Oral tricyclic antidepressants

*Abstracted from Hazell.[25]

patient versus out-patient treatment; (iv) the effectiveness of any treatment modality on relapse prevention; and (v) augmentation of antidepressant medication with a mood stabiliser or antipsychotic drug versus antidepressant medication alone for treatment resistant depression.

A systematic review has demonstrated the superiority of cognitive behaviour therapy (CBT) over non-specific supportive therapies for inducing remission in children and adolescents with mild-to-moderate depression. The educative approach used in CBT is generally well suited to children and adolescents, although some complain that participating in CBT is too much like doing schoolwork. Some of the higher order cognitions required to undertake CBT are only developing in mid-adolescence.[26] An example would be the capacity to differentiate fully theory from evidence. For this reason, CBT delivered to children needs to be tailored to individual need. A greater emphasis may need to be given to the behavioural components of the intervention. CBT appears to be equally effective whether it is delivered individually or in a group format. The evidence for other forms of psychotherapy is equivocal. CBT is probably most valuable for children with mild or even subclinical symptoms of depression. Although a promising treatment, few paediatricians have received the training necessary to deliver CBT to children. However, it may be possible to incorporate the following elements of CBT into brief counselling of children with depression: (i) encourage the child, with the help of parents, to schedule some pleasant activities each week; (ii) give the child the message that there are several possible solutions to most problems; and (iii) challenge excessively negative perceptions.

Selective serotonin re-uptake inhibitors (SSRIs) are the only class of antidepressant medication for which there is evidence of efficacy in children and adolescents. The evidence, however, is weaker than that for adults, with only a small number of published trials involving two agents (fluoxetine and paroxetine), a somewhat smaller risk difference (percentage responding to active treatment minus percentage responding to placebo) than adult studies, and a tendency for symptom reduction to be detected by clinicians, but not by the patients.[25] Fluoxetine is longer acting than the other SSRI drugs. While this may expose the patient to a greater risk of side-effects, an advantage for young people is that the occasional missed dose is less likely to disrupt treatment, or to cause a discontinuation syndrome. Although some guidelines recommend introducing fluoxetine in lower doses than used with adults,[27] many children and adolescents will tolerate an 'adult' dose of 20 mg. Some young people will require daily doses of up to 60 mg to achieve remission. It is important to persist with treatment for at least 6 weeks before deciding that it has been ineffective. A trap for the inexperienced is to change a patient to another, possibly less effective treatment, before the first-line treatment has taken effect. Treatment should be continued for at least as long as one would for adults (9–12 months).[27] If there is a recurrence of depressive symptoms upon discontinuation of treatment, further maintenance treatment may be required. Such maintenance treatment will be tailored to the need of the patient, and could continue from 1 year to indefinitely.[27]

Owing to the higher rate of switching to mania in young people with depression compared with adults, drug-induced mania is an important risk that should be discussed with the patient and family. Adverse effects are similar for all the SSRI drugs, are dose-dependent, and generally subside with time. Common side-effects include gastrointestinal symptoms, restlessness, sweating, headaches, initial insomnia and tremor. Fluvoxamine (for which no RCTs have been published for juvenile depression) is marketed on the basis of being sedating rather than activating; however, in two similar RCTs directed to children with obsessive compulsive disorder, the difference in rates of insomnia between active treatment and placebo was actually greater for fluvoxamine[28] than fluoxetine.[29] A more serious adverse effect is the serotonin syndrome, characterised by agitation, confusion and hyperthermia. In the paediatric setting, the syndrome could be misattributed to the primary medical condition, or to the effects of concurrent medication. Treatment is supportive, and the SSRI medication should be withheld. The risk of serotonin syndrome is increased in the presence of other serotonergic drugs including other antidepressants, St John's Wort, and tryptophan. SSRI drugs may also increase the plasma levels of other medications such as anticonvulsant drugs owing to competition for metabolic pathways. A discontinuation syndrome, characterised by flu-like symptoms lasting up to 2 weeks, has been reported following cessation or dose reduction of paroxetine.[30] The syndrome has not been reported with fluoxetine, possibly because its longer half-life means the drug is cleared more gradually from the body. In the paediatric setting, the discontinuation syndrome could be misattributed to a concurrent medical condition. The syndrome may be prevented by tapering the dose of SSRI over several weeks.

A systematic review of tricyclic drugs for depression in children and adolescents found evidence of no effect. The findings from an analysis of data from trials involving only adolescents were contradictory, with evidence of a small treatment effect on continuous measures of outcome, but no evidence of effect on categorical measures.[25] One interpretation of this apparent contradiction is that adolescents show a trend towards responding to tricyclic drugs in a manner similar to adults.

There are small and equivocal trials of the reversible monoamine oxidase inhibitor moclobemide, and the selective noradrenergic re-uptake inhibitor venlafaxine.[25] Neither drug should be considered first-line treatment for depression in young people. A small trial of lithium monotherapy for depression in young people with a parental history of bipolar disorder found no benefit over placebo. An open label trial of St John's Wort in 101 children under the age of 12 years with depression found global improvement after 6 weeks in all subjects with evaluable data (about three-quarters of the original sample).[31] It is hard to take such a claim of effectiveness seriously, and data from a properly conducted RCTs are needed.

In the event of a lack of response to an adequate trial of CBT and an SSRI, the diagnosis of depression should be reviewed and further consideration should be given to the presence of perpetuating factors such as intercurrent substance abuse or environmental stress. This may be an appropriate time to consider hospitalisation, or at least to increase the frequency of out-patient visits. If there is no other explanation for the absence of treatment response, then augmentation of the SSRI with a mood stabiliser or an antipsychotic may be considered, although the efficacy of such strategies has not been evaluated in controlled trials in children. Electroconvulsive therapy (ECT) should be considered if symptoms are severe and there has been minimal response to other treatments. Indications for ECT include prominent psychotic symptoms and life-threatening restrictions to food and fluid intake. Evidence of efficacy is available only from case studies, but it is unlikely that it will ever be possible to conduct randomised controlled trials comparing ECT with sham treatment in young people.

PREVENTION

Strategies to prevent the occurrence of depression among children and adolescents fall into two major categories. The first is concerned with early intervention directed to mother infant dyads at risk of attachment difficulties through problems such as maternal mental illness and economic disadvantage. Such intervention is often seen as being primarily directed to the prevention of child abuse and neglect or of the emergence of conduct symptoms in the child. However, it is likely that the fostering early attachment is also, indirectly, a protective factor against depression. Such prevention activity has often taken the form of home visiting and supportive counselling. There is some evidence that these interventions reduce the incidence of various social and mental health problems, but the direct impact on the occurrence of depression has yet to be evaluated. The second group of preventive activities centres around universal and indicated interventions directed to school students. The MindMatters programme introduced to some Australian schools combines whole of school activities directed to the reduction of problems such as bullying and harassment with classroom programmes that promote emotional resilience. The Resourceful Adolescent Program (RAP) is another universal curriculum-based programme directed to promoting resilience. A non-randomised controlled study has demonstrated that students exposed to RAP had lower levels of depressive symptoms at 10-month follow-up than students who were not exposed to the programme.[32]

While not always considered within a prevention framework, a further important strategy against the development of depression in teenagers is the effective treatment of conditions that may precede the onset of depression. Examples include anxiety disorders (including post-traumatic stress disorder), conduct problems, learning difficulties, chronic medical conditions and substance abuse. It has often been thought that substance abuse arises as a complication of depression (the self-medication hypothesis), but longitudinal research has shown that heavy marijuana use, for example, predisposes to the onset of depression.[33]

Key points for clinical practice

- Depression in children more often presents with irritability, anxiety or somatic symptoms than with low mood.

- Depression may occur in the aftermath of infectious disease and may be confused with or confounded by postviral fatigue syndromes.

- Depression is too common among children and adolescents to be considered the exclusive domain of specialist mental health services. Just as general practitioners treat many adults with mild-to-moderate depressive illness, paediatricians may increasingly provide a similar service to children and adolescents.

- Serial observation of the mental state over several visits may give a more reliable indication of depression than one cross-sectional assessment.

- Co-morbidity is the norm. Common co-occurring conditions include anxiety, obsessive compulsive disorder, disruptive behaviour and, in older patients, substance abuse.

- Most depressive illness in children and adolescents can be treated on an out-patient basis. Reasons for hospitalisation include a high level of suicidality, the need for complex investigation, a lack of response to out-patient treatment, and a need to provide the young person temporary protection from an adverse social environment.

- Mild-to-moderate depression may respond to cognitive behaviour therapy (CBT). Elements of CBT that may be incorporated into paediatric practice include; encouraging the child, with the help of parents, to schedule some pleasant activities each week, giving the child the message that there are several possible solutions to most problems, and challenging excessively negative perceptions.

- Moderate-to-severe depression is more likely to respond to a serotonin re-uptake inhibiting drug. It is important to ensure the child has been exposed to an adequate dose of medication before at least 4 weeks before ruling that a medication is ineffective.

Key points for clinical practice (continued)

- Augmentation of antidepressant medication with a mood stabiliser or an atypical antipsychotic is best supervised by a clinician with experience in the field.

- Antidepressant medication should be continued for about 12 months to protect against relapse.

- Caution should be taken to observe for a switch into a manic state, as there is evidence that this may occur more commonly in young people suffering depression than it does in adults.

- A secure home environment, a safe school environment, and adequate attention to health and learning difficulties may all protect against the onset of depression in young people.

References

1, Birmaher B, Ryan ND, Williamson DE *et al*. Childhood and adolescent depression: a review of the past 10 years. Part I. *J Am Acad Child Adolesc Psychiatry* 1996; **35**: 1427–1439.
2. Poznanski EO, Mokros HB. *Children's Depression Rating Scale-Revised*. Los Angeles, CA: Western Psychological Services, 1996.
3. Sawyer M, Arney FM, Baghurst PA *et al*. *The Mental Health of Young People in Australia*. Canberra, ACT: Mental Health and Special Programs Branch, Commonwealth Department of Health and Aged Care, 2000.
4. Lewinsohn PM, Essau CA. Depression in adolescents. In: Gotlib IH. (ed) *Depression in Special Populations*. New York: Guilford, 2002: 541–559.
5. Chen X, Rubin KH, Li BS. Depressed mood in Chinese children: relations with school performance and family environment. *J Consult Clin Psychol* 1995; **63**: 938–947.
6. Hankin BL, Abramson LY, Moffitt TE, Silva PA, McGee R, Angell KE. Development of depression from preadolescence to young adulthood: emerging gender differences in a 10-year longitudinal study. *J Abnorm Psychol* 1998; **107**: 128–140.
7. Sawyer MG, Arney FM, Baghurst PA *et al*. *The Mental Health of Young People in Australia*. Canberra, ACT: Mental Health and Special Programs Branch, Commonwealth Department of Health and Aged Care, 2000.
8. Costello EJ, Costello AJ, Edelbrock C *et al*. Psychiatric disorders in pediatric primary care: prevalence and risk factors. *Arch Gen Psychiatry* 1988; **45**: 1107–1116.
9. Dunn DW, Austin JK, Huster GA. Symptoms of depression in adolescents with epilepsy. *J Am Acad Child Adolesc Psychiatry* 1999; **38**: 1132–1138.
10. Tortenson O. The treatment of mood disorders in children and adolescents by general paediatricians. *Biol Psychiatry* 2001; **49**: 970–972.
11. Wells KB, Kataoka SH, Asarnow JR. Affective disorders in children and adolescents: addressing unmet need in primary care settings. *Biol Psychiatry* 2001; **49**: 1111–1120.
12. Porter SC, Fein JA, Ginsburg KR. Depression screening in adolescents with somatic complaints presenting to the emergency department. *Ann Emerg Med* 1997; **29**: 141–145.
13. Winter LB, Steer RA, Jones-Hicks L, Beck AT. Screening for major depression disorders in adolescent medical outpatients with the Beck Depression Inventory for Primary Care. *J Adolesc Health* 1999; **24**: 389–394.
14. Horwitz SM, Leaf PJ, Leventhal JM, Borsyth B, Speechley KN. Identification and management of psychosocial and developmental problems in community-based, primary care pediatric practices. *Pediatrics* 1992; **89**: 480–485.
15. Carter BD, Edwards JF, Kronenberger WG, Michalczyk L, Marshall GS. Case control study of chronic fatigue in pediatric patients. *Pediatrics* 1995; **95**: 179–186.
16. Garralda E, Rangel L, Levin M, Roberts H, Ukoumunne O. Psychiatric adjustment in adolescents with a history of chronic fatigue syndrome. *J Am Acad Child Adolesc Psychiatry* 1999; **38**: 1515–1521.

17. Harrington R. Childhood depression: is it the same disorder? In: Rapoport J. (ed) *Childhood Onset of 'Adult' Psychopathology*. Washington DC: American Psychiatric Press, 2000; 223–243.

18. Rice F, Harold G, Thaper A. The genetic aetiology of childhood depression: a review. *J Child Psychol Psychiatry* 2002; **43**: 65–79.

19. Todd RD, Botteron KN. Family, genetic, and imaging studies of early-onset depression. *Child Adolesc Psychiatric Clin North Am* 2001; **10**: 375–390.

20. Goodyer IM, Herbert J, Tamplin A, Altham PM. First-episode major depression in adolescents. Affective, cognitive and endocrine characteristics of risk status and predictors of onset. *Br J Psychiatry* 2000; **176**: 142–149.

21. Kaufman J, Martin A, King RA, Charney D. Are child-, adolescent-, and adult-onset depression one and the same disorder? *Biol Psychiatry* 2001; **49**: 980–1001.

22. Steingard RJ, Renshaw PF, Yurgelun-Todd D *et al.* Structural abnormalities in brain magnetic resonance images of depressed children. *J Am Acad Child Adolesc Psychiatry* 1996; **35**: 307–331.

23. Gladstone TR, Kaslow NJ. Depression and attributions in children and adolescents: a meta-analytic review. *J Abnorm Child Psychol* 1995; **23**: 597–606.

24. Duggal S, Carlson EA, Sroufe LA, Egeland B. Depressive symptomatology in childhood and adolescence. *Dev Psychopathol* 2001; **13**: 143–164.

25. Hazell P. Depression in children and adolescents. *Clinical Evidence* 2003; <www.clinicalevidence.com last> accessed March 2003.

26. Harrington R, Clark A. Prevention and early intervention for depression in adolescence and early adult life. *Eur Arch Psychiatry Clin Neurosci* 1998; **248**: 32–45.

27. American Academy of Child and Adolescent Psychiatry. Practice parameters for the assessment and treatment of children and adolescents with depressive disorders. AACAP. *J Am Acad Child Adolesc Psychiatry* 1998; **37 (Suppl 10)**: 63S–83S.

28. Riddle MA, Reeve EA, Yaryura-Tobias JA *et al.* Fluvoxamine for children and adolescents with obsessive-compulsive disorder: a randomized, controlled, multicenter trial. *J Am Acad Child Adolesc Psychiatry* 2001; **40**: 222–229.

29. Geller DA, Hoog SL, Heiligenstein JH *et al.* Fluoxetine treatment for obsessive-compulsive disorder in children and adolescents: a placebo-controlled clinical trial. *J Am Acad Child Adolesc Psychiatry* 2001; **40**: 773–779.

30. Diler RS, Avci A. Selective serotonin reuptake inhibitor discontinuation syndrome in children: six case reports. *Curr Ther Res Clin Exp* 2002; **63**: 188–197.

31. Hübner WD, Kirste T. Experience with St John's Wort (*Hypericum perforatum*) in children under 12 years with symptoms of depression and psychovegetative disturbances. *Phytother Res* 2001; **15**: 367–370.

32. Shochet IM, Dadds MR, Holland D, Whitefield K, Harnett PH, Osgarby SM. The efficacy of a universal school-based program to prevent adolescent depression. *J Clin Child Psychol* 2001; **30**: 303–315.

33. Patton GC, Coffey C, Carlin JB, Degenhardt L, Lynskey M, Hall W. Cannabis use and mental health in young people: cohort study. *BMJ* 2002; **325**: 1159–1198.

Timothy J. David

15

Paediatric literature review – 2002

ALLERGY

de Jong MH *et al*. The effect of brief neonatal exposure to cows' milk on atopic symptoms up to age 5. Arch Dis Child 2002; 86: 365–369. *Early brief exposure to cows milk in breast fed children is not associated with atopic disease or allergic symptoms.*

Hourihane JO *et al*. Impact of repeated surgical procedures on the incidence and prevalence of latex allergy: a prospective study of 1263 children. J Pediatr 2002; 140: 479–482. *Previous surgery increased the odds by 13 times. See also pp. 370–372.*

Macdougall CF *et al*. How dangerous is food allergy in childhood? The incidence of severe and fatal allergic reactions across the UK and Ireland. Arch Dis Child 2002; 86: 236–239. *Prescribing an epinephrine autoinjector requires a careful balance of advantages and disadvantages.*

Schoetzau A *et al*. Maternal compliance with nutritional recommendations in an allergy preventive programme. Arch Dis Child 2002; 86: 180–184. *Non-compliance is an important potential confounder.*

Sears MR *et al*. Long-term relation between breastfeeding and development of atopy and asthma in children and young adults: a longitudinal study. Lancet 2002; 360: 901–907. *Breastfeeding does not protect children against atopy and asthma and may even increase the risk. See also pp. 887–888.*

Prof. T.J. David MD PhD FRCP FRCPCH DCH
Booth Hall Children's Hospital, Charlestown Road, Blackley, Manchester M9 7AA, UK
Tel: +44 161 220 5536; Fax: +44 161 904 9320; E-mall: t.david@netcomuk.co.uk

Sherriff A *et al*. Hygiene levels in a contemporary population cohort are associated with wheezing and atopic eczema in preschool infants. Arch Dis Child 2002; 87: 26–29. *High levels of hygiene at 15 months of age were independently associated with wheeze and eczema.*

Vanderhoof JA *et al*. Probiotics in pediatrics. Pediatrics 2002; 109: 956–958. *Review.*

Watura JC. Nut allergy in schoolchildren: a survey of schools in the Severn NHS Trust. Arch Dis Child 2002; 86: 240–244. *Schools are insufficiently informed.*

CARDIOVASCULAR

Ferrieri P *et al*. Unique features of infective endocarditis in childhood. Pediatrics 2002; 109: 931–943. *Review.*

Fleisher BE *et al*. Infant heart transplantation at Stanford: growth and neurodevelopmental outcome. Pediatrics 2002; 109: 1–7. *Difficulties with growth and development.*

COMMUNITY

Bagust A *et al*. Economic evaluation of an acute paediatric hospital at home clinical trial. Arch Dis Child 2002; 87: 489–492. *Unlikely to reduce NHS costs but significantly increase patient and carer satisfaction. See also pp. 371–375.*

Cook P *et al*. Bereavement support following sudden and unexpected death: guidelines for care. Arch Dis Child 2002; 87: 36–39. *Review.*

Dennison BA *et al*. Television viewing and television in bedroom associated with overweight risk among low-income preschool children. Pediatrics 2002; 109: 1028–1035. *Association between TV viewing and being overweight.*

Emond A *et al*. An evaluation of the first parent health visitor scheme. Arch Dis Child 2002; 86: 150–157. *No clear advantage over conventional health visiting.*

Garrett M *et al*. Locomotor milestones and babywalkers: cross sectional study. BMJ 2002; 324: 1494. *Babywalkers are associated with delay in achieving normal locomotor milestones.*

Halliday HL. Early postnatal dexamethasone and cerebral palsy. Pediatrics 2002; 109: 1169–1170. *Review.*

Hiscock H *et al*. Randomised controlled trial of behavioural infant sleep intervention to improve infant sleep and maternal mood. BMJ 2002; 324: 1062–1065. *Significantly reduces infant sleep problems at two but not four months.*

Jennings P. Should paediatric units have bereavement support posts? Arch Dis Child 2002; 87: 40–42. *Review.*

Packman A *et al*. Searching for the cause of stuttering. Lancet 2002; 360: 655–656. *Review.*

ACCIDENTS

James LP *et al*. Predictors of outcome after acetaminophen poisoning in children and adolescents. J Pediatr 2002; 140: 522–526. *Paracetamol ingestion warrants observation for 48 hours. See also pp. 495–498.*

Riordan M *et al*. Poisoning in children 1: general management. Arch Dis Child 2002; 87: 397–399. *Review. See also pp. 397–410.*

Sibert JR *et al*. Preventing deaths by drowning in children in the United Kingdom: have we made progress in 10 years? Population based incidence study. BMJ 2002; 324: 1070–1071. *There is a small reduction but 100 children a year still die from drowning. See also pp. 1049–1050.*

Wickham T *et al*. Head injuries in infants: the risks of bouncy chairs and car seats. Arch Dis Child 2002; 86: 168–169. *Dangerous if placed inappropriately.*

CHILD ABUSE

Barber MA *et al*. Fits, faints, or fatal fantasy? Fabricated seizures and child abuse. Arch Dis Child 2002; 86: 230 *Review.*

Benger JR *et al*. Simple intervention to improve detection of child abuse in emergency departments. BMJ 2002; 324: 780–782. *A flowchart to increase awareness.*

Carter R. Non-accidental head injury in children: gathering the evidence. Lancet 2002; 360: 271–272. *Review.*

Champion MP *et al*. Duodenal perforation: a diagnostic pitfall in non-accidental injury. Arch Dis Child 2002; 87: 432–433. *Report of 3 cases.*

Dubowitz H *et al*. Child neglect: outcomes in high-risk urban preschoolers. Pediatrics 2002; 109: 1100–1107. *Psychological neglect is significantly related to reported behaviour problems.*

Dunstan FD *et al*. A scoring system for bruise patterns: a tool for identifying abuse. Arch Dis Child 2002; 86: 330–333. *Whether the scoring system will be any use in other populations is unknown.*

HANDICAP

Halliday HL. Early postnatal dexamethasone and cerebral palsy. Pediatrics 2002; 109: 1169–1170. *Review.*

Hutton JL *et al*. Effects of cognitive, motor, and sensory disabilities on survival in cerebral palsy. Arch Dis Child 2002; 86: 84–90. *Survival rates decrease as the severity of cognitive, motor, and sensory disabilities increased.*

Pharoah POD *et al*. Cerebral palsy in twins: a national study. Arch Dis Child 2002; 87: F122–F124. *Like-sex twins are at greater risk of cerebral palsy.*

IMMUNISATION

Andrews N et al. Recall bias, MMR, and autism. Arch Dis Child 2002; 87: 493–494. *Recall bias is responsible for some claims of a causal link between immunisation and autism.*

Davies P et al. Antivaccination activists on the world wide web. Arch Dis Child 2002; 87: 22–25. *Parents are likely to encounter antivaccination activists.*

Finn A et al. Should the new pneumococcal vaccine be used in high-risk children? Arch Dis Child 2002; 87: 18–21. Review.

Freed GL et al. The process of public policy formulation: the case of thiomersal in vaccines. Pediatrics 2002; 109: 1153–1159. *Review.*

Jodar L et al. Development of vaccines against meningococcal disease. Lancet 2002; 359: 1499–1508. *Review.*

Madsen KM et al. A population-based study of measles, mumps, and rubella vaccination and autism. N Engl J Med 2002; 347: 1477–1482. *Strong evidence against hypothesis that MMR causes autism.*

Offit PA et al. Addressing parents' concerns: do multiple vaccines overwhelm or weaken the infant's immune system? Pediatrics 2002; 109: 124–129. *Review.*

Pichichero ME et al. Mercury concentrations and metabolism in infants receiving vaccines containing thiomersal: a descriptive study. Lancet 2002; 360: 1737–1741. *Ethylmercury seems to be eliminated from blood rapidly via the stools after parenteral administration of thiomersal in vaccines.*

Taylor B et al. Measles, mumps, and rubella vaccination and bowel problems or developmental regression in children with autism: population study. BMJ 2002; 324: 393–396. *Further evidence against involvement of MMR vaccine in the initiation of autism.*

Wolfe RM et al. Anti-vaccinationists past and present. BMJ 2002; 325: 430–432. *Review.*

INFANT FEEDING

Black RE *et al*. Optimal duration of exclusive breast feeding in low income countries. BMJ 2002; 325: 1252–1253. *Review.*

Bryant P *et al*. Cytomegalovirus transmission from breast milk in premature babies: does it matter? Arch Dis Child 2002; 87: F75–F77. *Review.*

Laing IA *et al*. Hypernatraemia in the first few days: is the incidence rising? Arch Dis Child 2002; 87: F158–F162. *The condition is under-reported.*

Wright KS *et al*. Infant acceptance of breast milk after maternal exercise. Pediatrics 2002; 109: 585–589. *Exercise does not impede acceptance of breast milk.*

SCREENING AND SURVEILLANCE

American Academy of Pediatrics. Red reflex examination in infants. Pediatrics 2002; 109: 980–981. *Review.*

Elliman DAC *et al*. Newborn and childhood screening programmes: criteria, evidence, and current policy. Arch Dis Child 2002; 87: 6–9. *Review*.

Grimes DA *et al*. Uses and abuses of screening tests. Lancet 2002; 359: 881–884. *Review*.

Laing GJ *et al*. Evaluation of a structured test and a parent led method for screening for speech and language problems: prospective population based study. BMJ 2002; 325: 1152–1154. *Ineffective approach*.

Leonard JV. Screening for inherited metabolic disease in newborn infants using tandem mass spectrometry. BMJ 2002; 324: 4–5. *Further assessment of performance and outcome is needed*.

Maxwell SL *et al*. Clinical screening for developmental dysplasia of the hip in Northern Ireland. BMJ 2002; 324: 1031–1033. *Improvements to screening processes could reduce late presentation*.

Williams C *et al*. Amblyopia treatment outcomes after screening before or at age 3 years: follow up from randomised trial. BMJ 2002; 324: 1549–1551. *Early treatment leads to a better outcome*.

SIDS

Buchino JJ et al. Sudden unexpected death in hospitalized children. J Pediatr 2002; 140: 461–465. *Review of all causes of sudden unexpected death*.

Froen JF et al. Comparative epidemiology of sudden infant death syndrome and sudden intrauterine unexplained death. Arch Dis Child 2002; 87: F118–F121. *Different risk factors suggest different aetiology*.

Malloy MH. Trends in postneonatal aspiration deaths and reclassification of sudden infant death syndrome: impact on the 'Back to Sleep' program. Pediatrics 2002; 109: 661–665. *No evidence of an increased risk of death from aspiration as a result of the 'Back to Sleep' program*.

Vestergaard M et al. Febrile convulsions and sudden infant death syndrome. Arch Dis Child 2002; 86: 125–127. *No support for the shared susceptibility hypothesis*.

DERMATOLOGY

Anonymous. Getting rid of athlete's foot. Drug Ther Bull 2002; 40: 53–54. *Review*.

Barnetson RSC *et al*. Childhood atopic eczema. BMJ 2002; 324: 1376–1379. *Review*.

Carter MC *et al*. Paediatric mastocytosis. Arch Dis Child 2002; 86: 315–319. *Review*.

Leaute-Labreze C *et al*. Pulsed dye laser for Sturge-Weber syndrome. Arch Dis Child 2002; 87: 434–435. *8 patients treated, all with at least some benefit*.

Reyes ML *et al.* Bone metabolism in children with epidermolysis bullosa. J Pediatr 2002; 140: 467–469. *Evaluation needed in severe cases.*

Roberts RJ. Head lice. N Engl J Med 2002; 346: 1645–1650. *Review.*

Sheridan RL *et al.* Long-term consequences of toxic epidermal necrolysis in children. Pediatrics 2002; 109: 74–78. *The most common involve the eyes, the skin, and the nails.*

Thomas KS *et al.* Randomised controlled trial of short bursts of a potent topical corticosteroid versus prolonged use of a mild preparation for children with mild or moderate atopic eczema. BMJ 2002; 324: 768–771. *Both are equally effective, but in the long term are they equally safe?*

Williams H. New treatments for atopic dermatitis. BMJ 2002; 324: 1533–1534. *Review.*

ENDOCRINOLOGY

Charmandari E *et al.* Why is management of patients with classical congenital adrenal hyperplasia more difficult at puberty? Arch Dis Child 2002; 86: 266–269. *Review.*

Drake AJ *et al.* Symptomatic adrenal insufficiency presenting with hypoglycaemia in asthmatic children with asthma receiving high dose inhaled fluticasone propionate. BMJ 2002; 324: 1081–1082. *Report of 4 alarming cases.*

Eid N *et al.* Decreased morning serum cortisol levels in children with asthma treated with inhaled fluticasone propionate. Pediatrics 2002; 109: 217–221. *Inhaled fluticasone, even at conventional doses, may have greater effects on the adrenal function than previously recognized.*

Grummer-Strawn LM *et al.* Precocious puberty in girls and the risk of a central nervous system abnormality: the elusive search for diagnostic certainty. Pediatrics 2002; 109: 139–142. *Review.*

Hindmarsh PC. Optimisation of thyroxine dose in congenital hypothyroidism. Arch Dis Child 2002; 86: 73–75. *Review.*

O'Sullivan E *et al.* Precocious puberty: a parent's perspective. Arch Dis Child 2002; 86: 320–321. *Not easy for parents.*

Ogilvy-Stuart AL. Neonatal thyroid disorders. Arch Dis Child 2002; 87: F165–F171. *Review.*

Perry RJ *et al.* Cushing's syndrome, growth impairment, and occult adrenal suppression associated with intranasal steroids. Arch Dis Child 2002; 87: 45–48. *Report of 9 cases.*

Reilly JJ *et al.* Obesity: diagnosis, prevention, and treatment; evidence based answers to common questions. Arch Dis Child 2002; 86: 392–395. *Review.*

Saenger P. Growth hormone in growth hormone deficiency. BMJ 2002; 325: 58–59. *Review.*

Todd GRG *et al.* Survey of adrenal crisis associated with inhaled corticosteroids in the United Kingdom. Arch Dis Child 2002; 87: 457–461. *Hypoglycaemia and convulsions the most common symptoms in 33 cases – see also pp. 455–456.*

Whincup PH *et al.* Early evidence of ethnic differences in cardiovascular risk: cross sectional comparison of British South Asian and white children. BMJ 2002; 318: 655–668. *The relation between adiposity and insulin concentrations was stronger among South Asian children.*

DIABETES

Barera G et al. Occurrence of celiac disease after onset of type 1 diabetes: a 6 year prospective longitudinal study. Pediatrics 2002; 109: 833–838. *There is an increased incidence of coeliac disease in diabetes.*

Hanas R et al. Indwelling catheters used from the onset of diabetes decrease injection pain and pre-injection anxiety. J Pediatr 2002; 140: 315–320. *The pain when injecting insulin can be significantly decreased by indwelling catheters.*

Inward CD et al. Fluid management in diabetic ketoacidosis. Arch Dis Child 2002; 86: 443–445. *Review.*

Schultz CJ et al. Markers of microvascular complications in insulin dependent diabetes. Arch Dis Child 2002; 87: 10–12. *Review.*

Sinha R et al. Prevalence of impaired glucose tolerance among children and adolescents with marked obesity. N Engl J Med 2002; 346: 802–810. *Highly prevalent in severe obesity. See also pp. 854–855.*

GROWTH

Anonymous. Why give a child growth hormone? Drug Ther Bull 2002; 40: 17–20. *Review.*

Wright CM *et al.* Growth reference charts for use in the United Kingdom. Arch Dis Child 2002; 86: 11–14. *Review.*

ENT

Baguley DM *et al.* Current perspectives on tinnitus. Arch Dis Child 2002; 86: 141–143. *Review.*

Jegoux F *et al.* Chronic cough and ear wax. Lancet 2002; 360: 618–619. *Case report.*

Paradise JL *et al.* Tonsillectomy and adenotonsillectomy for recurrent throat infection in moderately affected children. Pediatrics 2002; 110: 7–15. *Modest benefit does not justify the risks.*

Rubenstein JT. Paediatric cochlear implantation: prosthetic hearing and language development. Lancet 2002; 360: 483–485. *Review.*

Tanner K *et al. Haemophilus influenzae* type B epiglottis as a cause of acute upper airways obstruction in children. BMJ 2002; 325: 1099–1100. *3 cases in fully immunised children.*

Tasker A *et al.* Reflux of gastric juice and glue ear in children. Lancet 2002; 359: 493 *Finding pepsin in middle ear fluid suggests an association.*

GASTROENTEROLOGY

Book LS. Diagnosing celiac disease in 2002: who, why, and how? Pediatrics 2002; 109: 952–954. *Review.*

Duro D *et al.* Association between infantile colic and carbohydrate malabsorption from fruit juices in infancy. Pediatrics 2002; 109: 797–805. *Apple juice may worsen colic in some infants.*

Gereige RS *et al.* Is it more than just constipation? Pediatrics 2002; 109: 961–965. *Constipation due to the Currarino triad (anal malformation, sacral abnormality, presacral mass).*

Godbole P *et al.* Limitations and uses of gastrojejunal feeding tubes. Arch Dis Child 2002; 86: 134–137. *Best confined to short-term use.*

Holmes GKT. Screening for coeliac disease in type 1 diabetes. Arch Dis Child 2002; 87: 495–499. *Review.*

Kawahara H *et al.* Intravenous atropine treatment in infantile hypertrophic pyloric stenosis. Arch Dis Child 2002; 87: 71–74. *Applicability uncertain.*

Nager AL *et al.* Comparison of nasogastric and intravenous methods of rehydration in pediatric patients with acute dehydration. Pediatrics 2002; 109: 566–572. *Both methods have their place.*

Peter CS *et al.* Gastroesophageal reflux and apnea of prematurity: no temporal relationship. Pediatrics 2002; 109: 8–11. *Reflux does not cause apnoea.*

Shanahan F. Crohn's disease. Lancet 2002; 359: 62–69. *Review.*

Swingler G *et al.* Seasonal plasma electrolyte fluctuations in childhood diarrhoea. Arch Dis Child 2002; 87: 426–427. *The prevalence of hypernatraemia was 2.5% in February and 10.8% in August.*

GENETICS AND MALFORMATIONS

GENETICS

Gardiner RM. The human genome project: the next decade. Arch Dis Child 2002; 86: 389–391. *Review.*

Guttmacher AE *et al.* Genomic medicine – a primer. N Engl J Med 2002; 347: 1512–1520. *Review.*

MALFORMATIONS

Astley SJ *et al*. Application of the fetal alcohol syndrome facial photographic screening tool in a foster care population. J Pediatr 2002; 141: 712–717. *Photographic screening can work.*

Botto LD *et al*. Occurrence of omphalocele in relation to maternal multivitamin use: a population-based study. Pediatrics 2002; 109: 904–908. *Periconceptional multivitamin use was associated with a 60% reduction in the risk for non-syndromic omphalocele.*

HAEMATOLOGY

Anie KA *et al*. Coping and healthy service utilisation in a UK study of paediatric sickle cell pain. Arch Dis Child 2002; 86: 325–329. *Pain accounted for about 24% of hospital service use.*

Cox Gill J *et al*. Evaluation of high concentration intranasal and intravenous desmopressin in pediatric patients with mild hemophilia A or mild-to-moderate type 1 von Willebrand disease. J Pediatr 2002; 140: 595–599. *Desmopressin enhances haemostasis.*

Qian XH *et al*. Aplastic anaemia associated with parvovirus B19 infection. Arch Dis Child 2002; 87: 436–437. *Parvovirus caused aplastic anaemia in 6/30 cases.*

INFECTIOUS DISEASE

Carrol ED *et al*. Procalcitonin as a diagnostic marker of meningococcal disease in children presenting with fever and a rash. Arch Dis Child 2002; 86: 282–285. *A more sensitive and specific predictor than CRP white cell count.*

Crowcroft NS *et al*. Whooping cough – a continuing problem. BMJ 2002; 324: 1537–1538. *Review.*

Crowcroft NS *et al*. Deaths from pertussis are underestimated in England. Arch Dis Child 2002; 86: 336–338. *33 deaths in period 1994–1999.*

Hackett SJ *et al*. Meningococcal bacterial DNA load at presentation correlates with disease severity. Arch Dis Child 2002; 86: 44–46. *Admission bacterial load is significantly higher in patients with severe disease.*

Hall S *et al*. Second varicella infections: are they more common than previously thought? Pediatrics 2002; 109: 1068–1069. *4.5% of cases in 1995 and 13.3% of cases in 1999 reported previous varicella.*

Kelly D *et al*. Hepatitis C-Z: recent advances. Arch Dis Child 2002; 86: 339–343. *Review.*

Merriman E *et al*. Toys are a potential source of cross-infection in general practitioners' waiting rooms. Br J Gen Pract 2002; 52: 138–140. *20% soft toys contaminated.*

Parry CM *et al*. Typhoid fever. N Engl J Med 2002; 347: 1770–1782. *Review*.

Pollard AJ *et al*. The meningococcus tamed? Arch Dis Child 2002; 87: 13–17. *Review*.

Robbins JB *et al*. Pertussis in developed countries. Lancet 2002; 360: 657–658. *Review*.

Thomas SL *et al*. Contacts with varicella or with children and protection against herpes zoster in adults: a case-control study. Lancet 2002; 360: 678–682. *Reduction of childhood varicella by vaccination might lead to increased incidence of adult zoster.*

Yolken RH. Nucleic acid amplification assays for microbial diagnosis: challenges and opportunities. J Pediatr 2002; 140: 290–292. *Review*.

MEDICINE IN THE TROPICS

Baquim AH *et al*. Effect of zinc supplementation started during diarrhoea on morbidity and mortality in Bangladeshi children: community randomised trial. BMJ 2002; 325: 1059–1063. *Substantial benefits.*

Bhandari N *et al*. Effect of routine zinc supplementation on pneumonia in children aged 6 months to 3 years: randomised controlled trial in an urban slum. BMJ 2002; 324: 1358–1361. *Supplementation substantially reduced the incidence of pneumonia in children who had received vitamin A.*

Biellik R *et al*. First 5 years of measles elimination in southern Africa: 1996-2000. Lancet 2002; 359: 1564–1568. *Regional measles elimination is considered feasible.*

Chai See Lum L *et al*. Risk factors for hemorrhage in severe dengue infections. J Pediatr 2002; 140: 629–631. *Prolonged duration of shock is a risk factor.*

Duke T *et al*. Hypoxaemia in acute respiratory and non-respiratory illnesses in neonates and children in a developing country. Arch Dis Child 2002; 86: 108–112. *Hypoxaemia is an under-recognised complication in children in non-industrialised countries.*

Gera T *et al*. Effect of iron supplementation on incidence of infectious illness in children: systematic review. BMJ 2002; 325: 1142–1144. *No apparent harmful effect.*

Gong YY *et al*. Dietary aflatoxin exposure and impaired growth in young children from Benin and Togo: cross sectional study. BMJ 2002; 325: 20–21. *Whether the association between aflatoxin exposure and impaired growth is a direct result of aflatoxin toxicity or reflects consumption of fungus affected food of poor nutritional quality is unknown.*

Osrin D *et al*. Cross sectional, community based study of care of newborn infants in Nepal. BMJ 2002; 325: 1063–1066. *Interventions need to focus on educating women about hygiene, encouraging early wrapping, and delaying bathing of newborn babies.*

Stitch A *et al*. Human African trypanosomiasis. BMJ 2002; 325: 203–206. *Review*.

Strand TA *et al.* Effectiveness and efficacy of zinc for the treatment of acute diarrhea in young children. Pediatrics 2002; 109: 898–903. *Substantially reduced the duration of diarrhoea.*

MALARIA

Adjuik M *et al.* Amodiaquine-artesunate versus amodiaquine for uncomplicated *Plasmodium falciparum* malaria in African children: a randomised, multicentre trial. Lancet 2002; 359: 1365–1372. *The combination improved treatment efficacy.*

Missinou MA *et al.* Fosmidomycin for malaria. Lancet 2002; 360: 1941–1942. *Safe and effective if given for 4 days or more.*

METABOLIC

Gahl WA *et al.* Cystinosis. N Engl J Med 2002; 347: 111–121. *Review.*

Landolt MA *et al.* Quality of life and psychologic adjustment in children and adolescents with early treated phenylketonuria can be normal. J Pediatr 2002; 140: 516–521. *Normal quality of life and psychological adjustment are achievable.*

Magee AC *et al.* Follow up of fetal outcome in cases of maternal phenylketonuria in Northern Ireland. Arch Dis Child 2002; 87: F141–F143. *Twelve out of 27 (44%) completed pregnancies produced babies with a congenital anomaly and/or developmental delay.*

Muntau AC *et al.* Tetrahydrobiopterin as an alternative treatment for mild phenylketonuria. N Engl J Med 2002; 347: 2122–2132. *Co-factor treatment may obviate the need for the most burdensome dietary restrictions in mild phenotypes. See also pp. 2094–2095.*

Walter JH *et al.* How practical are recommendations for dietary control in phenylketonuria? Lancet 2002; 360: 55–57. *Maintaining control is difficult.*

MISCELLANEOUS

Bridges SJ *et al.* Plagiocephaly and head binding. Arch Dis Child 2002; 86: 144–146. *Orthotic devices do not improve plagiocephaly.*

Burton JL *et al.* The Alder Hey affair. Arch Dis Child 2002; 86: 4–7. *Review of implications for pathology practice.*

Craig JV *et al.* Infrared ear thermometry compared with rectal thermometry in children: a systematic review. Lancet 2002; 360: 603–609. *Ear temperature is not a good approximation of rectal temperature.*

Cropper S *et al.* Managed clinical networks. Arch Dis Child 2002; 87: 1–5. *Review.*

de la Sierra Antona M *et al*. Estimation of the length of nasotracheal tube to be introduced in children. J Pediatr 2002; 140: 772–774. *Formula to allow rapid calculation.*

Downes AJ *et al*. Prevalence and distribution of petechiae in well babies. Arch Dis Child 2002; 86: 291–292. *One or two petechiae are common.*

Ebbeling CB *et al*. Childhood obesity: public-health crisis, common sense cure. Lancet 2002; 360: 473–482. *Review.*

Henderson AJ *et al*. Risk adjusted mortality of critical illness in a defined geographical region. Arch Dis Child 2002; 86: 194–199. *Children with a high initial risk of mortality were significantly more likely to survive in a tertiary paediatric intensive care unit than in general intensive care units.*

Jean-Mary M *et al*. Limited accuracy and reliability of infrared axillary and aural thermometers in a pediatric outpatient population. J Pediatr 2002; 141: 671–676. *No substitute for rectal measurement if accurate measurement of fever is needed.*

Leung DYM *et al*. Prevalence of superantigen-secreting bacteria in patients with Kawasaki disease. J Pediatr 2002; 140: 742–746. *No significant difference between patients and controls.*

Moller H. Testicular cancer risk in relation to use of disposable nappies. Arch Dis Child 2002; 86: 28–29. *No association.*

Stanley TV *et al*. Classical Kawasaki disease in a neonate. Arch Dis Child 2002; 86: F135–F136. *Report of a case in a 2-week-old, with coronary artery aneurism on day 5.*

Tingle JH. Do guidelines have legal implications? Arch Dis Child 2002; 86: 387–388. *Review.*

Tuffrey C *et al*. Use of the internet by parents of paediatric outpatients. Arch Dis Child 2002; 87: 534–536. *In a middle class area, 1 in 5 parents looked up their child's condition before coming to clinic.*

NEONATOLOGY

Agarwal R *et al*. Antenatal steroids are associated with a reduction in the incidence of cerebral white matter lesions in very low birthweight infants. Arch Dis Child 2002; 86: F96–F101. *Halves the incidence of white matter lesions.*

Amin HJ *et al*. Arginine supplementation prevents necrotizing enterocolitis in the premature infant. J Pediatr 2002; 140: 425–431. *Reduces the incidence of all stages of necrotizing enterocolitis.*

Boylan GB *et al*. Phenobarbitone, neonatal seizures, and video-EEG. Arch Dis Child 2002; 86: F165–F170. *Often ineffective as a first line anticonvulsant.*

Briscoe L *et al*. Can transcutaneous bilirubinometry reduce the need for blood tests in jaundiced full term babies? Arch Dis Child 2002; 86: F190–F192. *Inaccurate.*

da Costa DE *et al*. Do not resuscitate orders and ethical decisions in a neonatal intensive care unit in a Muslim community. Arch Dis Child 2002; 86: F115–F119. *It is argued that in this group it is better to make decisions for parents rather than asking them to be responsible.*

Dimitriou G *et al*. Effect of posture on oxygenation and respiratory muscle strength in convalescent infants. Arch Dis Child 2002; 86: F147–F150. *Superior oxygenation in the prone posture was noted.*

Draper ES *et al*. A confidential enquiry into cases of neonatal encephalopathy. Arch Dis Child 2002; 87: F176–F180. *Significant or major episodes of suboptimal care were identified for 64% of the encephalopathy cases and 75% of the deaths.*

Glinianaia SV *et al*. Fetal or infant death in twin pregnancy: neuro-developmental consequence for the survivor. Arch Dis Child 2002; 86: F9–F15. *The risk of cerebral palsy is increased.*

Gray L *et al*. Breastfeeding is analgesic in healthy newborns. Pediatrics 2002; 109: 590–593. *A potent analgesic.*

Gressens P *et al*. The impact of neonatal intensive care practices on the developing brain. J Pediatr 2002; 140: 646–653. *Review.*

Heuchan AM *et al*. Perinatal risk factors for major intraventricular haemorrhage in the Australian and New Zealand Neonatal Network, 1995–97. Arch Dis Child 2002; 86: F86–F90. *Five antenatal and early perinatal factors alone can predict the rate of grade 3–4 IVH with reasonable accuracy.*

Johnson AH *et al*. High-frequency oscillatory ventilation for the prevention of chronic lung disease of prematurity. N Engl J Med 2002; 347: 633–642. *Benefits uncertain.*

Johnson LH *et al*. System-based approach to management of neonatal jaundice and prevention of kernicterus. J Pediatr 2002; 140: 396–403. *Review of 90 cases.*

Katumba-Lunyenya JL. Neonatal/infant echocardiography by the non-cardiologist: a personal practice, past, present, and future. Arch Dis Child 2002; 86: F55–F57. *Review.*

Kumazaki K *et al*. Placental features in preterm infants with periventricular leukomalacia. Pediatrics 2002; 109: 650–655. *Examining the placenta is important.*

Levene M. The clinical conundrum of neonatal seizures. Arch Dis Child 2002; 86: F75–F77. *Review.*

Liet JM *et al*. Dopamine effects on pulmonary artery pressure in hypotensive preterm infants with patent ductus arteriosus. J Pediatr 2002; 140: 373–375. *Effects are variable.*

Lipkin PH *et al*. Neurodevelopmental and medical outcomes of persistent pulmonary hypertension in term newborns treated with nitric oxide. J Pediatr 2002; 140: 306–310. *Adverse outcomes were the same in NO and control groups.*

Littlefield TR *et al*. Multiple-birth infants at higher risk for development of deformational plagiocephaly: II. Is one twin at greater risk? Pediatrics 2002; 109: 19–25. *The lower in utero infant is at increased risk.*

Mei-Zahav M *et al.* Convulsions in retinal haemorrhage: should we look further? Arch Dis Child 2002; 86: 334–335. *Out of 153 children, one had retinal bleeding after a convulsion.*

Nuntnarumit P *et al.* Efficacy and safety of tolazoline for treatment of severe hypoxemia in extremely preterm infants. Pediatrics 2002; 109: 852–856. *Effective treatment for severe resistant hypoxemia.*

Rapaport R. Thyroid function in the very low birth weight newborn: rescreen or reevaluate? J Pediatr 2002; 140: 287–289. *Review. See also pp. 311–314.*

Rauch F *et al.* Skeletal development in premature infants: a review of bone physiology beyond nutritional aspects. Arch Dis Child 2002; 86: F82–F85. *Review.*

Schrag SJ *et al.* A population-based comparison of strategies to prevent early-onset group B streptococcal disease in neonates. N Engl J Med 2002; 347: 233–239. *Routine screening for group B streptococcus during pregnancy prevents more cases of early-onset disease than the risk-based approach. See also pp. 280–281.*

Stoll BJ *et al.* Changes in pathogens causing early-onset sepsis in very low birth weight infants. N Engl J Med 2002; 347: 240–247. *Uncommon but potentially lethal.*

Toet MC *et al.* Comparison between simultaneously recorded amplitude integrated electroencephalogram (cerebral function monitor) and standard electroencephalogram in neonates. Pediatrics 2002; 109: 772–779. *Cerebral function monitor can miss some abnormalities.*

Tommiska V *et al.* Parental stress in families of 2 year old extremely low birthweight infants. Arch Dis Child 2002; 86: F161–F164. *Stress mostly abated by 2 years.*

Watkinson M. Hypertension in the newborn baby. Arch Dis Child 2002; 86: 78–81. *Review.*

Whitelaw A *et al.* Posthaemorrhagic ventricular dilation. Arch Dis Child 2002; 86: F72–F74. *Review.*

Wisewell TE *et al.* A multicenter, randomized, controlled trial comparing surfaxin (lucinactant) lavage with standard care for treatment of meconium aspiration syndrome. Pediatrics 2002; 109: 1081–1087. *Safe and potentially effective. See also pp. 1167–1168.*

NEPHROLOGY

Coulthard MG et al. Outcome of reaching end stage renal failure in children under 2 years of age. Arch Dis Child 2002; 87: 511–517. By school age, most infants treated for end stage renal failure will have a functioning transplant, reasonable growth, and will attend a normal class.

Garcia FJ et al. Jaundice as an early diagnostic sign of urinary tract infection in infancy. Pediatrics 2002; 109: 846–851. *A UTI was found in 7.5% of asymptomatic, afebrile, jaundiced infants younger than 8 weeks old.*

Ronkainen J et al. The adult kidney 24 years after childhood Henoch-Schonlein purpura: a retrospective cohort study. Lancet 2002; 360: 666–670. *Can cause renal impairment or end-stage renal disease later in life.*

NEUROLOGY

Emery AEH. The muscular dystrophies. Lancet 2002; 359: 687–695. *Review.*

Lynch JK *et al*. Report of the National Institute of Neurological Disorders and Stroke Workshop on Perinatal and Childhood Stroke. Pediatrics 2002; 109: 116–123. *Review.*

Morgan T *et al*. Intracranial hemorrhage in infants and children with hereditary hemorrhagic telangiectasia (Osler-Weber-Rendu syndrome). Pediatrics 2002; 109: e12. *An uncommon but disastrous complication.*

Stafstrom CE *et al*. The usefulness of children's drawings in the diagnosis of headache. Pediatrics 2002; 109: 460–472. *Drawings contained features that were claimed to be highly specific for migraine (vs other types of headache). Needs confirmation in other populations.*

Stewart JM. Orthostatic intolerance in pediatrics. J Pediatr 2002; 140: 404–411. *Review.*

EPILEPSY

Kossoff EH et al. Efficacy of the ketogenic diet for infantile spasms. Pediatrics 2002; 109: 780–783. *Safe, well-tolerated, and possibly effective.*

Koutroumanidis M. Panayiotopoulos syndrome. BMJ 2002; 324: 1228–1229. *Review of 2 seizure syndromes.*

Pedley TA et al. Sudden death in epilepsy: a wake-up call for management. Lancet 2002; 359: 1790–1792. *Review.*

OPHTHALMOLOGY

Gaili H *et al*. Exogenous *Pseudomonas endophthalmitis*: a cause of lens enucleation. Arch Dis Child 2002; 86: F204–F206. *Devastating if not recognised.*

O'Connor AR *et al*. Long-term ophthalmic outcome of low birth weight children with and without retinopathy of prematurity. Pediatrics 2002; 109: 12–18. *Visual impairments are associated with low birth weight per se.*

Rahl JS *et al*. Risk, causes, and outcomes of visual impairment after loss of vision in the non-amblyopic eye: a population-based study. Lancet 2002; 360: 597–602. *Risk greater than previously assumed. See also pp. 621–622.*

Wheatley CM *et al*. Retinopathy of prematurity: recent advances in our understanding. Arch Dis Child 2002; 87: F78–F82. *Review.*

ORTHOPAEDICS

Astrom E *et al*. Beneficial effect of long term intravenous bisphosphonate treatment of osteogenesis imperfecta. Arch Dis Child 2002; 86: 356–364. *An efficient symptomatic treatment.*

Edgar M. A new classification of adolescent idiopathic scoliosis. Lancet 2002; 360: 270–271. *Review.*

Ferguson LP *et al*. Osteomyelitis in the well looking afebrile child. BMJ 2002; 324: 1380–1381. *Osteomyelitis should be considered even if there is a history of trauma.*

PSYCHIATRY

Arseneault L et al. Cannabis use in adolescence and risk for adult psychosis: longitudinal prospective study. BMJ 2002; 325: 1212–1213. *Using cannabis in adolescence increased the likelihood of experiencing symptoms of schizophrenia in adulthood.*

Black C et al. Relation of childhood gastrointestinal disorders to autism: nested case-control study using data from the UK General Practice Research Database. BMJ 2002; 325: 419–421. *No evidence that children with autism were more likely than those without to have had defined gastrointestinal disorders at any time before the diagnosis of autism.*

Fazel M et al. The mental health of refugee children. Arch Dis Child 2002; 87: 366–370. *Review.*

Goodman R et al. Mental health problems of children in the community: 18 month follow up. BMJ 2002; 324: 1496–1497. *Childhood psychopathology is often persistent.*

Hawton K et al. Deliberate self harm in adolescents: self report survey in schools in England. BMJ 2002; 325: 1207–1211. *Far more common in females.*

Kroll L et al. Mental health needs of boys in secure care for serious or persistent offending: a prospective, longitudinal study. Lancet 2002; 359: 1975–1979. *Boys in secure care have a high rate of psychiatric morbidity.*

Leckman JF. Tourette's syndrome. Lancet 2002; 360: 1577–1586. *Review.*

Patterson J et al. Improving mental health through parenting programmes: block randomised controlled trial. Arch Dis Child 2002; 87: 472–477. *Might be helpful. See also pp. 468–471.*

Woolfenden SR et al. Family and parenting interventions for conduct disorder and delinquency: a meta-analysis of randomised controlled trials. Arch Dis Child 2002; 86: 251–256. *Beneficial effects on reducing time spent in institutions and criminal activity.*

Abul-Ainine A *et al*. Short term effects of adrenaline in bronchiolitis: a randomised controlled trial. Arch Dis Child 2002; 86: 276–279. *No improvement*.

Bush A *et al*. Primary ciliary dyskinesia. Arch Dis Child 2002; 87: 363–365. *Review*.

Butler CC *et al*. Management of suspected acute viral upper respiratory tract infection in children with intranasal sodium cromoglicate: a randomised controlled trial. Lancet 2002; 359: 2153–2158. *Not useful*.

Gendreau MA *et al*. Responding to medical events during commercial airline flights. N Engl J Med 2002; 346: 1067–1073. *Useful advice concerning fitness to travel and respiratory (and other) disease*.

Grigg J. The health effects of fossil fuel derived particles. Arch Dis Child 2002; 86: 79–83. *Review*.

Marcus CL *et al*. Clinical practice guideline: diagnosis and management of childhood obstructive sleep apnea syndrome. Pediatrics 2002; 109: 704–712. *Review*.

Martinon-Torres F *et al*. Heliox therapy in infants with acute bronchiolitis. Pediatrics 2002; 109: 68–73. *Beneficial in moderate-to-severe cases*.

Schroeder K *et al*. Should we advise parents to administer over the counter cough medicines for acute cough? Systematic review of randomised controlled trials. Arch Dis Child 2002; 86: 170–175. *No more effective than placebo*.

Tan TQ *et al*. Clinical characteristics of children with complicated pneumonia caused by *Streptococcus pneumoniae*. Pediatrics 2002; 110: 1–6. *Complicated disease is increasing*.

Turner SW *et al*. Reduced lung function both before bronchiolitis and at 11 years. Arch Dis Child 2002; 87: 417–420. *The mechanism for wheeze and reduced lung function after bronchiolitis appears to be related to premorbid lung function and not bronchiolitis per se*.

Zach MS *et al*. Adult outcome of congenital lower respiratory tract malformations. Arch Dis Child 2002; 87: 500–505. *Review*.

ASTHMA

Allen DB. Inhaled corticosteroid therapy for asthma in preschool children: growth issues. Pediatrics 2002; 109: 373–380. *Review*.

Child F *et al*. Inhaler devices for asthma: do we follow the guidelines? Arch Dis Child 2002; 86: 176–179. *Large numbers of children are given inhalers they cannot use*.

Ekins-Daukes S *et al*. Burden of corticosteroids in children with asthma in primary care: retrospective observational study. BMJ 2002; 324: 1374 *60–80% of children were on high doses of steroids.*

Lemanske RF. Inflammation in childhood asthma and other wheezing disorders. Pediatrics 2002; 109: 368–372. *Review.*

Martinez FD. Development of wheezing disorders and asthma in preschool children. Pediatrics 2002; 109: 362–367. *Review.*

Skoner DP. Outcome measures in childhood asthma. Pediatrics 2002; 109: 393–398. *Review.*

Skoner DP. Balancing safety and efficacy in pediatric asthma management. Pediatrics 2002; 102: 381–392. *Review.*

Strunk RC. Defining asthma in the preschool-aged child. Pediatrics 2002; 109: 357–361. *Review.*

CYSTIC FIBROSIS

Bines JE et al. Energy metabolism in infants with cystic fibrosis. J Pediatr 2002; 140: 527–533. *No evidence for a defect of energy metabolism.*

Burns JL. Emergence of new pathogens in CF: the devil we know or the devil we don't know? J Pediatr 2002; 140: 283–284. *Review.*

Casaulta C et al. Images in paediatrics. Unilateral exophthalmos in a 2.5-year-old girl. Arch Dis Child 2002; 86: 343 *Mucocoele infected with Pseudomonas.*

Dobson L et al. Clinical improvement in cystic fibrosis with early insulin treatment. Arch Dis Child 2002; 87: 430–431. *4 cases with normal glucose tolerance. Anecdotal.*

Eubanks V et al. Effects of megestrol acetate on weight gain, body composition, and pulmonary function in patients with cystic fibrosis. J Pediatr 2002; 140: 439–444. *Short-term use results in significant weight gain. See also pp. 393–394.*

LiPuma JJ et al. An epidemic Burkholderia cepacia complex strain identified in soil. Lancet 2002; 359: 2002–2003. *B. cepacia genomovar III is found in soil.*

Orenstein DM et al. Cystic fibrosis: a 2002 update. J Pediatr 2002; 140: 156–164. *Review.*

Pencharz PB et al. There is no evidence of a primary defect in energy metabolism in subjects with cystic fibrosis. J Pediatr 2002; 140: 498–499. *Review.*

Prince AS. Biofilms, antimicrobial resistance, and airway infection. N Engl J Med 2002; 347: 1110–1111. *Review.*

Stutman HR et al. Antibiotic prophylaxis in infants and young children with cystic fibrosis: a randomized controlled trial. J Pediatr 2002; 140: 299–305. *Did not support use of cephalexin.*

Walsh NM et al. Risk factors for Burkholderia cepacia complex colonization and infection among patients with cystic fibrosis. J Pediatr 2002; 141: 512–517. *Contact with patients with B. cepacia, in hospital or at camp, is a major risk factor. See also pp. 467–469.*

Wyatt HA et al. Serum hyaluronic acid concentrations are increased in cystic fibrosis patients with liver disease. Arch Dis Child 2002; 86: 190–193. *Suggests high concentrations are due to a failure of hepatic clearance rather than overproduction in the lung.*

SURGERY

Gatrad AR *et al.* Religious circumcision and the Human Rights Act. Arch Dis Child 2002; 86: 76–78. *Review.*

Ludman L *et al.* Hirschsprung's disease: functional and psychological follow up comparing total colonic and rectosigmoid aganglionosis. Arch Dis Child 2002; 86: 348–351. *The proportion of patients with faecal incontinence 7–17 years after definitive surgery was high in both groups.*

Swenson O. Hirschsprung's disease: a review. Pediatrics 2002; 109: 914–918. *Review.*

THERAPEUTICS

Berde CB *et al.* Analgesics for the treatment of pain in children. N Engl J Med 2002; 347: 1094–1103. *Review.*

Clarkson A *et al.* Surveillance for fatal suspected adverse drug reactions in the UK. Arch Dis Child 2002; 87: 462–467. *Medicines most frequently mentioned were anticonvulsants (65 deaths), cytotoxics (34 deaths), anaesthetic agents (30 deaths), and antibiotics (29 deaths). The individual drug most frequently mentioned was sodium valproate (31 deaths).*

Eichenfield LF *et al.* A clinical study to evaluate the efficacy of ELA-Max (4% liposomal lidocaine) as compared with eutectic mixture of local anesthetic cream for pain reduction of venipuncture in children. Pediatrics 2002; 109: 1093–1098. *Equally safe and effective.*

TROPICAL MEDICINE see MEDICINE IN THE TROPICS

Index

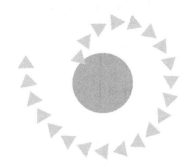